DEPARTMENT OF EMERGENCY MEDICINE

PREVENTION AND TREATMENT OF ALCOHOL PROBLEMS:
RESEARCH OPPORTUNITIES

Report of a Study by a Committee of the

INSTITUTE OF MEDICINE

Division of Mental Health and Behavioral Medicine

The work on which this publication is based was performed pursuant to Contract No. ADM 281-87-0003 with the National Institute on Alcohol Abuse and Alcoholism of the Department of Health and Human Services. Additional support for this study was provided by The Pew Charitable Trusts and by the National Research Council Fund.

2101 Constitution Avenue, N.W.
Washington, D.C. 20418

(202) 334-2328

Publication IOM-89-13

Library of Congress catalog Card No. 89-63865
International Standard Book Number 0-309-04182-1

Additional copies of this report are available from:

National Academy Press
2101 Constitution Avenue, NW
Washington, DC 20418

S071
Printed in the United States of America

First Printing, February 1990
Second Printing, September 1990

INSTITUTE OF MEDICINE
Division of Mental Health and Behavioral Medicine

Committee to Identify Research Opportunities
in the Prevention and Treatment of
Alcohol-Related Problems

[Steering Committee]

ROGER EMIL MEYER, Co-Chair, Professor and Chair, University of Connecticut Health Center, Farmington, Connnecticut.

ROBERT F. MURRAY, JR., Co-Chair, Professor of Pediatrics, Medicine, Oncology, and Genetics, Howard University School of Medicine, Washington, D.C.

THOMAS F. BABOR, Professor of Psychology, University of Connecticut Health Center, Farmington, Connecticut.

JOHN W. FARQUHAR, Professor of Medicine, Director, Stanford Center for Research in Disease Prevention, Stanford University, Stanford, California.

MERWYN R. GREENLICK, Vice President Kaiser Foundation Hospitals, and Director, Health Care Research, Portland, Oregon.

JOHN E. HELZER, Department of Psychiatry, Washington University School of Medicine, St. Louis, Missouri. (Currently, Professor and Chair of Psychiatry, University of Vermont School of Medicine, Burlington, Vermont.)

HAROLD D. HOLDER, Director, Prevention Research Center, Berkeley, California.

SHEPPARD G. KELLAM, Professor and Chairman, Department of Mental Hygiene, Johns Hopkins University, School of Hygiene and Public Health, Baltimore, Maryland.

TING-KAI LI, Professor of Medicine and Biochemistry, Department of Medicine, Indiana University Medical Center, Indianapolis, Indiana.

GEORGE E. WOODY, Chief, Substance Abuse Treatment Unit, Philadelphia V.A. Medical Center and Clinical Professor of Psychiatry, University of Pennsylvania, Philadelphia, Pennsylvania.

Study Staff

Study Director: Alice H. Fraenkel
Division Director: Fredric Solomon
Research Assistants: Jay Sternberg, Karen Goldberg
Editor: Leah Mazade
Secretaries: Angela Parlor, Katherine B. Edsall, Elizabeth Kitsinger, Elaine Lawson

INSTITUTE OF MEDICINE
Division of Mental Health and Behavioral Medicine

Panel on Opportunities for Research on
Treatment of Alcohol Problems

ROGER EMIL MEYER, Chair, Professor and Chair, University of Connecticut Health Center, Farmington, Connnecticut.

THOMAS F. BABOR, Professor of Psychology, University of Connecticut Health Center, Farmington, Connecticut.

RICHARD K. FULLER, Assistant Chief of Gastroenterology Service, Cleveland V.A. Medical Center, Cleveland, Ohio.

MERWYN R. GREENLICK, Vice President, Kaiser Foundation Hospitals, and Director, Health Care Research, Portland, Oregon.

JOHN E. HELZER, Department of Psychiatry, Washington University School of Medicine, St. Louis, Missouri. (Currently, Professor of Psychiatry, University of Vermont School of Medicine, Burlington, Vermont.)

BARBARA S. McCRADY, Associate Professor of Psychology and Clinical Director, Center for Alcohol Studies, Piscataway, New Jersey.

A. THOMAS McLELLAN, Research Professor, Department of Psychiatry, Philadelphia V.A. Medical Center, Philadelphia, Pennsylvania.

WILLIAM R. MILLER, Professor of Psychology and Psychiatry, and Director of Clinical Training, Department of Psychology, University of New Mexico, Albuquerque, New Mexico.

GEORGE E. WOODY, Chief, Substance Abuse Treatment Unit, Philadelphia V.A. Medical Center and Clinical Professor of Psychiatry, University of Pennsylvania, Philadelphia, Pennsylvania.

PREFACE

Problems related to the use of alcohol continue to exact a dreadful toll on individuals and societies. In the United States, alcohol use is involved in nearly 100,000 deaths every year and plays a major role in numerous medical and social problems from liver disease to homelessness. The National Institute on Alcohol Abuse and Alcoholism (NIAAA), has been given responsibility by Congress for fostering biomedical and behavioral research on alcohol problems. In 1986, NIAAA asked the Institute of Medicine (IOM) to undertake a study to assess the current state of knowledge about alcohol-related problems and identify important and promising avenues for research.

NIAAA identified three broad areas of research progress and needs for IOM to review: (1) causes and consequences of the misuse of alcohol, (2) prevention, and (3) treatment. An IOM committee completed the first phase of this study in 1987 with the release of the report Causes and Consequences of Alcohol Problems: An Agenda for Research. The present report, which deals with research in the prevention and treatment of alcohol-related problems, was prepared by a different committee; it represents the second and final phase of that effort. Together, the two reports comprise an update of the 1980 IOM study, also commissioned by NIAAA, Alcoholism, Alcohol Abuse and Related Problems: Opportunities for Research. Additional support for this study was provided by the Pew Charitable Trusts.

In some cases, the material in this volume updates or amplifies topics that were reviewed in Causes and Consequences of Alcohol Problems. For instance, Chapter 2 on epidemiology does not aim at comprehensiveness but rather at enhancing, with recent research results and in some cases more extensive coverage, some of the information that appeared in the earlier report. One example is the information that has become available recently on the role of alcohol in injuries; this report is able to treat that subject more fully than was possible in 1987. In those areas of research that have seen little change, however, the committee refers the reader to discussions in the earlier volume.

Throughout their deliberations, committee members maintained the view that alcohol problems constitute a continuum ranging from occasional misuse by social drinkers to chronic misuse by individuals suffering from alcohol dependence syndrome. The adoption of such a perspective introduces the issue of terminology to describe the various points along the continuum. This thorny problem often arises in any attempt to write about the alcohol field; it is dealt with in various ways (e.g., see IOM, 1987, pp.16-18). Except when discussing particular studies (in which the terminology used by researchers is retained), the committee employs three general levels of reference in this report to distinguish areas along the continuum of alcohol problems. The first level, the least severe in the committee's scheme, consists of alcohol-related problems, which may involve undesirable health, personal, or societal consequences. This terminology appears most conspicuously in Part I, the prevention section of the report. The second level is heavy drinking; this category constitutes a more severe level of problems arising from the injudicious or risky use of alcohol but stops short of dependence or addiction. The third level of reference comprises the most severe alcohol problems, which may be described by the term alcoholism or, more often, alcohol dependence. This report reviews a wide range of research efforts whose targets of interest represent a myriad of points along the continuum and are described in terms of these levels of problem severity.

Such a broad perspective and scope prompt mention of three limitations that should be understood to govern the committee's presentation. First, the research cited in the report is illustrative of recent progress but is not intended to be comprehensive or exhaustive. Second, this is not a policy document. Although the committee's presentation of the current state of research into alcohol-related problems might be used to inform policymaking, its focus, as established by NIAAA's mandate and IOM's subsequent charge, is to identify promising avenues of research. The committee thus did not consider the formulation of policy recommendations based on research results to be properly part of its task nor could it have done so, given the constraints of time and other resources. Some may find the report disappointing in this respect. For a thorough discussion of policy in the field of alcohol-related problems, the committee would refer the reader to the National Research Council report Alcohol and Public Policy: Beyond the Shadow of Prohibition (Moore and Gerstein, 1981) and to the forthcoming IOM report Broadening the Base of Treatment for Alcohol Problems (in press).

Third, the committee limited its scope of work in that it made no attempt to rank its recommendations. Given the large number of areas of research and the multiple perspectives of multiple disciplines involved in the study of alcohol-related problems, it would not be useful to try to prioritize recommendations across so many different approaches to prevention and treatment. The field is still relatively new; there has often been little substantive or replicative evaluation of many of the approaches, and it is too soon to draw conclusions about the most promising areas of research. Consequently, the committee has refrained from any system of prioritization of its recommendations and instead identifies what it considers to be the most promising approaches within each of the areas under discussion.

Following the framework of its charge, the committee's report is divided into three parts. Part I examines prevention research, taking as its conceptual framework a public health model of alcohol-related problems. The model proposes three interacting elements: the "agent" (alcohol); the "host" or individual (traits that affect an individual's susceptibility or vulnerability to problem outcomes); and the "environment" (a multifaceted concept involving such varied milieus as the broad legal environment--minimum drinking age laws or zoning decisions to exclude bars from neighborhoods--and the normative environment--general attitudes and beliefs regarding alcohol--as well as the "micro" environments of family and peer groups). The committee examines current prevention research using the interactive points of the model as an organizing framework and also moves beyond it to identify work in other disciplines that holds promise for application to alcohol-related problems. Part II of the report delineates the research picture for the treatment of alcohol-related problems and opportunities for advancement in this area. Part III, the shortest section, briefly discusses funding mechanisms and the necessary infrastructure to carry out prevention and treatment research on alcohol-related problems.

The steering committee was greatly assisted in its efforts by the IOM staff, under the leadership of Alice Fraenkel, who served as study director, and Fredric Solomon who provided overall supervision of the project. Its deliberations were enriched by the contributions of several consultants and, especially, by two panels--one on prevention research and one on treatment research. The committee itself, however, is responsible for the final report.

REFERENCES

Institute of Medicine. Alcoholism, Alcohol Abuse and Related Problems: Opportunities for Research. Washington, DC: National Academy Press, 1980.

Institute of Medicine. Causes and Consequences of Alcohol Problems: An Agenda for Research. Washington, DC: National Academy Press, 1987.

Institute of Medicine. Broadening the Base of Treatment for Alcohol Problems. Washington, DC: National Academy Press, in press.

Moore, M and D. Gerstein, eds. Beyond the Shadow of Prohibition. M. Moore and D. Gerstein, eds. Washington, DC: National Academy Press, 1981.

CONTENTS

Part I: Research Opportunities in the Prevention of Alcohol-Related Problems

Introduction

Problems with alcohol con   :ieties. In the
United States, alcohol use i   and plays a major
role in numerous medical ana social problems. The National Institute on Alcohol Abuse
and Alcoholism (NIAAA), which was given responsibility by Congress for fostering research
on the prevention and treatment of alcoholism, asked the Institute of Medicine (IOM) to
undertake a study to assess the current state of knowledge about alcohol-related problems
and to identify the most important and promising avenues for research into (a) their causes
and consequences, (b) their prevention, and (c) the treatment of those who suffer the ill
effects of alcohol misuse. IOM completed the first phase of this study in 1987, releasing
a committee report entitled Causes and Consequences of Alcohol Problems: An Agenda
for Research. The present report, which deals with research in the prevention and
treatment of alcohol-related problems, represents the second and final phase of that effort.

The report is divided into three parts. In the first part, the committee examines the social
and personal aspects of alcohol-related problems toward which prevention efforts are
directed; delineates the features of a public health orientation that it deems most
appropriate for the prevention task; discusses individual vulnerability to alcohol misuse;
reviews genetic, developmental, and social learning perspectives on prevention; and indicates
how various perspectives both differ from and complement each other. Also examined are
relevant initiatives that have been undertaken at the community level in other health-related
fields. The committee concludes by making recommendations for promising research
opportunities that should be pursued.

In Part II, which is devoted to treatment research, the committee begins its discussion
with a brief historical introduction and then presents a review of recent research and future
research opportunities. In doing so, it considers the underlying philosophical issues as well
as the formidable methodological problems in conducting treatment research. Central to
this is a broad review of available treatment modalities and the methodological difficulties
involved in developing effective patient-treatment matching schemes. Noting the similarities
between alcohol and other substance abuse disorders, the committee reviews advances in
research on smoking cessation and dependence on other drugs. Part II also presents an
overview of recent studies on the treatment of various medical sequelae of alcohol abuse,
concluding with a discussion of research on cost considerations and related issues that are
important to the formulation of public policy for the provision of alcohol treatment
services. The committee identifies research opportunities in each area explored.

In the final part of the report, the committee concludes that cooperative multisite research
efforts are indispensable to the implementation of the research directions it recommends.
It also offers recommendations to NIAAA concerning the kinds of funding mechanisms
deemed most suitable for achieving the agency's goals.

Throughout their deliberations, committee members clearly expressed the view that alcohol
problems constitute a continuum that ranges from occasional misuse by social drinkers to
chronic misuse by individuals suffering from alcohol dependence syndrome. This report
considers numerous points along that continuum. The prevention part of the report, with

its strong orientation toward primary prevention (i.e., preventing the onset of problems), emphasizes the environmental influences that can interact with genetic, constitutional, and biological vulnerabilities of the individual and eventually result in a variety of harmful behaviors. Prevention research thus includes social, legal, and community-wide interventions that might alter the behavior not only of individuals but of entire societies. Treatment research is concerned with individuals who are at a point on the continuum at which they can be identified as having an actual alcohol problem.

RESEARCH OPPORTUNITIES IN THE PREVENTION OF ALCOHOL PROBLEMS A PUBLIC HEALTH PERSPECTIVE

The wide distribution of alcohol problems in the population has strong implications for the direction prevention research should take. Until recently, the prevailing model emphasized prevention of the extreme problem of alcoholism or alcohol dependence. Now, however, that focus has expanded to a broader interest in alcohol-related problems, a concept that encompasses a far greater range of individuals and necessarily expands the range of prevention activities to include not only drinking behavior but also the medical, personal, and social consequences of alcohol use.

As a conceptual framework for organizing its discussion of current prevention research and future research opportunities, the committee found a public health perspective to be particularly useful. The public health model posits three elements that interact to produce or attenuate specific problems. These elements are the agent (alcoholic beverages); the individual, or "host," who has the problem; and the environment (the physical, interpersonal, and social milieu surrounding the use of alcohol). The strength of the public health model is that it highlights the interactive nature of these elements in alcohol problems and illuminates the complexity that is now known to exist. Interventions based on such a view can thus take into account more of the possible factors or variables that are involved not only in the causation of problems but in their prevention.

Preventive interventions generally can be seen as attempts either to alter an agent, individual, or environmental factor that contributes to an alcohol problem or, conversely, to exploit a factor that reduces risk. Interventions can be universal (directed at an entire population), selected (directed at a subgroup considered to be at greater risk than others for a problem), or indicated (directed at specific individuals who actually show signs of possible problems with alcohol). The committee's use of the term prevention in Part I is limited largely to the prevention of the onset of problems; indicated interventions would be considered secondary prevention or early therapeutic intervention and are discussed in the treatment section of the report (Part II).

The committee uses this framework in its discussions of a number of aspects of alcohol problem prevention: the epidemiology of alcohol problems; the interactions among the elements noted above, focusing variously on the individual and the environment; community approaches to prevention in alcoholism and other fields; and methodological issues that affect the feasibility of research and the quality of evidence it produces. Part I concludes with the committee's overall recommendations on the future course of prevention research.

The Epidemiology of Alcohol-Related Problems

Alcohol use has been associated with a wide range of physical and social problems, including disease, accidental and intentional violence, homelessness, unemployment, and marital discord. Injuries are a leading cause of morbidity and mortality in the United States, and alcohol is involved in many of them. For example, up to 50 percent of fatal automobile crashes involve alcohol and result in more than 20,000 fatalities annually. Alcohol also has a demonstrated association with risk of injury from falls and drownings, and about half of all fire and burn deaths are associated with alcohol use.

Yet proving a causal role for alcohol in traumatic events or determining the magnitude of the relationship is difficult, owing to methodological problems in the designs of many of the studies used to support the contention of causality. Ideally, the most persuasive evidence would be provided by studies that compare exposure to alcohol (blood alcohol levels) among injury victims with exposure among comparable, uninjured persons who are selected for study when they appear at a later date at the same site and at the same time of day that the original incident occurred. Studies of this type, however, are logistically difficult to execute and therefore infrequently undertaken. Other methodological difficulties encountered with study designs include the proper determination of cases, measurement of the extent of alcohol exposure, distortion of results as a consequence of interviewer biases, and determination of the temporal sequence of exposure and incident.

These methodological problems also bedevil studies that have shown an association of alcohol with other physical and social problems. Alcohol is sometimes used by both perpetrators and victims of violent crimes and is often involved in unprofessional, unplanned property crimes. Moreover, some alcohol use is indicated in 35 percent of successful suicides. There is also a widespread belief that child abuse and neglect are associated with alcohol abuse; however, this association is unproven and should be investigated further. Similarly, studies are warranted on the influence of alcohol on sexually transmitted diseases and sexual activity, including early sexual activity and adolescent pregnancy.

One problem of particular concern has been the effects of alcohol on unborn children. Fetal alcohol syndrome (FAS) is a cluster of permanent physical deformities and mental retardation that result from drinking during pregnancy. There are one to three FAS babies for every 1,000 live births. In addition, some children exhibit mild physical and mental deficiencies following prenatal alcohol exposure; these kinds of abnormalities are called fetal alcohol effects (FAE).

The role of epidemiological research in the prevention of alcohol problems is important in defining the extent and prevalence of the various problems that need to be addressed. Also of value in prevention is a consideration of the interaction of the various factors researchers believe may contribute to the development of such problems. The discussion that follows describes three avenues of research that share a common focus on the individual in their exploration of antecedents of the heavy use of alcohol.

Individual-Environment Interactions: Focus on the Individual

There are obviously many possible approaches to prevention research from the point of view of the individual alone. The three chosen by the committee are illustrative of the interactive perspective it believes is most fruitful for further research, that is, the individual in the context of his or her environment, both the specific drinking milieu and the broader developmental setting of the maturing person.

The Life-Course Developmental Perspective

The first approach, the life-course or life-span developmental view of individual vulnerability, attempts to link age to drinking behavior and to specify the pathways and interactions that both predict and cause drinking problems. Researchers have used this concept to construct analytical frameworks to investigate individual vulnerability to alcohol problems and, in particular, the heavy use of alcohol. Recently, researchers have suggested that certain interactions between risk factors in an individual (e.g., neurophysiological variables, temperament, behavior) and factors in his or her environment (e.g., life events, family, peers, work) contribute to the development of alcohol problems. Identifying those risk factors is important for devising effective prevention programs.

Prospective studies of a cohort or generation of individuals offer a powerful tool for risk factor identification. Such studies follow a selected group of people, interviewing them at various points in their lives, to track the development or, often in later years, the lessening of alcohol problems. Several consistent findings have emerged from the few available prospective studies that have examined the antecedents of the heavy use of alcohol:

- antisocial behavior during childhood has been shown to be related to adult alcohol problems;
- aggressive behavior and the combination of aggressive and shy behavior in first grade have been found to predict heavy alcohol use at ages 16 and 17; and
- males judged to be shy as children were least likely to become alcoholics as adults.

Other factors that have frequently been found to predate adverse alcohol outcomes include difficulty in school achievement, inadequate parenting, hyperactive behavior, heightened marital conflict in the childhood home, and, among males, weak interpersonal ties.

Recommendations for the next stage of prospective research that would lead to improved approaches to developmentally oriented interventions include

- follow-up studies of cohort members to assess intermediate outcomes and stages along developmental paths;
- studies of the factors that influence heavy use and abuse of alcohol both within individuals and across different environments; and
- studies of transitions in stages of development as times of potential vulnerability to alcohol-related problems (e.g., going to school, entering the work force).

The committee also recommends continued maintenance and expansion of existing longitudinal data bases as particularly valuable to prospective research efforts.

Social Learning Models

The social learning perspective on prevention research is the second approach selected by the committee for detailed review. Social learning approaches rest on the processes by which individuals acquire and maintain behavior. They can be coordinated with other models of the avenues leading to alcohol abuse because they incorporate (1) the individual's innate biological vulnerability as well as the experience he or she acquires during the course of development; (2) immediate environmental antecedents and consequences of behavior; and (3) cognitive processes whose presence or absence can explain, or be used to prevent, some alcohol-related behaviors.

The central assumptions of the social learning perspective predict multiple pathways to alcohol use. They propose that alcohol use abuse and alcohol-related behavior are learned within a cultural context and superimposed on an individual's biologically determined predisposition to problems with alcohol, if any. One major part of this approach that sets it apart from many others is that the individual is viewed as an active agent in the learning process; thus, persons who have learned to misuse or abuse alcohol can also learn self-regulation of alcohol use. Specific cognitive information-processing mechanisms--an individual's beliefs, expectations, coping skills, and perceptions of self-efficacy--play a central role in regulating alcohol-related behavior. Understanding these mechanisms is essential for developing effective prevention programs.

Promising approaches for prevention include training in social and coping skills and in self-management techniques such as self-monitoring (e.g., to estimate blood alcohol levels) and cognitive restructuring. A behavioral approach can also be used: the behavioral model assumes that many individuals who do not have severe alcohol problems can learn to stabilize or reduce their drinking by acquiring alternative coping skills, changing life-style habits, and learning safe drinking practices. Individuals go through predictable stages of readiness to change; these stages can be exploited to teach people the basic principles of habit change by means of self-help or media-assisted protocols.

Research suggestions for testing the social learning model include the following steps, which are geared toward answering a number of specific questions that it raises:

- describe the reciprocal interactions among behavioral, cognitive, and environmental processes;
- design experiments that explore the role of beliefs and expectations in the acquisition of problem drinking practices, as well as the relevance of self-efficacy in prevention; and
- explore the motivational factors underlying the stages of readiness to change.

Genetic Determinants of Risk

Major research efforts are continuing on projects to identify the genetic factors that may predispose an individual to alcohol abuse or dependence. However, there have been no major developments since the publication of IOM's first report, Causes and Consequences of Alcohol Problems, in 1987. Progress toward identifying chromosomal markers and genes that confer vulnerability were discussed in that volume. At present, the single best predictor of alcohol dependence is family history, although not all children of alcoholics are at equal risk. The basis of the differential risk is not yet understood; consequently, research on targeted interventions does not appear to be indicated at this time.

A consideration of the genetic determinants of risk, as well as what can be learned from the life-course developmental and the social learning approaches to prevention research, focuses on the individual in the public health equation of the development of alcohol problems. A different vantage point next is provided: the role of the drinking environment in the interactions that lead to alcohol problems.

Individual-Environment Interactions:
Focus on the Environment

Many factors in the environment influence the choices that individuals make about their drinking practices. (In its use of the term environment here, the committee refers to the drinking setting and the cultural and economic milieu surrounding alcohol use.) The manipulation of these factors has been seen as useful in efforts to prevent alcohol-related problems. For example, there is a positive association between alcohol availability and consumption. Studies have shown that a higher minimum age of purchase can reduce consumption by young people and may reduce alcohol-related traffic accidents. (Actual reductions, however, appear to be a function of compliance by retail establishments and enforcement by authorities.) In addition, alcoholic beverage sales are sensitive to price, and a relationship exists among the price of alcoholic beverages, alcohol consumption, and alcohol-related problems. Researchers differ, however, in their estimates of the levels of price sensitivity of different beverages for purchasers of different ages.

Research opportunities to investigate aspects of environmental controls on the availability of alcoholic beverages include identifying the effect of retail price on heavy, high-risk drinking; investigating the role of location, density, and hours of sale of alcohol outlets; and determining the effect or effects of pricing strategies.

The standards of a community, both explicit and implicit, play a large role in shaping behavior and determining alcohol availability and consumption. The media play their parts in significantly affecting public perceptions of norms of alcohol use. Alcohol-related information is conveyed primarily through three modes: (1) public information campaigns, (2) commercial advertising by the alcohol industry, and (3) fictional television and movie programming that depicts drinking. The effective use of counteractive media can be an important component of a prevention effort, especially for young people who are major consumers of media offerings.

Other aspects of the so-called drinking environment can also be brought into play to prevent adverse consequences of alcohol use. For example, both the law and social pressure can be used to reduce the number of drivers who drink. Studies are needed to assess the effect of changes in speed limits on the number of drunk-driving accidents and to explain the decline in fatal crashes in the early 1980s. Another promising legal strategy that needs evaluation involves the drinking context. Several states or jurisdictions have passed server liability statutes, making those who serve alcoholic beverages liable for the actions of their patrons. This liability has led to server training in assessing patron consumption, interventions by servers, and planned changes in the drinking settings of establishments that serve alcoholic beverages.

The workplace as a drinking setting offers another promising avenue of prevention research--promising in terms of both the knowledge to be gained and the reduction of costs incurred when employees have alcohol problems. More studies of the social organization of the workplace are needed to explain differential rates of drinking problems. In considering the workplace as a setting for alcohol consumption, individual heavy drinking may be viewed as a cultural effect, a group response to work conditions, or a consequence of individual proclivities. Research should be directed toward discovering the extent to which occupational drinking groups evolve and the determinants of affiliation with such groups.

Focusing on the environmental influences that shape drinking behavior seems to lead naturally to the possibility of community-wide programs or strategies to reduce alcohol problems. Several large-scale programs have been developed for other aspects of health behavior, and their implementation has included an evaluation component. These approaches and their potential relevance to alcohol problems are discussed below.

Community Approaches and Perspectives from Other Health Fields

As a result of several community-wide prevention programs that incorporated sound research designs, significant changes have been made in the health behavior of program participants. Although the studies were conducted to alter unhealthful behaviors other than alcohol abuse, the lessons learned from these efforts and the strategies used may be applicable to the prevention of alcohol-related problems.

Two studies have attempted to alter community risk factor profiles for cardiovascular disease (CVD). The Stanford Three-Community Study conducted during the 1970s provided evidence that community-wide health education involving mass media and supplemental face-to-face instruction can be effective in changing behavior and thus reducing CVD risk factors. The study, which was conducted over three years, used the three communities as different experimental conditions: in the first town, the program was carried out through the mass media alone; in the second, mass media techniques were supplemented with intensive face-to-face instruction; and in the third, no program was instituted at all. The results of the educational program components were assessed over time by using a multiple logistic function that incorporated age, sex, plasma cholesterol, systolic blood pressure, relative weight, and smoking. During a two-year period, in those towns in which the program was presented, a statistically significant reduction was achieved in the community's composite risk score for CVD as a result of significant declines in blood pressure, smoking, and cholesterol levels. Even greater reductions were seen in the town in which face-to-face instruction was used.

The Stanford Five-City Project is an ongoing 13-year study involving two intervention and three control communities that began in 1978 as an outgrowth of the Three-Community Study. Although the primary goal of the Five-City Project is to reduce the risk of CVD, other important subsidiary goals include an analysis of the program's cost-effectiveness, development of educational and community organization methods, transfer of control to community organizations, and measurement of morbidity and mortality. Interim results of the project show a promising reduction in risk factors. The next step should be to learn how to replicate these results in disorders other than CVD.

The lessons learned from these studies can be summarized as follows:

• Theory should be used as a basis for program planning, implementation, and evaluation; in addition, drawing from several disciplines may increase the strength of the theoretical framework that eventually results.
• A comprehensive, integrated program is needed when the target of the intervention is an entire population rather than high-risk individuals alone.
• Formative and process evaluation is required. In the Stanford studies, such evaluation included needs analysis, pretesting of educational programs, and analysis of the implementation process following the introduction of the programs into the community.

• An extensive evaluation of outcome is essential and must be conducted using validated measures of the occurrence of risk-related behaviors and behavior change. These evaluations should include three levels of analysis: the individual, organizations, and the community.

There have also been successful campaigns in several other health-related areas. For example, a campaign to promote seat belt use indicated that legislation combined with work site-based incentives and education could promote some types of behavior change. A cancer prevention program sponsored by the National Cancer Institute in collaboration with the Kellogg Company provoked a demonstrable interest in dietary change. Some smoking prevention and cessation programs have achieved a degree of success. In addition, there have been several school-based programs that have apparently reduced adolescent pregnancies. The guiding principles offered by these campaigns, which may be applicable to programs to prevent alcohol problems, include the necessity to establish multiple outcome objectives and to design programs to meet the needs of the target population. Furthermore, these programs show that a potential exists for a beneficial, synergistic effect when several approaches are combined--for example, in the case of seat belt use, both legislation and education.

The growing evidence of success in these other fields makes it probable that the prevention of some alcohol problems can be effected through the use of similar methods. The generalization of principles from these efforts should be a carefully planned endeavor involving formative evaluation, pilot testing, behavioral analysis, and the critical review of research. In addition, the methodological issues noted below must be addressed.

Methodological Issues in Alcohol Prevention Research:
Conclusions and Recommendations

There is no single research design or analytical strategy that has characterized prevention research on alcohol problems. A variety of approaches can be used depending on the goals of the research, the setting afforded, and the amount and type of variation to be controlled or explained. A frequently encountered difficulty is that much prevention research must be conducted outside the laboratory, raising issues of feasibility, cost, precision, and validity. Yet both laboratory and field research are needed; in fact, the validity of conclusions is strengthened when consistency is demonstrated between the two approaches. In recent years, alcohol prevention research has made use of a variety of qualitative and quantitative methods in both of these research domains, including quasi-experimental designs, which are frequently used because of the difficulties involved in the random assignment of subjects in field research.

The committee formulated a number of recommendations for future alcohol prevention research programs that can be summarized as follows:

• Findings from biomedical research should be integrated with theories from the social sciences that seek to explain alcohol use and abuse. Integrated models can then be used to guide the development of prevention interventions.
• Theory-driven research should be promoted. Its development can be aided by borrowing theory-based analogues from studies in other health fields.
• Life-span considerations and developmental factors should be incorporated into comprehensive theories of research that draw on work in any of the fields applicable to alcohol problem prevention. If specific interactions between individual characteristics and

environmental or cultural demands are predicted to produce a group at risk, such predictions can be used to plan and test preventive strategies.

    • Collaboration among scholars from diverse fields should be encouraged in theory development. These fields might include the biomedical sciences, psychology, sociology, anthropology, clinical epidemiology, education, econometrics, and any other disciplines shown to be relevant.

    • Program planning and implementation should be integrated with evaluation. Pilot studies of untested components of programs (formative research) should be increased. One barrier to community prevention research has been the cost of collecting the data necessary to measure whether an intervention was effective. NIAAA may want to encourage local and county agencies to develop information management systems that can serve as data bases.

    • Long-term community trials of prevention strategies should be instituted.

    • Prevention research should inform policy formation. In particular, prevention research must develop the necessary methods and techniques to help prevention planners estimate the potential effects of various interventions, based on the best available research.

    • Prevention research should include a consideration of cost-effectiveness in evaluations of interventions.

Together, the committee's recommendations present an ambitious program for the coming years that, if implemented, may help to substantially reduce the human and economic burden of alcohol problems. The pursuit of such an outcome, however, also requires a complementary consideration of the research opportunities to be found in treatment of alcohol problems. These opportunities are discussed in Part II of the report.

RESEARCH OPPORTUNITIES IN THE TREATMENT OF ALCOHOL PROBLEMS

After brief mention of some of the historical factors in treatment research, the committee divides its discussion of treatment research opportunities into a number of areas: issues of assessment, methodology, and research design; treatment modalities; early identification and treatment; patient-treatment matching; advances in the treatment of other psychoactive substance-use disorders; the health consequences of alcohol abuse; and the public policy considerations that attend treatment costs, benefits, and cost offsets.

Historical Factors in Treatment Research

During the past few years, a variety of factors, many of them outside the realm of the academic scientific community, have influenced the course of alcohol treatment research. Some of these factors, which will continue to influence future research efforts, are described briefly below.

Federal involvement in alcohol treatment is changing. After a period in which it supported mainly biomedical and psychosocial research, NIAAA has indicated renewed interest in treatment research by creating the Division of Clinical and Prevention Research and by making new funds available for research projects.

New trends are emerging in the financing, size, and public/private ownership of alcoholism treatment services. These shifts include changes in reimbursement policy, the expansion of inpatient treatment, increases in the number of for-profit treatment providers, the growth of Alcoholics Anonymous (AA), and the emergence of nontraditional sources of recruitment into treatment (e.g., media advertising, employee assistance programs, drinking-driver programs).

Demographic trends in the general population have important implications for the demand for alcohol-related health services. Alcohol abuse and dependence reach their peak prevalence between the ages of 35 and 45. Maturing of the baby boom population means that an increasingly larger proportion of the population is passing through this period of greatest risk; moreover, alcohol problems already were among the most prevalent problem conditions, compared with other medical or mental disorders. Other demographic trends that may influence the demand for treatment services include changes in the nuclear family, increases in the number of homeless persons, aging of the population, and deinstitutionalization of psychiatric patients. The methods that are currently available for assessing a community's need for alcohol treatment services have improved but still require refinement.

Popular trends in treatment and referral may have a profound effect on the treatment-seeking population as well as on the treatments being delivered. The past decade has seen the emergence of public interest groups dedicated to the prevention and prosecution of drunk driving, Americans' increasing health consciousness, a decline in the public's preference for distilled beverages, and an increased awareness of the hazards of heavy drinking.

The emergence of the trends noted above, as well as the shifts or changes in those factors that have traditionally influenced treatment research, offer increased opportunities for policy-oriented studies. Such work might include research on the economic forces shaping the demand for, and provision of, treatment services; the geographic distribution of treatment; reliable and valid techniques of prevalence assessment; popular trends and concepts in the field; alternative treatment systems; and outcome monitoring of samples from multiple facilities. The development of data bases is another fruitful area: data are needed to track emerging trends in patient characteristics, population demographics, alcohol use, and utilization of services. There have already been notable achievements in the area of treatment evaluation. Some of these advances are discussed below, together with several of the major, unresolved evaluation research issues.

Conceptual and Technical Advances in Assessment

Alcohol dependence is now viewed as one core syndrome within a broader spectrum of alcohol-related problems. A distinction is made between alcohol dependence, which is seen as a coherent syndrome, and alcohol-related disabilities, which are considered to be a heterogeneous set of physical, psychological, and social impairments that occur independently of alcohol dependence. In research terms, this distinction means that assessments should focus both on dependence and on the problems that may or may not be associated with it. Alcohol dependence itself is viewed as a continuum from relatively mild to severe that can be measured by diagnostic criteria and by the use of assessment instruments.

Significant advances have been made in new techniques for screening, diagnosis, and differential assessment. The third edition of the American Psychiatric Association's Diagnostic and Statistical Manual of Mental Disorders (DSM-III) has had a major impact on the classification of mental and substance abuse disorders in general; in addition, it has fostered further development of structured diagnostic interviews as assessment instruments. Together, these two advances have had a significant effect on the way clinicians make diagnoses and have improved diagnostic reliability in the alcohol field.

In addition to progress in diagnosis, there have been advances in basic research that have begun to stimulate new approaches to assessment and patient treatment placement. Differential assessment requires a detailed evaluation of a patient's alcohol-use disorder including etiology, presenting symptoms, substance-use patterns, and alcohol-related problems. This is crucial to individualized treatment planning--the so-called matching of individuals to specific kinds of treatment. In the past decade there has been a growing interest in the development of questionnaires, interviews, performance tests, personality inventories, and biological tests designed to assess the extent of a patient's disorder and to quantify alcoholism as a multidimensional clinical disorder. Instruments have been developed that can generate reliable, standardized information for research.

Another assessment technology in which there has been great interest is the development of laboratory tests that detect alcohol consumption. The presence of alcohol in blood, urine, breath, or sweat is evidence of drinking. However, owing to the relatively short half-life of alcohol once it is ingested, alcohol tests using blood, breath, or urine cannot indicate chronic alcohol use. Other biological markers for drinking are currently being tested but are not yet sensitive enough to be used alone to monitor treatment outcome.

Questions have been raised about the validity of verbal data obtained from persons with alcohol problems. Such data are inherently neither valid nor invalid; they vary in validity with the methodological sophistication of data-gathering techniques and the personal characteristics of the respondent. Methodological problems with self-reported data span all of the disciplines that must rely on this technique; research is required to improve the procedures for gathering valid verbal report data.

Advances in assessment techniques have contributed to a more accurate estimation of the relative contributions of client characteristics, therapeutic interventions, program settings, and environmental variables to the success or failure of treatment, that is, to its outcome. Yet more research is needed to identify the active ingredients of traditional and experimental treatment interventions in order to match individuals to the treatment that will be the most effective (produce the best outcome) for them. There has been little evaluation of the short-term impact of specific treatment components (e.g., alcohol education, AA groups, individual counseling); consequently, there is a strong need to use newly developed techniques that specify treatment quality, process, and outcome in order to identify the active ingredients of treatment interventions.

In recent years, increasingly sophisticated methodological approaches have been developed for use in alcohol treatment evaluation. Research findings from preclinical, experimental, quasi-experimental, and descriptive research should lead to the identification of the active components of treatment. Indeed, evaluation research holds the key to advances in the therapeutic effectiveness of treatment for alcohol problems.

Effectiveness of Treatment Modalities: Studies of Process and Outcome

Since 1980 more than 250 new studies have been published reporting outcome data on various approaches to the treatment of alcohol problems. Some of the areas covered include pharmacotherapies (antidipsotropic, "effect-altering," and psychotropic medications), aversion therapies, psychotherapy and counseling, didactic approaches, mutual help groups, behavioral self-control training, conjoint therapies, broad-spectrum treatment strategies, and relapse prevention procedures. Behavioral self-control training is the single most studied modality since 1980, but the evidence for its effectiveness is mixed. Recent research on conjoint therapies suggests that interventions to improve the functioning of couples and families may enhance favorable outcomes. However, only couples therapy has been systematically evaluated; the effectiveness of whole-family therapy is unknown. Another promising direction is toward the use of appropriately planned broad-spectrum strategies. These methods address not only alcohol consumption but also other life problems and have been associated with lower rates of relapse to alcohol abuse.

Typically, alcohol treatment programs in the U.S. offer a <u>combination</u> of modalities that include detoxification and health care, AA groups, lectures and films, group therapy, individual counseling, recreational and occupational therapy, medication, and aftercare group meetings. High success rates for such programs are sometimes claimed, but scientific evaluation of these traditional, multicomponent endeavors is lacking. (It has been limited to uncontrolled studies, which are difficult to interpret). The absence of random assignment and control groups means that absolute effectiveness cannot be inferred. Increased attention should be devoted to the possibility of conducting controlled trials in a broad range of facilities.

One aspect of treatment research for which controlled trials have been conducted is the intensity and duration of treatment. Controlled studies of mixed (unselected) populations of alcoholics have found no differences in outcome based on these factors. Similarly, the overall effectiveness of treatment with unselected patients appears to be no different in residential or nonresidential programs. It seems likely that certain subpopulations of alcoholics would benefit differentially from longer, more intensive treatment or from hospital-based programs. For example, data suggest that intensive residential treatment may be warranted for socially unstable individuals or for those with more severe levels of alcohol dependence or psychopathology. They also show that aftercare designed to maintain the results of treatment has been shown to increase residential treatment effectiveness.

Whereas <u>outcome</u> research provides data on the overall impact of therapeutic interventions, <u>process</u> research investigates the underlying elements involved in treatment, that is, the active ingredients of treatment efficacy. Some of the variables that have been investigated in this regard are motivation, compliance, mandated treatment, and therapist skills and characteristics. One of the more interesting findings in this area indicates that for some individuals, change can occur with minimal interventions (i.e., brief treatment strategies).

The broader question being investigated through all of these studies is: Does treatment work? A meaningful answer must be sought from a number of different perspectives. Given the heterogeneity of treatment and the available research evidence, there is no doubt that <u>all</u> treatments for alcohol problems cannot be considered to be effective. If the question, however, is taken to mean, Are <u>any</u> of these treatments effective? then the answer is a more confident Yes. There is no guidance, however, from the literature indicating a single superior treatment approach for all persons with alcohol problems. The committee views the current array of treatment procedures optimistically and is encouraged by the opportunities for continued research to improve the effectiveness of treatment.

Early Identification and Treatment

Since 1980 increased attention has been given to the identification and treatment of individuals early in their development of alcohol problems. Low-cost interventions based on self-help manuals or brief counseling may be effective as a first attempt to intervene with a large number of people who drink heavily but who show little or no dependence on alcohol. Indeed, current data indicate that brief interventions are superior to no treatment or to waiting list status. Thus, in experimental study designs, the use of research-supported brief intervention comparison groups can circumvent the ethical dilemma of refusing treatment in order to form control groups. Brief and early interventions are also being investigated for use with pregnant women to prevent both fetal alcohol syndrome and fetal alcohol effects.

The development of early identification and treatment procedures implies that the reduction of alcohol consumption to low-risk levels--rather than abstinence--is a worthwhile goal within certain contexts and populations. Consistent with the picture of alcohol problems as a continuum from mild to severe, a goal of moderation is seen as being most feasible toward the milder end and abstinence most vital toward the severe end, with a large gray area between. The question of "appropriate" goals for treatment outcome is complex, however, as well as emotionally charged and highly controversial within the alcohol treatment community. The contraindications for specific treatment goals are an important area for future research.

Effective, inexpensive early interventions are still in the early stages of development. Whereas promising results have been reported from a few programs, there have been little rigorous evaluation and few studies on the behavioral processes that may underlie the effectiveness of such strategies. In addition to the research needed in these areas, further exploration of screening, recruitment, and implementation processes is important. For example, more research attention should be devoted to the evaluation of low-cost, rapid screening procedures that can be used routinely by primary care practitioners. In fact, if studies continue to show the effectiveness of early identification and treatment, the training of health care professionals in screening and brief intervention and the development of materials for continuing education are certainly warranted.

Patient-Treatment Matching and Outcome Improvement in Alcohol Rehabilitation

In the past 10 years, matching patients with treatments has been recognized as a sophisticated idea with as yet untapped possibilities for improving the effectiveness and efficiency of treatment. One major area of work on this topic has been the investigation of basic patient characteristics that generally predict outcome (i.e., the "success" or "failure" of treatment) across a variety of treatment modalities. Four patient variables appear to be generally predictive of treatment outcome: (1) social stability/social supports (fewer supports result in worse treatment response generally but especially in outpatient treatment); (2) psychiatric diagnosis including severity/number, duration, and intensity of symptoms (greater severity indicates generally worse treatment response); (3) severity of alcohol use/severity of alcohol dependence syndrome (greater severity means worse treatment response); and (4) presence of antisocial personality disorder (generally indicative of poor treatment response). From research of this kind have come matching strategies that (1) permit patients to select among alternative treatments (the "cafeteria" approach); (2) employ feedback designs which generate testable hypotheses (patients are assigned on the basis of "statistical hunches" to a particular treatment); and (3) test the effects of the addition of an element to the usual treatment.

Effective matching requires clear specification of the characteristics of individuals seeking treatment and of the components of particular treatment approaches. There have been a number of advances in such measurements, but more research is required. Analysis of defined stages of rehabilitation or treatment (rather than of detoxification or maintenance following treatment) offers great potential for refining the process of optimal treatment selection. Opportunities exist for matching before treatment or rehabilitation starts (i.e., in the treatment selection process), a point that might be particularly appropriate for such populations as adolescents, Native Americans, women, homeless men, the elderly, and so on. Matching to an appropriate level of treatment intensity can also take place at the initiation of treatment; matching to specific treatment components can occur during the treatment process. Some studies have already been conducted in these areas, but more efforts are needed to clarify and further refine existing data, particularly in the case of treatment components. Matching to a particular posttreatment environment for aftercare should also be investigated.

Advances in the Treatment of Other Psychoactive Substance-Use Disorders: Implications for Alcohol Treatment Research

There are many parallels between alcoholism and other addictive disorders, although treatment for alcohol problems has often developed in isolation. In addition, there is a significant comorbidity of dependence on alcohol with dependence on other psychoactive drugs, including nicotine. Both the presence of comorbidity and the parallels that are known to exist suggest the possibility of applying treatment methods used for other substance-use disorders to the treatment of alcohol problems. They also suggest the importance of research into the common processes that may underlie these dependence disorders and the need to develop effective approaches for treating multiple problems within the same treatment protocol.

Several common foci have characterized recent research in psychoactive substance-use disorders. Common theoretical issues include the processes and stages of change, relapse, coping skills, and conditioning factors. There are also several treatment approaches that have been applied to the treatment of more than one psychoactive substance-use disorder (e.g., combining pharmacotherapies with psychological treatments, using treatments based on social learning principles, brief physician interventions, and self-help groups).

There are a number of approaches that have been applied rather extensively in treatment of other substance-use disorders but that have yet to be studied in detail in relation to alcohol treatment. These methods include procedures for self-directed change, behavioral approaches, change process research, psychotherapy using state-of-the-art research methods and well-specified treatment protocols, and pharmacotherapeutic approaches to treatment. These studies offer reason for optimism in that (a) formal treatment makes a difference in the rate of successful change seen in individuals who undertake it, (b) differential effects of different treatments have been demonstrated, and (c) a variety of methods are being developed.

Health Consequences of Alcohol Abuse

Alcohol abuse has diverse deleterious effects on health, including those resulting from intoxication, the withdrawal syndrome, and many types of organ damage. Hepatic cirrhosis could be considered the most serious alcohol-related medical disease because it has the highest mortality. Yet the cognitive impairment induced by alcohol abuse is also a serious concern because it impedes daily functioning. The committee, in response to its charge, focused on opportunities for research on the treatment of alcohol-related illnesses. It reviewed research in such areas as pharmacological and nonpharmacological detoxification, treatment of seizures and delirium tremens, treatment of postwithdrawal symptoms (sleep disorders, nervous system effects), and cardiovascular and liver effects.

There has been some progress in treating certain alcohol-related illnesses, but other disorders still have no specific treatment. Generally, in treatment for alcohol-related illnesses, treatment of the abuse of alcohol is paramount for the prevention and containment of alcohol-related organ pathology, and abstention is essential to the possible reversal of organ damage and to inhibit the progression of cellular and tissue damage.

In some of the study areas noted above, multisite studies of treatments for alcohol-related health consequences are essential because the low frequency of illness results in insufficient numbers of study subjects. Alcoholic hallucinosis, pancreatitis, and cardiomyopathy are examples of disorders whose understanding might require multisite research efforts. Controlled treatment trials of detoxification or research on ways of limiting or reversing cognitive impairment could be carried out at either single or multiple sites.

Treatment Costs, Benefits, and Cost Offsets: Public Policy Considerations

The final topics in the committee's review of research opportunities related to alcohol treatment are cost and public policy considerations. Traditionally, the criteria used in studies of this kind have been those that measured changes in the potential of the system to cure disease. In the past 20 years, a counterinfluence has developed: the primary (or even exclusive) use of economic criteria. Neither of these approaches, however, is sufficient on its own to deal with the complexities of the policy issues that surround treatment for alcohol problems.

Public policy research can take a variety of forms. For example, policy analysis entails a review of what is known about a subject in order to consider policy alternatives systematically. There are few good policy analyses of the costs and benefits of alcohol abuse treatment, and more are needed. Another strategy is to foster the inclusion of cost of treatment as a variable within alcohol treatment evaluations, an approach that would lead to important research opportunities.

Cost offset studies measure posttreatment health care costs (including the cost of ongoing alcohol treatment) incurred by treated alcoholics and compare them with the total health care costs this group would have incurred if no alcohol treatment had been received. The studies using this method that have been conducted thus far suffer from certain methodological problems; nevertheless, they suggest that alcohol treatment contributes to sustained reductions in total health care utilization and costs. A question of great interest is the extent to which coverage for alcohol treatment might actually stimulate the use of other health care services, thereby improving the patient's condition and reducing his overall use of general medical services in the long run. An ideal cost-offset study to investigate such an issue would include no-treatment controls, but the legal, ethical, and methodological difficulties of conducting this type of effort are formidable. Still, research that moves as close as possible toward this true experimental strategy should be encouraged.

There are two other important areas of current policy interest in which practically no research has been conducted on the cost-effectiveness of treatment The first is insurance-related factors: the effect of different insurance benefits on entry into treatment, the selection of a specific treatment modality, consumer satisfaction, and the ultimate cost of the system. There is also a need for research that compares payment sources. For example, research on different benefit programs offered by a single employer is a promising area for comparison studies (by payment source) of the effect of treatment on utilization. In addition, employee assistance programs provide an opportunity to answer questions about the costs and effectiveness of certain treatments.

The other area in which almost no research has been conducted is managed care programs, an increasingly common addition to health care benefits. Managed care programs provide information to help in the selection of treatment options, typically through review procedures that specify the conditions under which treatment must be delivered, thus attempting to prevent unnecessary treatment. These specialized cost-containment procedures include hospital preadmission review, continued stay review, mandated second opinion programs, discharge planning, major case management, and alternate service recommendations. They may be provided by a peer review organization, by health insurance company staff, or by private case management companies.

The roles of public and private financing for alcohol treatment are an important policy question. Increased private expenditures for treatment may result in public cost offsets (e.g., decreased criminal justice costs, fewer motor vehicle accidents) but not necessarily in private cost offsets. More research is needed to provide policymakers with the necessary information to make financing decisions that promote the equitable provision of cost-effective, appropriate treatment services.

FUNDING MECHANISMS AND THE NECESSARY INFRASTRUCTURE FOR TREATMENT AND PREVENTION RESEARCH

Exploitation of the research opportunities identified by the committee in this report will depend on adequate funding and an appropriate research infrastructure (i.e., personnel, facilities). Over the past decade, there have been substantial increases in the federal alcohol research budget. NIAAA has relied on two mechanisms for funding treatment and prevention research, the investigator-initiated grant and the research center. Research support by NIAAA and the Veterans Administration (VA) has led to improvements in methodologyand theory, as well as an expansion of the pool of researchers and facilities. More remains to be done, however, and Part III of the the report discusses the issues involved in supporting the scientific research infrastructure.

Supporting the Scientific Infrastructure for Prevention Research

Prevention research now constitutes approximately 9 percent of NIAAA's total extramural research/research training budget. In earlier years, allocations for prevention research funds were based on NIAAA's perceptions of the effectiveness of various intervention strategies; because little effort was made to ensure sound evaluation, there was limited conclusive information forthcoming about outcomes or intervention efficacy. Yet much has been learned since the 1970s about outcome evaluation; the experiences of the National Heart, Lung, and Blood Institute (NHLBI) and the National Cancer Institute (NCI) with demonstration and educational research grants have yielded fresh insights into ways that future alcohol prevention programs might be designed, implemented, and evaluated.

In particular, the use of prevention trials to evaluate intervention effectiveness should become an established tradition at NIAAA. Significant opportunities now exist for NIAAA/National Institute on Drug Abuse (NIDA), and the Office of Substance Abuse Programs (OSAP) to conduct controlled prevention demonstration projects with well-designed prevention components. Furthermore, when funding of prevention demonstration projects is allocated in the future, money should be set aside for the joint design and evaluation of prevention trials by NIAAA, NIDA, and OSAP.

The various mechanisms currently in use by NIAAA for funding such research appear to be appropriate for most basic and applied prevention studies. Such investigations should include pilot projects, prototype studies, controlled intervention trials, and studies of defined populations. However, for major preventive trials (i.e., comprehensive, multiyear efforts that often involve several research sites or centers), the committee recommends the development of special funding mechanisms, such as a separate budget line item. Also required for all of these studies are certain infrastructure elements, for example, the development of expertise in outcome evaluation and a support mechanism responsive to community initiatives that represent new or unique research opportunities.

A research strategy that will lead to effective prevention programs will require collaborative designs and coordinated analyses. The committee suggests the development of a system that connects research groups in cooperative studies to combine individual strengths and support strong theoretical and methodological integration. It also suggests that NIAAA explore various mechanisms to provide leadership in this area. The committee recommends that NIAAA continue to promote collaborative prevention strategies and new prevention research initiatives.

Supporting the Scientific Infrastructure for Treatment Research

Although federal alcohol research funds in general have increased over the past decade, it was not until 1988 (when NIAAA created its new Division of Clinical and Prevention Research) that treatment research was accorded more stature in the overall federal alcoholism research program. As a consequence of the earlier lack of attention, there have been few controlled studies of treatment modalities or settings in relation to outcome. Treatment research methods are often shaped by the requirements of the treatment program, which may limit the rigor of the research design. Another limitation is the availability of trained researchers. The number of qualified treatment researchers needs to be increased by a variety of mechanisms, especially expanded support for postdoctoral training.

One mechanism that is already in place but that could be more effectively employed in treatment research is the program of grants to NIAAA's 12 research centers. Only one of these centers currently conducts alcohol treatment research. NIAAA might consider funding additional centers devoted to treatment research, in collaboration with another federal agency. The centers might also offer an avenue for increasing the number of research personnel: with the expansion of treatment research at the centers, NIAAA could budget funds for additional trained staff.

The committee commends the recent designation of set-aside funds within block grants for use in evaluating alcohol and drug abuse treatment programs and in assessing the quality of various forms of treatment. This policy could well encourage linkages among university-affiliated researchers, state agencies, and treatment facilities. One impetus for this change in focus is the fact that an appreciable proportion of alcoholism treatment now takes place in freestanding inpatient units that are largely unaffiliated with major academic or research centers. Strong interest has been generated in research on various treatment settings and the matching of individuals seeking treatment for their particular alcohol problem. However, to systematically examine treatment setting and treatment matching, it is essential to develop a pool of treatment facilities that are willing to participate in controlled treatment trials. Such trials also require that specific funds be set aside for thorough patient assessments at entry to treatment and at follow-up points; in addition, assessment reliability must be ensured both within and between sites. An excellent mechanism for this type of effort would be the Public Health Service's cooperative agreement. Indeed, the use of cooperative agreements to fund large-scale alcoholism treatment research should be encouraged. Staff of NIAAA could play a critical role in bringing together a network of investigators and a variety of treatment facilities from both the public and private sectors.

Another promising mechanism for systematic treatment evaluation is the VA's collaborative study. However, the VA recently announced plans to curtail the availability of alcohol treatment, a policy that will have a devastating impact on treatment research in the alcohol field. Given the high percentage of veterans with alcohol-related pathology who are hospitalized in medical/surgical units in VA hospitals, the committee urges the VA to reverse these actions and renew its commitment to both alcohol treatment and treatment research.

There appears to be sufficient flexibility in NIAAA's operational mechanisms to permit the implementation of most of the research opportunities outlined in this report. Over the years, the agency has developed a number of programs and activities that are capable of stimulating research and providing expert advice. As new funding and funding mechanisms are developed or become available, NIAAA should evaluate the experience of other agencies involved in clinical trials and large-scale collaborative studies. Their programs may serve as models for achieving some of NIAAA's goals; they may also indicate large areas of common interest. By coordinating activities among such interest groups as research centers, pharmaceutical companies, hospital chains, insurance companies, and state and federal agencies, NIAAA may be able to guide treatment research on alcohol problems along an increasingly coherent and productive path.

I

RESEARCH OPPORTUNITIES IN THE PREVENTION
OF ALCOHOL-RELATED PROBLEMS

Research related to prevention involves many different kinds of activities--from prospective cohort studies to studies of drinking environment and context, from studies of mass media campaigns to documentation of the effects of one-on-one counseling. Consequently, prevention researchers come from a number of different fields, bringing their own particular approaches and perspectives to an effort that is already multifaceted in terms of targets and methodology. As a way of organizing its work and providing a conceptual framework to examine a varied gathering of potentially fruitful avenues of research, the committee adopted a public health model in which three major elements--the individual, the agent (alcohol), and the environment-- all act together either to produce or attenuate alcohol-related problems.

In assessing progress and opportunities in prevention research, the committee placed special emphasis in its deliberations on the interactive aspects of the model--in particular, the interaction of the individual and the environment--as the central feature of its framework. This is similar to the approach advocated in the National Research Council's report, Alcohol and Public Policy: Beyond the Shadow of Prohibition (Moore and Gerstein, 1981). In keeping with the varied nature of prevention research, it surveyed a wide range of disciplines for potential research opportunities, focusing particularly on those strategies and efforts that involved an interactive approach or perspective.

With a scope of interest that encompasses a wide variety of disciplines and viewpoints, it is probably inevitable that conceptual differences are reflected in the problems that surround the use of certain terms. "Environment" is a case in point. In its discussions, the committee used this owrd to mean both "environment" in a specific sense--the drinking setting and the cultural and economic milieu surrounding the use of alcohol--as well as in the broader sense of the total developmental setting of a child. The committee has clarified whenever necessary its particular uses of this term.

The prevention section of the report, Part I, is divided into six chapters. Chapter 1 presents a brief discussion of the public health model used to organize the rest of the discussion in the other chapters, along with a typology of interventions by target (e.g., total population, selected groups, high-risk individuals). Chapter 2 is an update and, in some cases, an amplification of the research presented in Causes and Consequences of Alcohol Problems (IOM, 1987) on the wide range of physical and social problems associated with alcohol use. This material refers mainly to prevention and early identification of alcohol-related problems and not to research involving those who are already afflicted with severe problems or alcohol dependence. Chapters 3 and 4 present several intriguing avenues of research, concentrating particularly on those that explore the interaction of the elements proposed in the public health model. Chapter 3 uses the individual as the central organizing element, while Chapter 4 focuses on the environment. Chapter 5 details community approaches and perspectives from research in other fields; Chapter 6 discusses methodological issues in prevention research and offers several broad recommendations on research opportunities.

As noted in the introduction to the report, little attempt is made here to address the implications of the research presented here for policymaking or for prevention program implementation at the grass-roots level. The diversity and complexity of the prevention research field dictated the committee's strict focus on the mandate it received from NIAAA to identify opportunities for research rather than applications of research for policymaking and program development.

REFERENCES

202-354-2352

Institute of Medicine. Causes and Consequences of Alcohol Problems: An Agenda for Research. Washington, DC: National Academy Press, 1987.

Moore, M. and D. Gerstein, eds. Alcohol and Public Policy: Beyond the Shadow of Prohibition. M. Moore and D. Gerstein, eds. Washington, DC: National Academy Press, 1981.

($25) POD 299

1

A PUBLIC HEALTH PERSPECTIVE ON THE PREVENTION OF ALCOHOL PROBLEMS

Alcohol use is involved in nearly 100,000 deaths annually, and it plays a major role in numerous medical and social problems in the United States. A contributor to deaths from liver disease and certain cancers, it is also a demonstrated risk factor for vehicular injuries (Haddon et al., 1961; McCarroll and Haddon, 1962). Indeed, drinking is involved in nearly half the deaths from car crashes in this country (U.S. Department of Transportation, 1986). Alcohol use has also been associated with injuries resulting from falls (Honkanen et al., 1983; Hingson and Howland, 1987) and probably contributes to other intentional (Collins, 1981; Merrigan, 1988) and unintentional injuries as well (Howland and Hingson, 1987, 1988). In 1980 the costs from absenteeism, property damage, medical care, and other services that could be attributed to alcohol use were approximately $89.5 billion (NIAAA, 1987).

The amount and frequency of drinking combined with the characteristics of the social and physical environment can either increase or decrease the risks of drinking (Moore and Gerstein, 1981). For example, a very intoxicated person would be at greater risk for an alcohol-related problem outcome in a dangerous activity and environment (e.g., when operating machinery) and at lower risk in a safer pursuit and environment (e.g., at home watching television).

Because the level of intoxication of an individual who is drinking interacts with environmental factors to determine the risks of drinking, alcohol-related problems are not limited to heavy drinkers. Moderate drinkers who drink occasionally but in an unsafe environment are also at risk for an alcohol-related problem. Therefore, everyone who drinks can be at risk, and even people who do not drink are often the innocent victims of the effects of such alcohol-related problems as violent crimes and car crashes.

Drinking problems can be aligned along a continuum from none to moderate to severe alcohol dependence (see IOM, 1987, pp. 16-17). It is estimated that 10 percent of the adult U.S. population has a serious drinking problem or are alcohol dependent. Another 30 percent does not drink at all. The remaining 60 percent is classified as light to moderate drinkers (IOM, 1987). Although heavy drinkers may suffer from the most severe effects of drinking and experience a greater concentration of problems, they do not account for the full range of alcohol problems. Surprisingly, the greatest proportion of problems can be attributed to moderate drinkers because the number of people in this group is larger than the number of alcohol-dependent persons.

Despite the severe and far-reaching consequences of alcohol use, success in preventing these problems has been limited. The purpose of this chapter is to describe a public health model of prevention, which the committee has used as a framework to organize its discussion of promising avenues of prevention research. The model's emphasis on the interaction of factors related to problems with alcohol, as well as its ability to encompass a wide variety of intervention approaches, seems particularly useful.

As described in the National Research Council (NRC) report <u>Alcohol and Public Policy:</u> <u>Beyond the Shadow of Prohibition</u> (Moore and Gerstein, 1981), as well as in the Institute of Medicine report <u>Causes and Consequences of Alcohol Problems</u> (IOM, 1987), research in the field of alcohol abuse has expanded from the focus on clinical alcoholism to a broader interest in alcohol-related problems. There is now a relatively large body of literature for such a new field, and within the last 10 years there has been a rapid expansion in the number and type of studies that have been completed.

The scope and distribution of alcohol problems throughout the population have profound implications for prevention. It has been persuasively argued (Moore and Gerstein, 1981; Room, 1981) that the goal of prevention should be expanded to that of reducing the occurrence of alcohol-related problems rather than merely lowering the prevalence of clinical alcoholism. Even if it were possible to identify and treat everyone with a severe drinking problem, environmental factors guarantee that there would still be alcohol-related problems associated with moderate drinking. This expanded concept, however, changes the focus of prevention efforts from an exclusive emphasis on drinking behavior to one that seeks to prevent the medical, personal, and social consequences of alcohol use. Heretofore, much of the discussion of prevention has tended to focus on intoxication as the sole cause of alcohol problems and has not adequately included the contributory role of the environment. This report assumes that the goal of prevention is to reduce the incidence of alcohol-related problems and that efforts to induce widespread change in social norms and behavior are components of a larger strategy to reduce all of these problems, including clinical alcoholism.

A PUBLIC HEALTH MODEL OF ALCOHOL-RELATED PROBLEMS

As outlined in <u>Causes and Consequences of Alcohol Problems</u> (IOM, 1987), the growing body of epidemiological data and the corresponding increase in understanding have led us to see that alcohol problems arise through a complex interaction of individual, interpersonal, and social factors. It is no longer suggested that these problems stem from a single determining mechanism such as inherited susceptibility to alcohol dependence or the availability of alcoholic beverages.

To gain a perspective on the interaction of multiple factors, prevention specialists have adopted an epidemiological or public health model of alcohol-related problems (Figure 1-1). The model shows three major elements that act together either to produce or attenuate specific problems:

    1. the agent--alcoholic beverages or ethanol itself;

    2. the individual (host)--traits that affect a person's susceptibility or vulnerability to the effects of alcoholic beverages; and

    3. the environment--the physical, interpersonal, or social milieu surrounding the use of alcohol that either regulates the individual's exposure to the agent or mediates the risk that the agent poses to the individual. This concept includes both macro- and microenvironments, such as the legal environment (alcoholic beverage control [ABC] laws, laws regarding driving under the influence of alcohol, minimum purchase age laws, zoning); the economic environment (pricing, the excise tax rate, promotions); the normative environment (general attitudes and beliefs regarding alcohol, mass media effects); and the physical aspects of the drinker's immediate environment.

As the model suggests, a specific alcohol-related problem does not result from only one or the other of these sources. Rather, the model emphasizes the interaction of sometimes subtle forces that shape the type and magnitude of problematic outcomes. The etiology of the specific problem--whether it be intoxication, dependence, or driving after drinking--can often be understood best from a public health perspective by isolating the relevant individual, agent, and environmental variables that are contributing influences. The preventive trial offers one method for determining the influence of a particular variable and its implications for subsequent interventions to prevent problem outcomes.

A preventive trial refers to an intervention that is targeted to a well population in which a presumed risk factor is modified or eliminated in hopes of detecting a reduced incidence of disorder in those who receive the intervention. The goal of a preventive trial is to provide the rationale for large-scale public health prevention programs that have the capacity because an incidence rate in a large population.

Preventive trials can provide researchers with an experimental capacity in that an experimental manipulation that modifies a causal risk factor in a population enables a

Figure 1

Alcohol problems are understood as the result of an interactior among individuals, the agent alcohol and the environment.

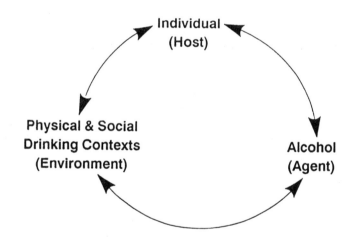

researcher to test an etiologic theory which may not be amenable to other sorts of empirical verification (a situation that is particularly applicable to human populations). These techniques enable prevention researchers to make a major contribution to an understanding of the etiology of a disorder. If experimentally induced changes in a risk factor are followed by a reduction in the incidence rate of disorder, one can be reasonably confident that the risk factor is part of the causal chain. Alternatively, well-designed and well-implemented preventive trials that fail to document a preventive effect cast doubt on established hypotheses concerning etiology.

In addition to serving as an experimental test of a causal hypothesis, a preventive trial allows an evaluation of (a) the feasibility of an intervention, (b) its potential interaction with individual and community variables, and (c) how its effect may vary across different settings and populations.

PREVENTION RESEARCH FROM A PUBLIC HEALTH PERSPECTIVE

The public health approach to primary prevention traditionally has been oriented toward lowering the rate of occurrence (incidence) of a disease or disorder in a defined population. Prevention interventions generally can be seen as attempts either to alter an agent, a host (individual), or an environmental factor that contributes to an alcohol problem or, conversely, to exploit a factor that reduces risk.

Broadening the scope of this traditional pattern somewhat, Gordon (1983) has proposed a novel conceptual scheme for preventive interventions, suggesting that they be considered universal, selected, or indicated in nature. Universal preventive interventions are directed at an entire population and not at subgroups that are presumed to be at heightened risk. Fluoridation of water, vitamin supplementation of bread and milk, and diphtheria-pertussis-titanus (DPT) immunization of infants are examples of preventive interventions that are deemed desirable for everyone. Selected interventions, on the other hand, are directed at a class of individuals who, by virtue of membership in a subgroup of the population, are presumed to be at greater risk for a problem outcome than those who are not part of the group. This presumption, which is typically the result of prior epidemiological findings, serves as a basis for designating certain individuals as appropriate candidates for preventive intervention. These individuals do not exhibit preclinical signs or report symptoms of disorder, but they do possess the factor that is presumed to heighten risk. The last interventions in Gordon's scheme, indicated interventions, are directed at specific individuals who are chosen because they exhibit indices of preclinical dysfunction.

The primary prevention of alcohol and other substance use-related problems, in the sense that this is generally understood to mean prevention of the onset of such problems, may be best achieved by using a combination of universal and selective approaches. (Indicated interventions would be considered secondary prevention; these approaches are discussed in the treatment section of the report.) Universal strategies, whether implemented through the mass media, legislation, community-wide interventions, or other types of efforts, can reach broad segments of the population. Selective procedures can target classes of individuals who have a high probability of developing a problem outcome with interventions of greater scope and intensity than would be necessary, practical, or affordable in a universal approach.

The model also helps us to visualize points that may be only peripherally related to the etiology of a specific problem but that nevertheless can be effective opportunities for interventions. Whether bars and taverns cause someone to become intoxicated, for example, is not as important as whether they can be designed or modified to prevent intoxication. In another case, although some individuals may be at greater risk of drinking and driving than others, the specific drinking context (e.g., a bar) may increase or decrease the given probability of the occurrence of alcohol-related problems. Similarly, certain normative environments (e.g., religious) may provide a high degree of protection to individuals who might otherwise be at risk.

The strength of the public health perspective is that it broadens our awareness and understanding of alcohol-related problems. It moves us beyond a focus on the drinker (host) alone and directs our attention to the interaction between the individual and the environment that results in a specific problem (Wallack, 1983). Recently, several strategies have been designed, and in some cases implemented, to reduce injuries and deaths from alcohol-impaired driving. For example, server interventions have been developed that encourage commercial servers of alcoholic beverages to intervene before a drinker can become intoxicated or before the drinker drives while intoxicated. In some jurisdictions, these interventions are used to supplement identification and treatment of alcoholics. Other suggestions to reduce deaths due to driving under the influence of alcohol include making roads and vehicles safer. No single prevention strategy is likely to be sufficient, however, given the complexity of the problem and the heterogeneity of drinkers and drinking situations.

The public health model also indicates the role played by the agent, alcoholic beverages. A lengthy discussion of the production, marketing, and wholesale or retail distribution of alcohol is beyond the scope of this report; however, it conveys a sense of the importance and complexity of the role of alcohol to say that, in the United States, a billion dollars a year is spent on advertising and marketing beer, wine, and spirits. Further research is needed to define and clarify the industry's role in the worldwide increase in per capita consumption (Ashley and Rankin, 1988). Research is also needed to delineate the ways in which economic factors affect the development of public policy in this area.

A SYSTEMS APPROACH

Although the perspective of the public health model provides a synthesizing overview of prevention goals, it is also necessary to apply theoretical models at the level of both the individual (micro) and the larger environment (macro) to design and evaluate effective prevention programs. Different theoretical constructs may apply at different levels of social complexity: individuals at different stages of the life course, social networks, organizations, communities, and regions. Optimally effective interventions require better integration of preventive efforts at several levels, and research is needed to permit the development of specific and comprehensive models that can bridge the gap between individual and societal factors.

Holder and Blose (1987) offer one solution to the need for integration. They contend that alcohol problem prevention efforts should be designed as a system rather than conceived of as isolated components; consequently, they call for concurrent use of several strategies that can result in synergistic effects. In this regard, valuable lessons may be learned from the community heart disease prevention trials (Farquhar et al., 1977, 1988); from studies of groups at high risk, using the methods of what has been called developmental epidemiology (Zucker and Gomberg, 1986; Kellam, in press); and from the school-based smoking and drug prevention programs (Flay, 1984; Perry, 1986) over several generations of studies.

Within the various levels of the social structure, distinct, unique elements may be isolated and employed to enhance or accelerate social change processes. For example, within the individual there are biological, cognitive, and behavioral factors that are thought to mediate individual behavior change. At the organizational level (e.g., school, work site), in addition to the individual and group levels, there are unique constructs that are relevant to the organization as a whole (e.g., social climate, work environment). It is possible to capitalize on these unique features both within and between levels of social structure so that additive and synergistic prevention effects can be obtained (Abrams et al., 1986).

In addition to the need to bridge the gap between micro and macrolevel approaches, it is important to consider a multidisciplinary approach. Insularity within disciplines does not promote theory building but results in a tendency to design interventions and select measures that are suboptimal. Priority should be placed on encouraging interaction among the disciplines that specialize in microlevel conceptualizations (biological markers, individual psychological factors) and macrolevel disciplines (mass media, social marketing, organizational and community change, health education, diffusion theory, policy, economics). It is also important to combine findings from disciplines focusing on the individual with those from such population-based disciplines as developmental and clinical epidemiology, anthropology, and sociology. In this manner, high-risk subgroups, subcultures, or critical developmental stages across the life span (e.g., puberty) can be identified. In addition, it is crucial to identify the relevant mediating mechanisms and behavioral end points for both theory development and evaluation of impact. A multidisciplinary approach will allow for appropriate selection of targets for prevention as well as the application of relevant theoretical models that will help to optimize the change process.

The chapters that follow review current research in the alcohol field and relevant lessons from other public health fields. They also raise some unanswered questions about the prevention of alcohol-related problems.

REFERENCES

Abrams, D. B., J. Elder, T. Lasater et al. A comprehensive framework for conceptualizing and planning organizational health promotion programs. In M. Cataldo and T. Coates, eds. Behavioral Medicine in Industry. New York: John Wiley and Sons, 1986.

Ashley, M. J., and J. G. Rankin. A public health approach to the prevention of alcohol related problems. Ann. Rev. Public Health 9:233-271, 1988.

Collins, J. J., Jr. Drinking and Crime: Perspectives on the Relationships Between Alcohol Consumption and Criminal Behavior. New York: Guilford Press, 1981.

Farquhar, J. W., N. Maccoby, P. D. Wood et al. Community education for cardiovascular health. Lancet 1:1192, 1977.

Farquhar, J., S. Fortmann, J. Flora et al. The Stanford Five-City Project: Results after 5 1/3 years of education. American Heart Association, Cardiovascular Disease Newsletter No. 43, abstract 27, Winter 1988.

Flay, B. R. What do we know about the social influences approach to smoking prevention? Review and recommendations. Pp. 67-112 in C. S. Bell and R. Battjes, eds. Prevention Research: Deterring Drug Abuse Among Adolescents and Children. NIDA Research Monograph No. 63. USDHHS Publ. No. (ADM)85-1334, Rockville, MD: National Institute on Drug Abuse, 1984.

Gordon, R. S. An operational classification of disease prevention. Public Health Reports 98:107-109, 1983.

Haddon, W., Jr., P. Valien, J. R. McCarroll, and C. J. A. Umberger. Controlled investigation of the characteristics of adult pedestrians fatally injured by motor vehicles in Manhattan. J. Chron. Dis. 14:655-678, 1961.

Hingson, R., and J. Howland. Alcohol as a risk factor for injury or death resulting from accidental falls: A review of the literature. J. Stud. Alcohol 48:212-219, 1987.

Holder, H. D., and J. O. Blose. The reduction of community alcohol problems: Computer simulation in three counties. J. Stud. Alcohol 48(2):124-135, 1987.

Honkanen, R., L. Ertama, P. Kuosmanen, et al. The role of alcohol in accidental falls, J. Stud. Alcohol 44:231-245, 1983.

Howland, J., and R. Hingson. Alcohol as a risk factor for injuries or death due to fires and burns: A review of the literature. Public Health Reports 102:475-483, 1987.

Howland, J., and R. Hingson. Alcohol as a risk factor for drownings: A review of the literature (1950-1985). Accid. Anal. Prev. 20:19-25, 1988.

Institute of Medicine. Causes and Consequences of Alcohol Problems: An Agenda for Research. Washington, DC: National Academy Press, 1987.

Kellam, S. G. Developmental epidemiological framework for family research on depression and aggression. In G. R. Patterson, ed. Depression and Aggression: Two Facets of Family Interactions. Englewood Cliffs, NJ: Lawrence Erlbaum Associates, in press.

McCarroll, J. R., and W. Haddon. A controlled study of fatal automobile accidents in New York City. J. Chron. Dis. 15:811-826, 1962.

Merrigan, D. The Link Between Alcohol and Child Abuse: A Review of the Literature. Social and Behavioral Sciences Section, School of Public Health, Boston University School of Medicine, 1988.

Moore, M. H., and D. R. Gerstein, eds. Alcohol and Public Policy: Beyond the Shadow of Prohibition. Washington, DC: National Academy Press, 1981.

National Institute on Alcohol Abuse and Alcoholism. Sixth Special Report to the U.S. Congress on Alcohol and Health. USDHHS Publ. No. (ADM)87-1519, Rockville, MD: NIAAA, 1987.

Perry, C. L. Community-wide health promotion and drug abuse prevention. J. School Health 56(9):359-363, 1986.

Room, R. The case for a problem prevention approach to alcohol, drug and mental problems. Public Health Reports 96(1):26-33, 1981.

U.S. Department of Transportation. Progress Report on Recommendations Proposed by the Presidential Committee on Drunk Driving. Washington, D.C., 1986.

Wallack, L. Alcohol advertising reassessed: The public health perspective. Pp. 243-248 in M. Grant, M. Plant, and A. Williams, eds. Economics and Alcohol: Consumption and Controls. London: and New York: Gardner Press, 1983.

Zucker, R., and E. Gomberg. Etiology of alcoholism reconsidered: The case for a biopsychosocial process. Am. Psychol. 41:783, 1986.

2

EPIDEMIOLOGY OF ALCOHOL-RELATED PROBLEMS

Alcohol use has been associated with a wide range of physical and social problems including disease, accidental and intentional violence, homelessness, unemployment, and marital discord. Awareness of the variety and magnitude of alcohol-related problems has led prevention research to move from a primary focus on severe problems of alcohol dependence toward the identification of multiple and interdependent mechanisms that underlie risks for specific problems. This can eventually lead to more effective approaches to early identification and preventive intervention.

For some problems (e.g., cirrhosis), the causal role of alcohol is well understood. In many other cases, however, little is known about the nature and extent of alcohol's contribution to problem outcomes. For example, many studies demonstrate that victims of trauma had a history of alcohol abuse or were exposed to alcohol when injury occurred; yet the process of developing effective interventions is constrained because the mechanisms through which alcohol use causes traumatic events are not thoroughly understood. Moreover, the inability to identify the specific risk attributable to alcohol use for such events as automobile crashes limits the ability to design evaluations for interventions.

In the sections that follow, the committee summarizes current knowledge about the epidemiology of a number of alcohol-related problems and identifies some of the gaps to be addressed in future research. The reader should note that this discussion is not meant to be comprehensive because many of these areas were discussed in the earlier report (IOM, 1987 see Chapters 3 and 10). Rather, as noted in the report's introduction, this chapter aims to update the earlier information or, in some cases, to augment the previous discussion of a topic with information that has recently become available.

INJURIES

Injuries are a leading cause of morbidity and mortality in the United States and the most frequent cause of death among children, adolescents, and young adults. Automobile crashes are the single largest cause of death involving alcohol and perhaps the most studied. In 1987 there were 41,435 fatal crashes nationwide. It is well documented that as many as 50 percent of fatal car crashes involve alcohol, resulting in more than 20,000 fatalities annually (Zobeck, 1986; NIAAA, 1987). People under the age of 25 are at particular risk for alcohol-related crashes. In 1984, 16 to 24 year olds constituted 20 percent of the population but accounted for 35 percent of drinking driver deaths (Zobeck, 1986). Alcohol also has a demonstrated association with the risk of injury from falls (Honkanen et al., 1983; Hingson and Howland, 1987a) and drowning (Howland and Hingson, 1988). Although estimates vary, evidence indicates that about half of all fire and burn deaths are associated with alcohol use, and from 25 to 50 percent of drowning may be the result of drinking.

Alcohol may contribute to injury in a number of ways. Drinking impairs judgment and therefore may result in incautious exposure to inherently dangerous situations (e.g., reckless

-31-

driving). Alcohol also impairs information processing and physical coordination, and can reduce an individual's ability to deal with threatening circumstances that are not necessarily attributable to his or her own actions. Finally, alcohol affects certain physiological functions (e.g., blood coagulation) and may contribute to the severity or outcome of an injury.

Methodological Problems in Studying Alcohol-Related Injuries

Determining the causal role of alcohol in traumatic events presents methodological difficulties. Investigations of the association between drinking and injury fall into four basic categories. Type I studies are descriptive and report alcohol exposure in a series of events (e.g., emergency room cases, coroner series, insurance-reported deaths). These studies provide no comparison groups and therefore no estimate of the risk associated with exposure. Type II studies compare the incidence of injury among populations being treated for alcohol abuse with the incidence among standard populations. Type III studies compare the frequency of the presence of alcohol in injury victims with the frequency of alcohol among cases of illness or death owing to natural causes. Type IV studies compare exposure to alcohol among injury victims with alcohol exposure among comparable, uninjured persons who are selected when they appear at the site of the injury at the same time of day as the injury occurred but at a later, predetermined time (e.g., one week later).

Although there is a sizable literature on the contribution of alcohol to injuries, inferences about causal linkage must be approached with caution. For example, Type I studies determine the frequency of exposure among victims but not among nonvictims. Let us assume that a study finds that 30 percent of cases of injury from a violent event are positive for alcohol. Without knowledge of alcohol exposure among a comparable group of noninjured persons, it is difficult to determine the extent to which alcohol contributed to the injuries, if at all. Thus, Type I studies provide only part of the evidence needed to establish causality. Unfortunately, these studies are often presented as proof of the alcohol-injury relationship.

Type II studies often provide evidence that individuals who abuse alcohol are more likely to experience injuries than the general population. In this case, the general population provides the comparison group missing from Type I studies. These outcomes may be confounded, however, because we cannot assume that alcohol abusers-- except for their drinking habits and their propensity for injury--are in all ways like the general population. For instance, persons who chronically abuse alcohol may have individual characteristics that both increase their likelihood of substance abuse and increase their likelihood of experiencing violence. Alcohol abuse may be associated with lower socioeconomic status, which in turn may be associated with living conditions (poor housing or poor neighborhoods) in which the likelihood of unintentional or intentional violence is greater than the living conditions of the general public, regardless of the victim's exposure to alcohol. Here, an association between alcohol abuse and injury may be spurious because both are caused by a third factor (i.e., economic status).

Type III studies use as controls those who died or accessed medical treatment because of illness as opposed to injury. Yet differences between the injured and the ill may be biased because ill persons may be less apt to consume alcohol than the general population. If this were so, the apparent association between alcohol and injury would be inflated.

Type IV studies provide the most persuasive evidence of the alcohol-injury linkage. By comparing the frequency of exposure among cases to that of controls (matched in terms of demographics and the circumstances under which the injury took place), the kinds of bias associated with studies of Type I, II, or III are reduced. Unfortunately, Type IV studies are rarely conducted, owing in part to their logistical difficulties. Nevertheless, some Type IV studies have been conducted and have helped to establish a causal association between alcohol and vehicular injury.

One problem in the study of the relationship between drinking and injury is the difficulty of determining with any degree of certainty the specific events or alcohol exposure involved in a given case. Event ascertainment is apt to be relatively complete for coroner studies (although this statement assumes that most victims of violence are located). However, in some jurisdictions, testing for alcohol at an autopsy is done at the coroner's discretion that is, when the coroner has reason to believe that alcohol contributed to the injury. If the only cases studied are those for which alcohol testing has been performed, it is possible that a disproportionate number of cases will be positive simply because only cases in which alcohol involvement was suspected were included. This bias would overestimate the alcohol-injury association. Similarly, in studies of emergency room patients, submitting to a test for alcohol is at the discretion of the victim. If a refusal to take the test was associated with alcohol exposure among injury cases (injuries often raise questions of responsibility for the event) but was less associated with alcohol among noninjured controls, the association between alcohol and injury would be understated. Another confounding factor is that inebriated persons may be less likely to seek medical attention for injuries, or more likely to delay seeking treatment, than injured persons who have not been drinking. In the first instance, alcohol-associated injuries would not be counted; in the second, some alcohol-related injuries would be incorrectly counted as no exposure to alcohol because the alcohol had been metabolized in the time during which treatment was delayed. In either case, the alcohol-injury association would again be understated.

Ascertaining both event and alcohol exposure is a particular problem in studies of intentional violence in which the object of the study is alcohol exposure among perpetrators. First, the perpetrator is often never apprehended and therefore cannot be tested for alcohol. Alternatively, apprehension may take time, during which the alcohol that was present at the event has been metabolized. On the other hand, inebriated criminals may be more likely to be caught, or to be caught quickly, because of impairments in judgment or mobility or because of other alcohol-related behaviors that draw attention to them. Thus, studies that show an association between intentional injury (e.g., assault or homicide) and alcohol exposure may actually be measuring the effect of alcohol on apprehension rather than an association between alcohol and the propensity for criminal violence.

There are also other methodological problems in studies to determine alcohol-injury association. For example, few studies of this kind are conducted "blind." More often than not, the observers are aware of the intent of the study and may unwittingly distort information. Moreover, the consistency of research results may vary greatly depending on how or if alcohol exposure is personalized. Some studies base exposure on self-reports, whereas others define measured exposure (breathalyser readings or blood alcohol levels) differently ("positive" may mean a trace of alcohol or exposure beyond a specified level).

Finally, few studies document carefully the temporal sequence of events, a lack that is important for several reasons. First, alcohol may have been ingested after the event (to "steady nerves" or "kill the pain") but before observation. Second, the length of time between exposure and observation will affect the level of exposure because alcohol is metabolized relatively quickly. Third, in cases of fatality, decomposition generates alcohols through fermentation. Sophisticated techniques are required to distinguish between these alcohols and ingested alcohols.

It may be concluded from the above discussion that, although it appears that alcohol consumption is causally related to excess numbers of injuries, any demonstration of the magnitude of that relationship presents very difficult methodological problems. Such difficulties include the determination of appropriate "cases," measurement of the extent of alcohol exposure, determination of the temporal sequence of exposure and incident, and distinguishing between the effect of alcohol on the likelihood of apprehension and its effects on the propensity to cause injury. The sections below present selected recent studies on the association between exposure to alcohol and the occurrence of various kinds of injuries.

Vehicular Injuries

Traffic crashes are the leading cause of death in the age group 1-34 years (Ross, 1982). From 1980 to 1985, fatal crashes declined 13 percent nationwide, from 45,284 in 1980 to 39,168 in 1985; in 1986, however, they increased 5 percent, to 41,062; and in 1987 they increased 6 percent to 41,435. Alcohol is unquestionably a major contributor to these crashes. In 1986, 23,987 traffic deaths, 52 percent of the total, involved a driver or pedestrian who had been drinking; 16,728, or 36 percent of the total, involved someone with a blood alcohol level above 0.10 percent (Fell and Klein, 1986). Many of the victims of drunk driving crashes were not drinking at the time of the events, and more than one-third of alcohol-related vehicular deaths were persons other than drinking drivers (i.e., passengers, other drivers, or pedestrians).

There is evidence that individuals who are at risk for drunk driving are also at risk for other behaviors that contribute to vehicular injury. For example, a survey of young (aged 18-25) New England drivers showed that 54 percent of drivers who reported driving in the last month after drinking four or more drinks also drove after marijuana use; only 11 percent of drivers who had not driven in the last month after drinking drove after marijuana use ($p < .001$) (Hingson and Howland, 1987b). In this study, only 1 percent of drivers who reported driving in the last month after drinking four or more drinks always wore seat belts; in comparison, 13 percent of drivers who had not driven in the last month after drinking always wore seat belts ($p < .001$). Almost half (45 percent) of drivers who reported driving in the last month after four or more drinks reported speeding (at least 20 miles per hour over the limit) in the past week; 21 percent of drivers who had not driven in the last month after drinking reported speeding during the past week ($p < .001$). Of drivers who reported driving in the last month after four or more drinks, 38 percent reported running at least one red light in the past week; this was true for only 14 percent of drivers who had not driven after drinking in the last month.

Falls

Each year, approximately 13,000 deaths in the United States are attributed to falls. Only motor vehicle crashes and firearms surpass falls as causes of fatal injuries (Baker, O'Neill, and Karpf, 1984). Laboratory studies have demonstrated several mechanisms by which alcohol could contribute to falls. For example, studies using the Romberg test (a technique used to study the neuromuscular effects of alcohol, which measures the ability to stand upright without swaying) have found that all individuals who were tested exhibited a significant amount of swaying at blood alcohol concentrations (BACs) greater than 100 mg/dl (milligrams per deciliter) or 0.1 gram percent; however, many were affected at much lower levels (Perrine, 1973). Other studies have shown that persons with BACs above 100 mg/dl have lowered divided attention performance, reduced visual acuity (Perrine, 1973), and reduced adaptation to brightness and glare (Adams and Brown, 1975). Moreover, alcohol is known to affect judgment and thus increase risk-taking behavior according to the National Highway Traffic Safety Administration (NHISA, 1985).

In related research, Smart (1969) has shown that chronic alcohol abusers experience higher than expected rates of vehicular injuries even when sober. This finding suggests that either some unidentified factor (e.g., personality) contributes to both accidents and alcohol abuse or that chronic abuse has long-term neurological or physiological effects that increase a person's risk of injury. On the basis of clinical observation, Summerskill and Kelly (1963), for example, have suggested that alcohol abuse contributes to osteoporosis. Thus, some sober alcoholics may fall as a result of spontaneous fractures.

Hingson and Howland (1987a) reviewed the English language literature on the alcohol-fall relationship. Twenty-one studies conducted in eight countries between 1950 and 1985 were identified. Most were Type I studies, reporting on the frequency of alcohol exposure among fall victims. Among these studies, the percentage of fatal falls involving alcohol ranged from 20 to 77 percent. The percentage of falls treated in emergency rooms (people alive on arrival) ranged from 17 to 53 percent.

Type II studies comparing the incidence of falls among treated alcoholics with the incidence among a standard population (adjusted for age, sex, and nationality) reported ratios (observed to expected rates of fatal falls) from 2.9 to 16. Type III studies comparing alcohol exposure among fall victims with alcohol exposure among cases of illness or death resulting from natural causes reported that fall victims were from 2.5 to 10 times more likely to have been drinking than nontrauma comparison cases.

There has been one casecontrol (i.e., Type IV) study of alcohol and falls (Honkanen et al., 1983). This study compared blood alcohol content (and other variables) among fall victims who were treated in emergency rooms with controls who were selected by visiting each accident site at the same time of day exactly one week after each event: 53 percent of patients injured in accidental falls in the evening in Helsinki--and 15 percent of time-, site-, and sex-matched control pedestrians--were alcohol involved. The relative risk (on a scale of 1.0 at zero BAC) did not increase at BACs less than 50 mg per 100 milliliters (ml) was about 3 at BACs of 50-100 mg/100 ml, about 10 at BACs of 100-150 mg/100 ml, and about 60 at BACs of 160 mg/100 ml or higher. The authors of this definitive study concluded that the risk at BACs above 100 mg/100 ml was so high that practically all cases with such BACs can be considered to have been caused by alcohol.

Drownings

In the United States, drowning ranks third among causes of accidental death (Baker, O'Neill, and Karpf, 1984). Approximately 7,200 Americans drown each year in a variety of settings (oceans, inland waters, bathtubs, swimming pools) and under a variety of circumstances (swimming, fishing, boating, diving, driving).

Several observations suggest that alcohol contributes to some of these drownings. For example, drowning are much more apt to involve powerboats than sailboats (Dietz and Baker, 1974), and powerboats involve speed and require skills that are similar to those required for driving. Because it is well documented that drinking increases the risk of vehicular injury, it is reasonable to suppose that alcohol also contributes to powerboat accidents. Similarly, because there is substantial evidence that alcohol contributes to falls, it is likely that alcohol contributes to drownings that result from falls into the water (from shore, boats, or piers). In addition, persons who drink may be less likely to wear life preservers (just as drunk drivers are less likely to wear safety belts).

Alcohol may also contribute to drowning in somewhat less direct ways. For example, it creates a sensation of warmth and may lead some swimmers to remain in the water too long and develop hypothermia. There is evidence that when the chest and abdomen are exposed to cold water, breathlessness and severe hyperventilation often result (Keatings and Evans, 1961). These reactions could limit a person's ability to swim or cause him or her to inhale water as a result of uncontrolled breathing. In addition, immersion in cold water increases venous pressure and pulse, and could lead to cardiovascular collapse through ventricular fibrillation (Giersten, 1970).

The Coast Guard has conducted tests demonstrating that environmental "stressors" (e.g., sun, wind, glare, vibrations, wave motion associated with water activities) may work synergistically with alcohol in degrading an individual's performance (Wright, 1985). Alcohol may also increase the risk of caloric labyrinthitis, an inner ear disturbance associated with sudden temperature drop. It has been suggested that this condition may cause a person who is unexpectedly submerged to become disoriented and swim down rather than up (Transportation Research Board, 1985).

Alcohol may retard laryngospasm when water is aspirated; it may also weaken the diving response or inhibit the body's response to increasing asphyxial blood-gas exchanges, or both (Gooden, 1984). Alcohol may heighten depression or anxiety in some individuals, thereby contributing to suicides by drowning. Finally, sober persons may drown as a result of the actions taken by others who are under the influence of alcohol.

A number of Type I studies of the frequency of alcohol exposure among drowning victims have been reported. The best of these suggest that 29 to 47 percent of the victims were exposed to alcohol (Howland and Hingson, 1988). Waller (1972) conducted a careful Type III study of nonhighway injury fatalities in Sacramento: 17 submersion deaths were included, of which 5 (29 percent) were positive for alcohol on autopsy. In the study, Waller matched injury fatalities with fatalities from nontraumatic cases. Of the matched controls, 67 (18 percent) of 371 were positive for alcohol. Thus, drowning victims were almost twice as likely as controls to have been drinking.

Fires and Burns

Fires and burns rank fourth among the causes of unintentional deaths in the United States. About 6,000 deaths annually are attributed to fires and burns (Baker, O'Neill, and Karpf, 1984) (this figure excludes approximately 500 deaths that result from vehicular and plane crash fires): 75 percent of fire and burn fatalities result from conflagrations, of which 85 percent are house fires (National Safety Council, 1984), and half of all house fires are blamed on cigarettes (Birky and Clarke, 1981). Drinking may thus contribute directly to fires when, for example, a victim becomes unconscious while smoking. Intoxication may also exert indirect effects by preventing a victim from hearing or correctly interpreting alarms of fires caused by others. Similarly, excessive alcohol consumption may impair the ability to escape from a fire once it has started.

Alcohol may contribute to fire and burn injuries in other ways. By decreasing a person's cognitive or neurological skills (e.g., balance), alcohol may also decrease his or her avoidance of inherently dangerous situations or cause burns as a result of falls into or against hot objects. There is some evidence that alcohol works synergistically with toxic gases, such as carbon monoxide, in accelerating behavioral incapacitation (Mitchell, Packham, and Fitzgerald, 1978). Finally, several studies suggest that hepatic dysfunction from chronic alcohol abuse decreases the probability of surviving serious burns (Rittenbury et al., 1965; Crikelair et al., 1968).

A number of studies (Type I) indicate the percentage of fire and burn victims who have been exposed to alcohol. Of these, the most reliable studies report that between 37 and 64 percent of fire or burn casualties had been drinking (Howland and Hingson, 1987). Two Type II studies provide estimates of risk for fire deaths among treated alcoholics in comparison with members of standard populations. One of these (Schmidt and deLint, 1972) found that alcoholics were almost 10 times more likely to die in fires than were members of a standard population of comparable age and sex. Another (Combs-Orme et al., 1983) found that male alcoholics were 9.2 times more likely to die in fires. For women, the risk for alcoholics was 9.8 times that of the comparable population. In a similar study, Stephens (1985) compared alcohol exposure among burn victims treated in an emergency room with alcohol exposure in patients presenting with illness. She reported that victims of fires and burns were 2.75 times more likely than patients who were ill to have been drinking.

A review of the literature on the role of alcohol in fire and burn deaths (Howland and Hingson, 1987) suggests that nearly half of those who die in fires are legally drunk at the time of their deaths. This observation is based on the relatively consistent results among 10 studies with complete blood alcohol testing. Although inferences about the causal role of alcohol in fire and burn injuries require some measure of exposure among noninjured persons, it seems clear that substantially less than 50 percent of the general population is intoxicated at any give time. Accordingly, there is convincing evidence that drinking is a risk factor in fire deaths.

CRIME

Studies indicate that alcohol is sometimes used by both the perpetrators and the victims of crimes immediately before the crime is committed. Alcohol is involved least in incidents of fraud, forgery, and embezzlement; it is most involved in homicides and assaults. In cases of violent crime (e.g., robbery, rape, homicide), the offender is more likely to have been drinking if the victim has been drinking. This association is stronger if the crime involves friends or acquaintances. For cases in which the crime occurs between strangers, the victim is more likely to have been drinking (Room, 1983). In property crimes, alcohol is most often involved in unprofessional and unplanned crimes, and most often in incidents in which there are multiple perpetrators (Cordelia, 1985).

SUICIDE

Suicide is one of the 10 leading causes of death in the United States for persons aged 34-54. Typically, some alcohol use is indicated in 35 percent of fatal suicides; 23 percent are intoxicated at the time of death (Roizen, 1982; U.S. Department of Health and Human Services, 1984; Abel and Zeidinberg, 1985). Reviews of follow-up studies of alcoholics show suicide rates of 8-21 percent (Kendall, 1983; Berglund, 1984). Yet many questions about the relationship between alcohol and suicide remain unanswered. There have been no studies comparing alcohol involvement among suicide attempters with alcohol involvement among suicide completers. Nor have studies assessed whether those committing suicide are more likely to drink than persons of comparable age, sex, and socioeconomic status (SES) who do not commit suicide. If, as seems likely, alcohol contributes to suicide, several questions come to mind. Is suicide attempted in part because the attempters are intoxicated and their judgment is impaired? Interviews with attempters could explore that question. Does chronic alcohol ingestion result in anxiety and depression that prompt suicidal thinking or in behavioral problems that socially isolate the potential suicide victim and reinforce a sense of guilt or worthlessness? It would be particularly useful to compare persons who are successfully treated for alcohol problems with those who are not successfully treated to see the extent to which the former may have lower subsequent suicide rates.

CHILD ABUSE

There is a widespread impression among direct service workers, which in turn is conveyed to the general public by the mass media, that child abuse and neglect are strongly associated with alcoholism and alcohol abuse. Literature reviews of this topic, however, indicate that research about possible associations between alcohol and child abuse has yielded contradictory findings (El-Guebaly and Offord, 1977; Epstein, Cameron, and Room, 1977; Hamilton and Collins, 1981; Orme and Rimmer, 1981). It is certainly plausible that alcohol use could contribute to child abuse in that alcohol inhibits mechanisms that normally control aggressive, hostile, or violent impulses (Bennett, Buss, and Carpenter, 1975). Alcohol use may also crowd out interpersonal relationships as a means of satisfying emotional need, and this could lead to child neglect. Alternatively, nonalcoholic parents or care givers with alcoholic spouses may be preoccupied with a spouse's drinking and exhaust energy that would otherwise be available for nurturing children.

On the other hand, several researchers have observed that some drinkers become pacified by alcohol (Coleman and Strauss, 1983). Unfortunately, there are no studies in the literature of interviewers who are blinded to the abuser status of those being interviewed. Without blinding, both interviewer and respondent bias may affect the interview results; either one might use alcohol to explain behavior that would have occurred even without it. Moreover, accurate measurements of drinking at the time of abuse are rarely, if ever, recorded.

Only a few studies have included control groups of child abusers and nonabusers. Five reports found no association between alcohol use and child abuse (Steele and Polloch, 1968; Smith, Hanson, and Nobel, 1973; Ellwood, 1980; Herman and Hirschman, 1981; Emslie and Rosenfeld, 1983). Four studies noted histories of alcohol abuse among child abusers (Bryant et al., 1963; Baldwin and Oliver, 1975; Rada, 1976; Ellwood, 1980), but this pattern was not significantly different from histories of alcohol use among nonabusers. Four other reports found alcohol abuse to be more pervasive among parents who abused children (Kaplan et al., 1983; Tarter et al., 1984; Famularo et al., 1986; Salzinger et al., 1986). These studies would seem to indicate that research on the association between alcohol and child abuse warrants focused attention and more rigorous investigation by using blinded interviewers, quantification of alcohol consumption, and more designs that use non-child abuser control groups.

SEXUALLY TRANSMITTED DISEASES

Since the AIDS epidemic began, more than 90,000 cases of AIDS have been reported, nearly one-half of whom have died. Alcohol may play a role in HIV infection either by reducing the likelihood that people will employ safer sex practices or by increasing the likelihood that persons who are offered intravenous (IV) drugs will accept those drugs and share needles when injecting. In an exploratory study of a sample of homosexual and bisexual men in San Francisco that was drawn from bathhouses, gay bars, and newspaper advertising, Stall (1986) reported that, after drinking or psychoactive drug use, the men in the study were more likely to engage in sex than when they had not been drinking. A low response rate (37 percent) and the nature of the sampling strategy preclude generalizing these findings to other gay men who are less open about their sexual orientation. Yet despite these caveats, the results of the study suggest other questions that warrant investigation--for example, whether these findings apply to the entire male population or whether the heterosexual population is more likely to engage in unprotected sex after drinking. Studies of the mechanism by which alcohol may influence such activity are also warranted. Are persons more uninhibited after drinking and less concerned about the risks of exposure to HIV or the consequences of infection? Does drinking make people less likely to inquire about partners' possibly risky behaviors? Do heavy drinkers underestimate their susceptibility to HIV or the consequences of HIV infection? Do they believe that condoms reduce sexual pleasure and performance? Do they believe condoms are effective in reducing transmission? Do they perceive greater obstacles to the use of condoms (e.g., cost, embarrassment) than persons who do not drink?

If an association between alcohol and HIV risk behavior becomes apparent, then educational programs that highlight the relationship of HIV to alcohol use and outline HIV risks to drinkers should be tested to see if they alter either drinking behavior or HIV risk-taking behavior after drinking.

EARLY SEXUAL ACTIVITY AND ADOLESCENT PREGNANCY

Various studies have shown a clustering of the variables of early sexual behavior in adolescents and early onset of the use of alcohol and tobacco (Jessor and Jessor, 1975; Jessor, 1983). Although a causal link from alcohol use to early sexual behavior has not been proven in these studies, the disinhibitory effects of alcohol and the expectancies associated with alcohol use could lead to a causal link. Further research might clarify this issue.

FETAL ALCOHOL SYNDROME AND FETAL ALCOHOL EFFECTS

Fetal alcohol syndrome (FAS), which was identified in the 1970s by researchers at the University of Washington, is a cluster of permanent physical deformities and mental retardation that results from drinking during pregnancy. There are approximately 1 to 3 FAS babies for every 1,000 live births resulting from alcohol misuse; among known alcoholic mothers, this rate increases to a range of 23 to 29 for every 1,000 live births (Hanson, Streissguth, and Smith, 1978; Sokol, Miller, and Reed, 1980; Rosett et al., 1983). Incidences as high as 19.5 for 1,000 live births have been reported among some Plains tribes of Native Americans (May et al., 1987).

Although the full spectrum of FAS-related birth defects occurs almost exclusively among alcoholic mothers, there has been no threshold level identified below which drinking during pregnancy could be considered safe. Lower levels of drinking during pregnancy result in more subtle birth defects that are more often neurobehavioral rather than physical (Hanson, Streissguth, and Smith, 1978; Sokol, Miller, and Reed, 1980; Rosett et al., 1983). Because women who drink heavily during pregnancy are also more likely to smoke cigarettes and to take psychoactive drugs during pregnancy, any deleterious effects of alcohol on the developing fetus may be superimposed on the adverse consequences of those other habits.

Studies of special strains of inbred mice and limited studies in humans suggest that genetic determinants in the mother probably influence maternal alcohol metabolism (Chernoff, 1980). In mice, the occurrence of malformations depends not only on the amount of ethanol consumed but also on the rate of alcohol metabolism. Preliminary studies of women showed that there is a tendency for blood alcohol and acetaldehyde levels to be higher in the first two hours after ingestion of a standard ethanol dose among women who had given birth to infants with FAS than in women in a control group (Cooper, 1984). These results do not provide definitive evidence that a metabolic marker for susceptibility to this syndrome can be identified. Rather, they suggest that specific genetic differences may some day be useful in identifying high-risk mothers. Meanwhile, combinations of alcohol ingestion with one or more other factors (e.g., parity, socioeconomic status, smoking, marital status, abuse of recreational drugs, deficient placental function) can be used to target the population of mothers at highest risk for FAS and to implement intensive programs designed to prevent this birth defect.

Babies who manifest the full range of FAS physical anomalies and mental retardation are readily recognized by physicians who are aware of the syndrome. However, some children may exhibit only mild growth deficiency and learning disabilities as indicators of prenatal alcohol exposure. These kinds of abnormalities are termed fetal alcohol effects (FAE). Thus, estimates of the frequency of deleterious prenatal alcohol exposure probably will have to be revised upward if clinicians can agree on the findings that should be designated as indicators of mild FAS (or FAE).

Several kinds of information are needed to develop prevention programs to reduce the frequency of FAS. Efforts should be mounted to develop epidemiological data for FAE. Research needs to further delineate the range of fetal problems that constitute this syndrome and identify the factors that place mothers at greatest risk of having babies with FAS. Further investigations should be undertaken of the bases for ethnic differences in the incidences of FAS and FAE.

The Anti-Drug Abuse Act of 1988 mandates that, as of November 18, 1989, warning labels be placed on all bottles and cans containing spirits. The warning labels will advise women not to drink alcoholic beverages during pregnancy because of the risk of ensuing birth defects. Attitudes concerning FAS and FAE should be assessed both before and after this law goes into effect.

Prospective studies are also needed to delineate the characteristic profile of high-risk mothers, especially those whose babies are affected by relatively small amounts of alcohol. In these women, genetic factors may play an important role in the susceptibility of the fetus to the toxic effects of alcohol.

REFERENCES

Abel, E. L., and R. Zeidinberg. Age, alcohol, and violent death: A postmortem study. J. Stud. Alcohol 46:228-231, 1985.

Adams, A. J., and B. Brown. Alcohol prolongs the time course of glare recovery. Nature 257:481-483, 1975.

Baker, S. P., B. O'Neill, and R. Karpf. The Injury Fact Book. Lexington, MA: Lexington Books, 1984.

Bako, G., W. C. MacKenzie, and E. S. O. Smith. The effect of legislated lowering of the drinking age on fatal highway accidents among young drivers in Alberta, 1970-1972. Can. J. Public Health 67:161-163, 1976.

Baldwin, J. A., and J. E. Oliver. Epidemiology and family characteristics of severely abused children. Br. J. Prev. Soc. Med. 29:205-221, 1975.

Bennett, R. M., A. H. Buss, and J. A. Carpenter. Alcohol and human physical aggression. Q. J. Stud. Alcohol 30(4):870-876, 1969.

Berglund, M. Suicide in alcoholism. Arch. Gen. Psych. 41:888-891, 1984.

Birky, M. M., and F. B. Clarke. Inhalation of toxic products from fires. Bull. N.Y. Acad. Med. 57:997-1013, 1981.

Bonnie, R. J. Regulating conditions of alcohol availability: Possible effects on highway safety. J. Stud. Alcohol, Suppl. No. 10:129-143, 1985.

Brown, D. B., and S. Maghsoodloo. A study of alcohol involvement in young driver accidents with the lowering of the legal age of drinking in Alabama. Accid. Anal. Prev. 13:319-332, 1981.

Bryant, J. D., A. Billingsley, G. A. Kerry, and W. K. Leafman. Physical abuse of children. Child Welfare 42:125-130, 1963.

Chernoff, G. F. The fetal alcohol syndrome in mice: An animal model. Teratology 22:71-75, 1980.

Coate, D., and M. Grossman. Effects of Alcoholic Beverage Prices and Legal Drinking Ages on Youth Alcohol Use. Cambridge, MA: National Bureau of Economic Research, 1986.

Coleman, D. H., and M. A. Strauss. Alcohol abuse and family violence. In E. Gottheil, ed. Alcohol, Drug Abuse and Aggression. Springfield, IL: Charles C. Thomas, 1983.

Combs-Orme, T., J. R. Taylor, E. B. Scott et al. Violent deaths among alcoholics. J. Stud. Alcohol 44:938-949, 1983.

Cook, P. J. The effect of liquor taxes on drinking, cirrhosis and auto accidents. Pp. 255-285 in M. Moore, and D. Gerstein, eds. Alcohol and Public Policy: Beyond the Shadow of Prohibition. Washington, DC: National Academy Press, 1981.

Cook, P. J., and G. Tauchen. The effect of minimum drinking age legislation on youthful auto fatalities, 1970-1977. J. Legal Studies 13:169-191, 1984.

Cooper, J. R. Maternal alcohol metabolism in fetal alcohol syndrome. Clin. Res. 32:113A, 1984.

Cordelia, A. Alcohol and property crime: Exploring the causal nexus. J. Stud. Alcohol 46:161-171, 1985. Also in NIAAA (1987).

Crikelair, G. F., F. C. Symonds, R. N. Ollstein et al. Burn causation: Its many sides. J. Trauma 8:572-582, 1968.

Dietz, P. E., and S. P. Baker. Drowning epidemiology and prevention. Am. J. Public Health 64:303-312, 1974.

El-Guebaly, N., and D. R. Offord. The offspring of alcoholics: A critical review. Am. J. Psych. 134:357-365, 1977.

Ellwood, L. Effects of alcoholism as a family illness on child behavior and development. Military Med. 145(3):188-192, 1980.

Emslie, G. S., and A. Rosenfeld. Incest reported by children and adolescents hospitalized for severe psychiatric problems. Am. J. Psych. 140(6):708-711, 1983.

Epstein, T., T. Cameron, and R. Room. Alcohol and family abuse. In M. Aarens et al. Alcohol Casualties and Crime. Special report prepared for NIAAA by the Social Research Group, University of California, Berkeley, 1977.

Famularo, R., K. Stone, R. Barnum, and T. Wharton. Alcoholism and severe child maltreatment. Am. J. Orthopsych. 56(3):481-485, 1986.

Fell, J. C., and T. Klein. The nature of the reduction in alcohol in U.S. fatal crashes. Society of Automotive Engineers Technical Paper Series 860038. Presented at the Society of Automotive Engineers Conference, Detroit, 1986.

Giersten, J. C. Drowning while under the influence of alcohol. Med. Sci. Law 10:216-219, 1970.

Gooden, B. Drowning and alcohol. Med. J. Aust. 141:478, 1984.

Hamilton, D. J., and J. J. Collins. The role of alcohol in wife beating and child abuse: A review of the literature. In J. J. Collins, ed. Drinking and Crime. New York: Guilford Press, 1981.

Hanson, J. W., A. P. Streissguth, and D. W. Smith. The effects of moderate alcohol consumption during pregnancy on fetal growth and morphogenesis. J. Pediatrics 92: 457-460, 1978.

Herman, J., and L. Hirschman. Families at risk for father-daughter incest. Am. J. Psych. 100:762-770, 1981.

Hingson, R., and J. Howland. Alcohol as a risk factor for injury or death resulting from accidental falls: A review of the literature. J. Stud. Alcohol 48:212-219, 1987a.

Hingson, R., and J. Howland. Prevention of drunk driving crashes involving young drivers: An overview of legislative countermeasures. Pp. 337-348 in T. Benjamin, ed. Young Drivers Impaired by Alcohol and Drugs. Royal Society of Medicine International Congress and Symposium Series No. 116. London: Royal Society of Medicine, 1987b.

Honkanen, R., L. Ertama, P. Kuosmanen et al. The role of alcohol in accidental falls. J. Stud. Alcohol 44:231-245, 1983.

Howland, J., and R. Hingson. Alcohol as a risk factor for injuries or death due to fires and burns: Review of the literature. Public Health Rep. 102:475-483, 1987.

Howland, J., and R. Hingson. Alcohol as a risk factor for drowning: A review of the literature, 1950-1985. Accid. Anal. Prev. 20:19-25, 1988.

Institute of Medicine. Causes and Consequences of Alcohol Problems: An Agenda for Research. Washington, DC: National Academy Press, 1987.

Jessor, R. Adolescent problem drinking: Psychosocial aspects and developmental outcomes. Paper presented at the Alcohol Research Seminar held as part of the international ceremony designating the NIAAA as a Collaborative Center of the World Health Organization, Washington, DC, November 2, 1983.

Jessor, R., and S. Jessor. Adolescent development and the onset of drinking: A longitudinal study. J. Stud. Alcohol 36:27-51, 1975.

Kaplan, S. J., D. Pelcovitz, S. Salzinger, and D. Ganeles. Psychopathology of parents of abused and neglected children and adolescents. J. Am. Acad. Child Psych. 22(3):238-244, 1983.

Keatings, W. R., and M. Evans. The respiratory and cardiovascular response to immersion in cold and warm water. Q. J. Exp. Physiol. 46:83-94, 1961.

Kendall, R. E. Alcohol and suicide. Substance and Alcohol Actions/Misuse 4:121-127, 1983.

May, P. A., K. S. Hymbaugh, J. H. Aase, and J. H. Samet. Epidemiology of fetal alcohol syndrome among American Indians of the southwest. In Alcohol and Health: Sixth Special Report to the U.S. Congress from the Secretary of Health and Human Services. Washington, DC: NIAAA, January 1987.

Mitchell, D. S., S. C. Packham, and W. E. Fitzgerald. Effects of ethanol and carbon monoxide on two measures of behavioral incapacitation of rats. Proc. West. Pharmacol. Soc. 21:427-431, 1978.

National Highway Traffic Safety Administration. Alcohol and Highway Safety 1984: A Review of the State of the Art. DOT HS 806-569. Washington, DC: NHTSA, 1985.

National Institute on Alcohol Abuse and Alcoholism. Sixth Special Report to the U.S. Congress on Alcohol and Health. DHHS Publ. No. (ADM) 87-1519. Rockville, MD: NIAAA, 1987.

National Safety Council. Accident Facts. Chicago: National Safety Council, 1984.

Orme, R. C., and J. Rimmer. Alcoholism and child abuse: A review. J. Stud. Alcohol 42:273-287, 1981.

Perrine, M. W. Alcohol influences on drinking-related behavior: A critical review of laboratory studies of neurophysiological, neuromuscular and sensory activity. J. Safety Res. 5:165-184, 1973.

Rada, R. T. Alcoholism and the child molester. Ann. N.Y. Acad. Sci. 273:492-496, 1976.

Rittenbury, M. S., F. H. Schmidt, R. W. Maddox et al. Factors significantly affecting mortality in burn patients. J. Trauma 5:587-600, 1965.

Roizen, J. Estimating alcohol involvement in several events. In National Institute on Alcohol Abuse and Alcoholism. Alcohol Consumption and Related Problems. Alcohol and Health Monograph No. 1. DHHS Publ. (ADM) 82-1190. Washington, DC: Government Printing Office, 1982.

Room, R. Alcohol and crime: Behavioral aspects. In S. H. Kadish, ed. Encyclopedia of Crime and Justice, vol. 1. New York: Free Press, 1983. Also in NIAAA (1987).

Rosett, J. L., L. Weiner, A. Lee, et al. Patterns of alcohol consumption and fetal development. Obstetrics and Gynecology 61:539-546, 1983.

Ross, H. L. Deterring the Drinking Driver: Legal Policy and Social Control. Lexington, MA: DC Heath and Co., 1982.

Salzinger, S., C. Samit, R. Krieger et al. A controlled study of the life events of mothers of maltreated children in suburban families. J. Am. Acad. Child Psych. 25(3):419-426, 1986.

Schmidt, W., and J. deLint. Causes of death of alcoholics. Q. J. Stud. Alcohol 33:171-185, 1972.

Smart, R. G. Are alcoholics' accidents due solely to heavy drinking? J. Safety Res. 1:170-173, 1969.

Smith, S. M., R. Hanson, and S. Nobel. Parents of battered babies: A controlled study. Br. Med. J. 3:17-32, 1973.

Sokol, R. J., S. I. Miller, and G. Reed. Alcohol abuse during pregnancy: An epidemiologic study. Alcoholism Clin. Exp. Res. 4:135-145, 1980.

Stall, R. D. A comparison of alcohol and drug use patterns of homosexual and heterosexual men: Working paper. Berkeley, CA: Alcohol Research Group, 1986.

Steele, B., and C. Polloch. A psychiatric study of parents who abuse infants and small children. In R. E. Helfer and C. H. Kempe, eds. The Battered Child. Chicago: University of Chicago Press, 1968.

Stephens, C. J. A study of alcohol use and injuries among emergency room patients. San Francisco: Medical Research Institute of San Francisco, 1985.

Summerskill, W. H. J., and P. J. Kelly. Osteoporosis with fractures in anicteric cirrhosis: Observations supplemented by micro- radiographic evaluation of bone. Mayo Clin. Proc. 38:162-174, 1963.

Tarter, R. E., A. M. Hegedus, G. Goldstein et al. Adolescent sons of alcoholics: Neurological and personality characteristics. Alcoholism Clin. Exp. Res. 8:216-222, 1984.

Transportation Research Board. Proceedings of the Workshop on Alcohol-Related Accidents in Recreational Boating. Washington, DC: National Academy Press, 1986.

U.S. Department of Health and Human Services. Fifth Special Report to the U.S Congress on Alcohol and Health. DHHS Publ. No. (ADM) 84-1291. Washington, DC: Government Printing Office, 1984.

Waller, J. A. Non-highway injury fatalities. I. The role of alcohol and problem drinking, drugs and medical impairment. J. Chron. Dis. 25:33-45, 1972.

Wright, S. J. SOS: Alcohol, drugs and boating. Alcohol Health Res. World 9:28-33, 1985.

Zobeck, T. Trends in Alcohol-Related Fatal Traffic Accidents, United States: 1977-1984. Surveillance Report No. 1. Washington, DC: U.S. Department of Health and Human Services, 1986.

3

INDIVIDUAL-ENVIRONMENT INTERACTIONS: FOCUS ON THE INDIVIDUAL

This chapter describes three avenues of research into antecedents of the heavy use of alcohol and possible interventions to prevent such use. The three perspectives share a common focus on the individual.

There are obviously many possible approaches to prevention research from the point of view of the individual alone. A number of these research avenues are presented in IOM's 1987 report, Causes and Consequences of Alcohol Problems. The approaches chosen by the committee for inclusion in Part I are illustrative of the interactive perspective the committee believes would be most fruitful for prevention research in alcohol-related problems: that is, the individual in the context of the environment, both the specific drinking environment and the broader, total developmental setting.

The first research approach uses life-course development and individual vulnerability as a framework for research to identify individuals, early in their lives, who may be at high risk of heavy alcohol use during adolescence. The section also discusses indicators of future problems with alcohol. Conclusions from this line of research could be used to design prevention efforts targeted to populations that are identified as being vulnerable. A second research avenue involves the use of social learning models, which can accommodate genetic, developmental, and environmental factors in their investigation of etiology and antecedents. The committee suggests several lines of intervention using this approach that may prevent problems with alcohol by teaching individuals to alter their behavior. The final research perspective, the genetic influences on the risk of developing severe alcohol problems or dependence, is discussed briefly; the committee notes that understanding of these effects is in an early stage and refers the reader to the first phase of this study (IOM, 1987) for a more complete treatment of the subject.

Despite their common focus on the individual, some differences among the three perspectives will be obvious to the reader. Nevertheless, it will become clear that they are complementary and that insights from each can be useful in preventing the heavy use of alcohol.

LIFE-COURSE DEVELOPMENT, VULNERABILITY, AND PREVENTION RESEARCH

The perspective on prevention research described in this section is derived primarily from epidemiological and developmental research and builds on advances in biological, behavioral, and sociological research. Its main tool is the prospective study, which follows cohorts or samples of individuals to map, in this case, developmental pathways to the heavy use of alcohol.

This approach to alcohol problem prevention, with its focus on the development of the individual, is based on research that searches for those physiological and psychological factors that interact with life events to produce "high-risk" populations who may be especially vulnerable to alcohol-related problems. The research findings on which the life-course developmental approach rests--and the implications of this model for preventive interventions--are presented here with research suggestions that may assist in future prevention program design and policy development.

The Developmental Approach: Rationale and Definitions

The research avenue described in this section stems from the assumption that a developmental perspective may be fruitful both for risk-factor research and for preventive trials in the areas of alcohol and substance use. As stated by Zucker and Noll (1982:316):

A developmental view of behaviors, including that related to alcohol use and abuse, in its simplest form implies the ability to link age to drinking phenomena in an orderly way. The complexity of the problem, however, lies in the ability to trace out the vagaries of this process, and to specify the exact pathways and interactions that both anticipate and produce the drinking behavior and problem or nonproblem sequelae. This implies the ability to trace out unfolding and maturational phenomena for the individual, as well as ongoing physiological, psychological, social, and sociocultural events as they affect the unfolding and are in turn affected by it.

Development is seen as a life-long process that occurs as a result of biological and environmental determinants and their interaction. Researchers have used this concept to construct analytical frameworks for the investigation of individual vulnerability to the heavy use of alcohol. A number of these frameworks are described briefly below.

The Life-Course Events Approach

This perspective (Baltes, Reese, and Lipsitt, 1980) sees behavioral development as shaped by three major systems of influence:

1. normative age-graded, or ontogenetic, influences--events that occur in very similar ways for all individuals in a culture or subculture (e.g., biological maturation, age-determined socialization events involving aspects of the family life cycle, entrance into and progression through the educational system, entrance into the work force, etc.),
2. normative history-graded influences, or cohort effects-- events that occur to most members of a given generation (a cohort) in a similar manner, although the actual experience of a history-graded event (e.g., a war or economic depression) may differ for members of the same as well as different generations, and
3. nonnormative life events--events vary across individuals and that are not shared across a population (e.g., divorce, loss of a job, having an alcoholic parent).

These three types of influences--age-graded, history-graded, and nonnormative--vary in their relative effect on an individual at different stages in the life span.

The life-event perspective posits that behavior involving the heavy use of alcohol will be influenced by all three categories of events. Such normative events as entering high school or college, leaving home to live on one's own, retirement, and death of a spouse may have a measurable effect on an individual's substance use. Similarly, history-graded events may have an impact on a subpopulation or a particular cohort. For example, Prohibition and its subsequent repeal in the United States during the early part of the twentieth century influenced the population's use of alcohol. In contrast, the cohort of teenagers and young adults during the late 1960s, the "Woodstock generation," experienced greater acceptance of drug experimentation and usage, an effect that was not as strongly felt by individuals who were older or younger. Finally, an individual's use of alcohol will be influenced by nonnormative or stressful life events that put severe burdens on his or her capacity to cope with life circumstances and change.

Social Fields

At each stage of life, individuals are involved in a few major social fields. In the early years, the dominant field of influence is the family of orientation, followed by school and classroom influences, and shortly thereafter by the peer group. The intimate social field develops through adolescence and becomes the marital social field later in the life course. In adulthood, the work field develops in importance, as does the individual's family of procreation. There are, altogether, a fairly small number of such social fields, and their influences vary at each stage of life.

Within each social field, significant people, or "natural raters" (e.g., schoolteacher, parent, spouse, work supervisor), define social tasks, evaluate efforts, and give feedback to an individual based on performance expectations. These natural raters can be asked by researchers to gauge an individual's social adaptational status (SAS), which can be defined as adequacy of performance in a particular social field at a particular stage of life (Kellam et al., 1975). Some childhood SAS ratings have been shown to predict later teenage outcomes involving the use of alcohol and other substances (Kellam et al., 1983). Examples of SAS predictors of later heavy alcohol use include poor school achievement and shy and aggressive classroom behavior, as rated by teachers (Kellam et al., 1975, 1983).

Risk Factors: Intraindividual and Environmental Domains

A number of researchers have considered prevention from the vantage of intraindividual differences that are associated with the heavy use of alcohol. These differences can be broken down into more specific risk-factor categories:

- neurophysiological variables (Tarter, Alterman, and Edwards, 1985; Heibrun et al., 1986; Baribeau, Ethier, and Braun, 1987);
- temperament (Tarter, Alterman, and Edwards, 1985);
- personality variables (Goodwin et al., 1975; Cantwell, 1978; Gaines and Connors, 1982; Folsom et al., 1985; Brooks et al., 1986; Labouvie and McGee, 1986);
- behavior variables (McCord and McCord, 1960, 1962; Robins, 1966; Jones, 1968, 1971; Vaillant, 1983); and
- social adaptational status variables (Kellam, Ensminger, and Simon, 1980; Knop et al., 1985).

It is also possible to make more fine-grained distinctions within each of these groupings. Furthermore, some research has indicated that there may be a genetic contribution to the etiology of alcoholism, possibly mediated through one or more neurophysiological, temperament, personality, or behavioral variables (Partanen, Bruun, and Markkanen, 1966; Goodwin et al., 1973, 1974; Begleiter et al., 1984; Cadoret, Troughton, and O'Gorman, 1987; Cloninger, 1987).

Factors that may influence drinking behavior have also been linked to various environmental domains:

- the family (Zucker and Barron, 1973; Ablon, 1976; Wolin, Bennett, and Noonan, 1979; Wolin and Bennett, 1980; Barnes, Farrell, and Cairns, 1986; Beardslee, Son, and Vaillant, 1986; Burnside et al., 1986; MacDonald and Blume, 1986; Needle et al., 1986);
- the peer group (Straus and Bacon, 1953; Alexander and Campbell, 1967; Needle et al., 1986; Selnow and Crano, 1986);
- the work setting (Smart, 1979);
- the community (Gibbons et al., 1986); and
- broader societal culture (Berger and Snortum, 1986; Dawkins, 1986; Gliksman and Rush, 1986; Linsky, Colby, and Straus, 1986; Vaillant, 1986).

Individual-Environment Interaction

Recently, researchers have suggested that certain interactions between risk factors in an individual and factors in the environment may contribute to the etiology of alcoholism. For example, a poor match between a child's temperament and parental behavior and style may heighten the risk for later alcoholism (Tarter, Alterman, and Edwards, 1985). A genetic vulnerability combined with particular environmental influences could also determine whether an individual exhibits problem drinking (Tarter, Alterman, and Edwards, 1985; Zucker and Gomberg, 1986; Cadoret, Troughton, and O'Gorman, 1987; McCord, 1988a). Indeed, the diathesis-stress concept that hypothesizes an etiology of schizophrenia spectrum disorders based on the notion of individual-environment interaction may be relevant to an understanding of the development of alcohol problems in some individuals.

A further area of research in individual-environment interactions involves the role of developmental transitions (e.g., entrance into college) in creating conditions that may lead to problem drinking (see Jessor and Jessor, 1975, 1977). The majority of individuals progress through developmental transitions without complications. Why some individuals are susceptible to episodes of problem drinking or other adverse outcomes during periods of heightened stress and change is a research question that can be addressed within a conceptual framework of individual-environment interaction. To carry out this kind of research, information about both the individual and his or her environment must be gathered during the planning stage of a study to detect interactions between the two. Developmental transitions should be seen as potential periods during which environmental influences may have more pronounced additive or interactive effects on individual characteristics.

Social adaptational status (SAS) ratings reflect a different kind of individual-environment interaction. An individual's behavioral response to social task demands within a specific social field will influence a natural rater's evaluation of performance adequacy. Poor SAS ratings can serve as markers of an etiologic process that may be leading to a problem outcome.

The Prospective Study: Characteristics and Advantages

The goal of the life-course developmental approach to prevention is to identify specific risk factors that may be useful in devising effective primary prevention programs. Prospective epidemiological studies that follow a cohort of individuals as they progress through developmental stages in the life course are a particularly important research strategy for risk-factor identification. Such studies also allow a more complete understanding of the developmental progression from antecedents to first use, to initiation, to heavy use, to abuse or dependency on a substance. Earlier work in this area (Kellam et al., 1975, 1983; Kellam, Ensminger, and Simon, 1980; Kellam, Brown, and Fleming, 1982; Kellam and Werthamer-Larsson, 1986; Kellam, in press) has combined the advantages of a life-course, developmental orientation and epidemiologically based research to map the developmental paths to the heavy use of alcohol within defined populations over significant portions of the life course. Kellam and colleagues have termed this approach developmental epidemiology.

The prospective study of a cohort of individuals is a major methodological advance over earlier studies that examined only clinical populations, either at a single point in time or through retrospective reports (e.g., Vaillant, 1966; Ball and Chambers, 1970; Stephens and Cottrell, 1972; El-Guebaly and Offord, 1977). As Kandel (1980) has pointed out, clinical populations of addicted individuals seen in hospitals or even outpatient clinics represent very special subgroups of the population of alcohol and other substance users; the risk factors identified among such groups may not be generalizable to other groups or populations.

The primary objective of a prospective epidemiological study involving a cohort is to identify, along developmental pathways, risk factors that heighten the probability of a problem outcome. A prospective epidemiological research strategy first requires that a researcher gain the cooperation of an epidemiologically defined population. If possible, participants should be enrolled early in their development--before initiating alcohol use--to facilitate the disentanglement of cause from effect. The temporal sequence of such factors as aggressive or antisocial behavior and heavy alcohol use, which has been hard to determine in cross-sectional or retrospective studies, is easier to discern when the prospective method is used and begins with a childhood cohort.

The prospective research strategy also allows for follow-up of multiple-problem outcomes. In the area of alcohol and other substance use, this capability is especially important because the heavy use of multiple substances combined with other problem outcomes is not uncommon (e.g., the co-occurrence of alcohol and drug abuse, of heavy alcohol use and major depression, and of substance abuse with schizophrenia spectrum disorders). Multiple-problem follow-up allows researchers to assess the specificity of an antecedent for a particular outcome; it can also help in gauging the impact of a preventive trial.

A prospective epidemiological methodology eliminates some of the problems of cross-sectional studies by enabling the same sample to be studied as it progresses through different developmental stages. Factors that are related to the initiation of alcohol use may not be the same as factors related to continuing problem use and abuse (Zucker and Gomberg, 1986). Continuities and discontinuities over time, both in the development of attitudes about drinking and in drinking behavior, can be described with the prospective approach (Christiansen, Goldman, and Brown, 1985); furthermore, factors that predict which subgroups will progress through different stages of drinking behavior leading to alcohol-related problems can be isolated. Multiple pathways leading to similar-appearing outcomes probably exist, and various theoretical models may be necessary to explain these different developmental paths (McCord, 1988b).

Findings from Prospective Risk-Factor Research

The few available prospective studies that examine the antecedents of heavy alcohol use or problem drinking have made important contributions to our understanding of the etiology of these problems. Based on the review by Zucker and Gomberg (1986), consistent findings that have emerged from this research are noted below.

Antisocial behavior during childhood has been shown to be related to adult alcohol problems (McCord and McCord, 1960; Robins, Bates, and O'Neal, 1962; Robins, 1966; Jones, 1968, 1971; Monnelly, Hartl, and Elderkin, 1983; Vaillant, 1983). In studies of the Woodlawn community in Chicago, aggressive behavior and the combination of aggressive and shy behavior in the first grade both were found to predict heavy alcohol use at ages 16 and 17 (Kellam, Brown, and Fleming, 1982; Kellam et al., 1983). In a finding analogous to those results, McCord (1988b) found that males who were judged to be shy as children were least likely to become heavy alcohol users or to engage in criminal behavior as adults, but those who were rated as both shy and aggressive as children were most likely to become heavy alcohol users or criminals. In a similar finding, Block, Block, and Keyes (1988) report an increased risk of later teenage drug use among 3-to 4-year-old children who displayed aggressive behavior.

Other factors that have consistently predated alcohol problems across many of these prospective studies include difficulty in school achievement (Robins, Bates, and O'Neal, 1962; Robins, 1966; Jones, 1968, 1971; Monnelly, Hartl, and Elderkin, 1983; Vaillant, 1983), inadequate parenting (McCord and McCord, 1960; Robins, Bates, and O'Neal, 1962; Robins, 1966; Jones, 1968, 1971; Monnelly, Hartl, and Elderkin, 1983; Vaillant, 1983), marital conflict in the childhood home (McCord and McCord, 1960; Robins, Bates, and O'Neal, 1962; Robins, 1966; Jones, 1968, 1971; Vaillant, 1983), ethnicity (McCord and McCord, 1960; Robins, Bates, and O'Neal, 1962; Robins, 1966; Vaillant, 1983), hyperactive behavior (McCord and McCord, 1960; Jones, 1968, 1971), and among males, weak interpersonal ties (Robins, Bates, and O'Neal, 1962; Robins, 1966; Jones, 1968, 1971; Monnelly, Hartl, and Elderkin, 1983; Hagnell et al., 1986). Finally, in their prospective study, Hagnell and colleagues (1986) found a greatly increased relative risk of alcoholism among men in their thirties who had used alcohol with their peers 20 years earlier--when they were less than 14 years of age.

Limitations in Existing Prospective Research

There are several important limitations in the prospective studies noted above. Often, the study samples were not drawn from a representative community population. This problem limits the generalizability of results, particularly with regard to women and minorities who have traditionally been underrepresented in such samples. In addition, most samples were not followed from early childhood; thus, the etiologic role of a host of factors that predate adolescence is unclear. Moreover, the relative importance and interrelationships of the various risk factors remain unclear.

Another problem in these studies has been that follow-up contact has not occurred with sufficient regularity to document continuity or discontinuity in developmental course prior, during, and subsequent to heavy use. In a recent review of the literature concerning "spontaneous remission" from alcohol problems, Fillmore and colleagues (1988) describe variability across the life course by age and sex and suggest that cultural factors may play an important role in structuring observed patterns over multiple generations. Generally, this observation is consistent with research that suggests that early problems with alcohol are not necessarily predictive of later problems with alcohol; periodic problem drinking is much more common than continuous abuse (Vaillant, 1983; Fillmore and Midanick, 1984).

Certain childhood factors are definitely associated with increased risk either for heavy drinking in adolescence or for serious alcohol problems in adult life. Yet in the majority of cases there is no continuity between adolescent problem drinking and alcohol problems later in life. About 50 to 60 percent of adolescent males and about 75 percent of adolescent females have been found to "remit" or "mature out" of their problem drinking patterns. It remains to be learned what the factors are that determine which adolescents remain vulnerable to continued difficulty with alcohol (Temple and Fillmore, 1985).

The theories, research approaches, and preventive interventions described in other parts of this report will generally focus on variables during adult life that are determinants of drinking behavior, whether or not an enduring vulnerability exists in the drinking individual. Naturally, when such a vulnerability to problems with alcohol is present, these determinants (e.g., situational factors) will be all the more powerful.

Research on Preventive Trials: Implications from Prospective Research

Although more sophisticated prospective studies are needed to better understand the etiology of alcohol problems, there is already sufficient knowledge to direct preventive trials at specific modifiable antecedents of, and risk factors for, heavy alcohol use and other substance-related problem outcomes. These preventive trials can test the efficacy of specific interventions in field settings and, like prospective cohort research, can inform etiologic theory by experimentally testing plausible causal models.

Chapter 1 of this report presented a threefold model for preventive interventions composed of universal preventive interventions (directed at the entire population), selected interventions (directed at a subgroup presumed to be at greater risk for a problem outcome), and indicated interventions (directed at specific individuals who exhibit indices of preclinical dysfunction). Universal and selected interventions are considered primary prevention; indicated preventive interventions are considered secondary prevention (see Chapter 10).

The life-course development approach suggests that targeting subgroups which are at greater risk to receive a preventive intervention may make that intervention more efficient. (A preventive intervention becomes more efficient as the percentage of program recipients increases who, but for the intervention, would have developed the disorder.) The identification of a risk factor that can be linked to a large proportion of cases with the problem outcome (i.e, a risk factor with a high attributable risk) is a prerequisite for an efficient, selected prevention study.

Under the selected intervention assumptions, the life-course developmental approach suggests certain principles that should be applied to the design of interventions to be tested for the prevention of alcohol and substance-use disorders: (1) interventions should be designed to conform to the developmental pathways taken by cohorts at each major stage of life; (2) vulnerable or high-risk individuals may need to participate in more than one intervention, both within a particular life stage (e.g., adolescence) and across life stages (e.g., adolescence-young adulthood); and (3) interventions should be embedded within or influence the social fields of family, school, work, and community in which a target population is active.

A number of studies suggest that there are potentially modifiable targets for selective approaches to preventive intervention. Tarter, Alterman, and Edwards (1985) integrate various psychological and biological characteristics associated with vulnerability to alcohol abuse, using a multidimensional concept of temperament. Variables that characterize the temperament dimensions linked to heightened risk for alcohol abuse include (1) a high activity level, (2) a deficit in attention-span persistence, (3) low soothability, (4) high emotionality, and (5) a disinhibited, impulsive manner of sociability.

Tarter's findings (1985) also present research evidence supporting the hypothesis that there may be a central nervous system (CNS) dysfunction present in some individuals prior to the onset of alcohol problems, that influences behavior. If such a CNS dysfunction is part of a developmental path leading to heavy alcohol use for these individuals, the potential effectiveness of traditional preventive interventions is questionable. Rather than attempt to modify the implicated risk factor directly, a "prosthetic" preventive approach could be taken. This approach would involve development (and testing) of a set of skills and cognitive coping strategies that a vulnerable individual would be taught or given, much like a prosthesis, to help compensate for or counteract a temperamental predisposition to abuse alcohol. Specific temperamental traits that an individual could be taught to control include impulsive behavior, activity level, and emotional arousal. Additionally, individuals could learn relaxation and other stress management techniques, as well as problem-solving skills, that might help prevent the heavy use of alcohol during periods of heightened stress.

As noted earlier, early aggressive behavior in the classroom has consistently been found to predict heavy alcohol use in late adolescence and early adulthood (Kellam, Brown, and Fleming, 1982; Kellam et al., 1983), and childhood antisocial behavior has been found to be a risk factor for alcohol abuse (McCord and McCord, 1960; Robins, Bates, and O'Neal, 1962; Robins, 1966; Jones, 1968, 1971; Monnelly, Hartl, and Elderkin, 1983; Vaillant, 1983). Should it be the case for the majority of individuals vulnerable to heavy alcohol use that these behaviors are learned responses rather than the product of a CNS dysfunction, it would be possible to develop and test preventive interventions that could be directed at modification of the behaviors themselves, modification of the environmental contingencies that reinforce and maintain the behaviors, or both.

Apart from individual characteristics that play a role in the development of alcohol-related problems, there are influences from various environmental domains. The family is an important source of influence, as well as an important setting within which preventive intervention could occur. Wolin, Bennett, and Noonan (1979) and Wolin and Bennett (1980) have found evidence to support the hypothesis that children from alcoholic families that have not maintained important family rituals during periods in which there is severe parental drinking are more likely to develop alcohol problems than are children from families with an alcoholic parent that have been able to maintain their rituals.
In a prospective study, McCord (1988b) examined the intergenerational transmission of alcoholism and found evidence that men with alcoholic fathers were more likely to become alcoholics themselves if the mother seemed to accept her husband's intoxicated behavior and to hold him in high esteem. These findings suggest that one developmental path to alcoholism in children of alcoholics may stem, in part, from family acceptance of an alcoholic parent's intoxicated behavior. Preventive interventions targeted to children who are at risk by virtue of having an alcoholic parent could be designed to modify those family

dynamics that lead to the disruption of important family rituals and to family overacceptance or unwillingness to confront intoxicated behavior in a parent.

The peer group is another source of environmental influence for alcohol and other substance use that is most salient during the adolescent stage of development (Alexander and Campbell, 1967; Biddle, Bank, and Marlin, 1980; Needle et al., 1986). Research findings suggest that membership in structured, goal-directed groups may protect teenagers against adolescent substance use (Selnow and Crano, 1986). The element that appears to be critical to the protective influence of formal groups is a group norm that does not expect or approve of substance use. Adolescent participation in nonstructured, informal peer groups without such a norm appears to increase the risk of substance use.

Pronounced sex differences in vulnerability to alcohol and other substance use remain unexplained and may have major importance in understanding the origins and paths leading to problem outcomes. Femaleness as well as shyness appear to be strong inhibitors of both adolescent delinquency and substance use, and both variables are important to an understanding of the evolution of these outcomes.

The following are opportunities for the next stage of prospective research into the etiology of heavy alcohol use from a developmental/epidemiological perspective:

- The next stage of prospective research on heavy alcohol use and alcohol-related problems should be integrated with research into other problem outcomes (e.g., drug use, suicide, delinquency, mental disorders). This integration would foster the development of theoretical models that explain the appearance of both single and multiple problem outcomes. These models can then be used for planning targeted prevention strategies for specific subgroups.
- Prospective studies should define and assess intermediate outcomes and stages along the developmental paths of cohort members. For example, observation at the preschool stage of development could assess genetic, family, and temperament variables. At the grade-school stage, researchers might investigate the behavioral responses that are either known or hypothesized to be antecedents of later alcohol-related problems. At follow-up in the preadolescent stage, a relevant outcome for assessment could be the initial use of alcohol; at the adolescent stage, it might be heavy use, whereas in young adulthood the outcomes of interest might include heavy use, abuse, and dependence. This approach entails repeated waves of follow-up study and multivariate modeling.
- The factors that influence the heavy use of alcohol should be considered within intraindividual domains and across environmental domains for their separate and joint contributions to the etiology of alcohol-related problems. Research should focus not only on measuring intraindividual and environmental factors that influence an individual's use of alcohol but also on the interaction of these two categories of influence.
- Particular attention should be paid to transitions among stages of development (e.g., transition to school, leaving home, entrance into the work force) as times when intraindividual factors may interact with conditions in certain environmental domains to produce alcohol-related problems. Researchers will need to examine how the development of drinking-related behavior is influenced by such age-graded, normative influences as the transition to high school and college, as well as such life events as the loss of a job or divorce.
- Cohort effects (e.g., a period of greater cultural tolerance or intolerance of substance use) must be taken into account to understand the etiology of alcohol and other

substance-use problems for a specific cohort of a particular culture in a given historical period.

   • Multistage sampling provides the needed bridge for linking large-scale, prospective research to studies based on more frequent or precise observations of smaller samples. Probability samples can be drawn from a defined population, or the entire population or cohort may be used for assessment, followed by a second sample drawn from the first. This second-stage sample can be drawn to represent the strata of the first sample, as well as the total population that was originally sampled. A third-stage sample can be drawn from the second sample, which represents strata from the second and the first. This method allows increasingly intensive assessments to be done on suitably small but representative subsamples.

Importance of Longitudinal Data Bases

The longitudinal data on which life-course developmental research now rests are extremely important as a national resource for the next stage of prevention research. Yet some longitudinal data sets are in immediate jeopardy of disappearing due to a lack of funding. There is now no mechanism other than the individual research grant by which to ensure the continued survival of these data. One proposal that has been discussed is to send data tapes to a central repository. However, this approach would not include information concerning documentation, specification of constructs, software languages, and the conditions under which the data were collected, all of which are necessary for researchers to be able to draw the most accurate inferences. Therefore, it seems most prudent to find mechanisms to support and maintain--as well as expand--existing longitudinal data bases, and to find ways of increasing their accessibility to the research community.

In the search for predictors of future problems with alcohol, there are other possible sources of data that could be exploited and correlated with longitudinal data bases. For example, most prevention intervention trials have been carried out separately from prospective epidemiological research. Yet these prevention trials have yielded data that can be further analyzed to determine which subgroups are affected by particular kinds of interventions and how they are affected. Further analysis would add to our ability to experimentally test the effects of specific predictors. Moreover, the particular subgroups to be targeted for preventive interventions could be identified by early predictors that have already been found in prospective epidemiological research.

The following are opportunities for research with expanded longitudinal data bases:

   • Analyses of potential predictors of later risk behaviors should be extended to as early in the life span as possible. Sex differences should be investigated much more intensively, and the populations that are studied should be described better.
   • Researchers should actively seek opportunities to use a profile of multiple outcomes rather than the single outcome of problematic alcohol use. To construct such a profile, data bases other than those specifically related to alcohol use should be included, and parallel agencies to NIAAA should be enlisted for help whenever possible.

SOCIAL LEARNING MODELS

As discussed in the section concerning life-course development and vulnerability, theoretical models that account for the behavior of individuals may be useful in designing population-based prevention programs because, ultimately, individual behavior change is necessary for prevention. Prevention research should therefore be directed toward elucidating those factors within an individual that underlie the drinking behavior and that may aid or retard the processes of change (Prochaska and DiClemente, 1982; Miller and Heather, 1986).

There are several useful models of alcohol use and abuse that focus on the individual and derive from biological and psychological processes (Blane and Leonard, 1987). To varying degrees, these models are based on biobehavioral, cognitive-emotional, and perceived sociocultural factors that contribute to the development of alcohol-related problems. These same factors can be used as a guide to intervention strategies.

A variety of antecedent variables have been proposed as predictors or mediators of behavior in the context of broader theoretical models. These models include problem behavior theory (Jessor and Jessor, 1977; Jessor, 1984), drug-use stress and drug-use coping skills hypotheses (Kandel, Kessler, and Margulies, 1978; Abrams, 1983), and models based on cognitive social learning theory (Bandura, 1977, 1986; Blane and Leonard, 1987). Alcohol-related problems have been conceptualized as resulting from low self-esteem and poor self-concept; moral deficiencies; underlying biochemical imbalances; inappropriate social norms within subcultures; or deficiencies in knowledge, attitudes, intentions, and alternative coping behaviors (Azjen and Fishbein, 1980; Perry, 1986). Yet the various biopsychosocial factors involved in alcohol-related problems, factors that could become important targets for prevention research and intervention design, are often underemphasized in prevention program planning. Those who design and implement intervention programs are often more explicit about their objectives than about the cause of the process in which they want to intervene (Goodstadt, 1986).

Among existing conceptual models, those based on a social learning perspective have generated a great deal of interest and are discussed in this section. Because social learning approaches delineate the processes by which individuals acquire and maintain behavior, they are useful for conceptualizing alcohol prevention research. In addition, social learning models can be coordinated with other models because they incorporate (a) the innate biological vulnerabilities of the individual, as well as the experience he or she acquires during the course of development; (b) immediate (proximal) environmental antecedents and consequences of behavior; and (c) cognitive-behavioral processes that are relevant to an individual's understanding of how to self-regulate alcohol use and alcohol-related behaviors (Abrams, 1983; Pomerleau and Pomerleau, 1984).

A number of studies have focused on social learning theory as it relates to alcohol use and abuse (Bandura, 1969, 1977, 1986; P. M. Miller, 1976; W. R. Miller, 1980; Marlatt and Gordon, 1985; Abrams and Niaura, 1987; Blane and Leonard, 1987; Nathan and Niaura, 1987; Wilson, 1987, 1988; Marlatt et al., 1988). The central concept of the social learning perspective is reciprocal determinism. Like the life-course developmental approach, reciprocal determinism emphasizes the interaction between individuals and their environment and can provide a bridge between microlevel (individual) and macrolevel (social network, organizational, community, and population) models. Abrams and Niaura (1987) have summarized the way social learning theorists view the development of problems of alcohol abuse:

• Learning to drink alcohol is an integral part of psychosocial development and socialization within a culture. Youthful drinking behaviors, beliefs, attitudes, and expectancies concerning alcohol are formed mainly through the social influences of culture, family, and peers. Much learning takes place before the child or adolescent consumes any alcohol. This learning influence is exerted indirectly through attitudes and expectancies and directly by the models of alcohol consumption provided by peers and family, by media portrayals of drinking, and by other mechanisms through which culturally acceptable or unacceptable habits are inculcated.

• Individual differences that predispose a person toward alcohol-related problems may interact with the influence of socializing agents and situational determinants. Such factors may be general (e.g., sensitivity or excessive reactivity to stressful stimuli, mood disorders) or alcoholspecific (e.g., differential vulnerability to alcohol effects, genetic determinants). Predisposing psychosocial factors may include deficits in coping skills or such behavioral excesses as problems with managing emotions (e.g., anger). The absence of normal-drinking role models or the presence of abusive-drinking role models may also result in deficits in an individual's self-regulation of drinking. These factors may increase the risk of alcohol abuse in vulnerable persons.

• Direct experience with alcohol becomes important when experimentation with alcohol begins (increasingly early in adolescence). At this point, continued alcohol use may be determined by the direct reinforcing and aversive effects of alcohol and such other proximal determinants as peer pressure and alcohol's stress-reducing properties or the belief that it enhances social interaction. Many of these effects will be mediated by modeling and by socially learned expectations, which may be the predominant determinants of the effects of alcohol (as opposed to pharmacological disinhibition processes).

• To the extent that any predisposing individual differences or social learning history factors interact with current situational demands, a person's perception of self-efficacy and coping may be undermined, and alcohol abuse rather than normal use may occur. The probability of continued drinking and eventual abuse is high if the individual is unable to develop alternative and more adaptive ways of coping with immediate (proximal) situational demands. In essence, the major immediate determinants of problematic drinking are high levels of external demand or strain that develop because (a) environmental stresses are exceeding an individual's coping capacity, (b) there is low self-efficacy for alternative coping behaviors, and (c) there are high outcome expectations that alcohol will produce the desired results, while (d) there is minimization or denial of the long-term negative consequences. Individual variations exist in the severity of the immediate proximal demands, the social learning history and genetic vulnerability of the person, the availability of alcohol, the repertoire of current cognitive and behavioral coping skills, and the probability of perceived positive or negative consequences following behavior. Depending on these variables, the individual will abstain, control drinking, have episodic abuse, display problem behaviors, or develop alcohol dependence.

• If alcohol use is sustained, an individual will develop a tolerance to its direct reinforcing properties (e.g., stress dampening) that will promote the ingestion of greater quantities to achieve similar effects. Thus, acquired tolerance and other pharmacological factors relating to dependence and withdrawal symptoms will come to control a person's behavior more powerfully than proximal environmental-cognitive interactions. Alcohol consumption can now be independently, negatively reinforced to avoid withdrawal symptoms, and increasing dependence can ensue. Classical conditioning factors, including conditioned cues and the sight and smell of alcohol, can themselves become environmental demands that result in a form of cognitive craving experienced as a desire or urge to drink (see Niaura et al., 1988).

• Any episode of alcohol abuse or problem behavior results in reciprocal individual and social consequences that can affect person-environment interactions in the future. Examples of reciprocal consequences include marital discord, loss of employment, and other changes in social supports. These changes, in turn, may create additional stress that further exacerbates drinking problems.

• Recovery after episodes of abusive drinking will require interventions that are different from those used to prevent or reduce the likelihood of problems developing initially (e.g., relapse prevention coping skills training).

Implications of Social Learning Theory for Research on Prevention

The central assumptions of a social learning perspective on the prevention of alcohol-related problems suggest various opportunities for prevention research. With respect to prevention, these assumptions place greater emphasis on the here-and-now (proximal) person-environment interactions than on those occurring in the more distant past. Furthermore, the individual is an active agent in the learning process, not a passive recipient. The specific emphasis of prevention activities may differ, depending on the stages of the life span and other factors, but in the social learning view, desirable self regulation of alcohol use and even modulation of behavior when intoxicated are thought to be primarily the result of interaction between current (proximal) individual and situational factors.

Specific cognitive information-processing mechanisms (beliefs, expectations, coping skills, self-efficacy) play a central role in regulating alcohol-related behavior (Bandura, 1977, 1986; Marlatt and Gordon, 1985; Wilson, 1987, 1988; O'Leary and Wilson, 1988). For the most part, health education and health belief models based on knowledge and attitude change can be incorporated into research on cognitive mechanisms, but they are poorly related to behavior and are therefore regarded as necessary but insufficient for change (Goodstadt, 1986). Selected examples of key concepts requiring more research include self-efficacy, vicarious learning or modeling, and the importance of beliefs and expectations of reward.

A social learning perspective assigns central importance to the construct of self-efficacy to explain how behavior patterns are acquired and how they are maintained in the face of external pressures and temptations (Bandura, 1977, 1986). Self-efficacy refers to an individual's perception of his or her capability to execute a particular course of action and his or her confidence in the mastery of the skills required to cope with a situation (Abrams and Niaura, 1987; Wilson, 1987, 1988). Efficacy judgments are thought to influence a person's choice of action, effort expended, perseverance in the face of resistance, and quality and strength of performance in a specific situation.

There are four mechanisms (listed here in order of power or importance) that can alter efficacy expectations: (1) actual performance accomplishments and corrective feedback that result in a change in behavior (e.g., skills training in a specific situation); (2) modeling or vicarious learning--observing others and their success or failure, as well as the similarity between the role model and oneself (e.g., identification with a sports star); (3) social persuasion (e.g., psychotherapy, verbal admonitions, or attempts at knowledge or attitude change); and (4) direct physiological changes during task performance (e.g., tension reduction or experiences of pleasure). More research is needed to determine the various ways these basic principles can be applied to alcohol prevention research and its applications.

Observational learning, both modeling and imitation, is considered to be of central importance in understanding such factors as peer pressure to drink, media influences, and the development of perceived social norms and expectations of what is appropriate and inappropriate behavior when intoxicated. MacAndrew and Edgerton (1969) relied heavily on learning through modeling in their anthropological account of drunken behavior. They noted that the wide variation in drinking rituals across cultural groups and ethnic groups could not be explained by biological or pharmacological factors alone (e.g., disinhibition models). Collins and Marlatt (1981) have summarized the modeling literature and concluded that "modeling has a powerful effect wherein the individual's consumption of alcohol will vary to match that of the model."

An understanding of the strong influence of modeling on behavior is essential to develop prevention programs, especially among youth and adolescents. Unfortunately, many traditional educational efforts in this area have been ineffective or actually counterproductive because of problems in either their content or their form (Nathan, 1983). For example, values clarification approaches or educational messages that are designed to modify knowledge or attitudes about alcohol can actually be counterproductive if they heighten an individual's curiosity about drinking without providing specific role models and guidelines on how to self-regulate behavior (e.g., Schlegel, cited in Best et al., 1988). Nathan (1983) and Wilson (1988) draw attention to a social learning analysis of media portrayals of drinking that is relevant for prevention research (see Chapter 4).

Another important element in social learning theory is that of learned expectancies and expectancy sets. Marlatt (1976, 1984) has postulated that people learn to expect short-term positive consequences from drinking and to minimize the longer term negative consequences. Also, as part of its stress-dampening effect, alcohol forestalls negative emotional reactions in many individuals because it blocks the memory of adverse consequences (Sher and Levenson, 1982). As Marlatt (1984) states, "Freed from the pressures of past painful memories and the anxious anticipation of future negative consequences, the heavy drinker experiences a narrowing of attention to the here and now and increased responsivity to immediate external cues to the exclusion of other past or future events." Thus, expectancies about drinking enable individuals to transform negative feelings into positive feelings or to reduce such negative emotional states as depression, anger, or anxiety.

An individual's beliefs and outcome expectations are often better predictors of behavior than the actual consequences of action (Marlatt and Rohsenow, 1980). A person's expectancy of reward, therefore, is a critical mediating variable that governs alcohol use and abuse, as well as problem behaviors when intoxicated (e.g., violence). It is by now well accepted that many "out-of-control" behaviors displayed by individuals when intoxicated are the result of beliefs, expectations, and attributions that are derived from perceived cultural norms. Expectancy theory has significant implications for prevention both in adolescents (Goldman, Brown, and Christiansen, 1987) and in adults.

Social learning theory has been used in numerous studies to show that response-contingent positive consequences (reinforcement) increase drinking and negative consequences (punishment) decrease drinking. Based on the principles of operant conditioning, studies in controlled laboratory settings (Cohen et al., 1971; Nathan and O'Brien, 1971) have shown that alcoholics will restrict their drinking to less than 5 ounces a day if this behavior is positively reinforced. It is thought that the combined effects of social influence that result from modeling and differential reinforcement patterns within the social network of the individual can account for most of the differing rates of alcoholism among different ethnic groups. Vaillant (1983) reports findings which suggest that drinking patterns may be modified by differentially rewarding moderate drinking; they may also change when cultures display immediate, consistent, and predictable disapproval of drunkenness or inappropriate behavior when intoxicated. More research of this type is needed to determine to what extent the principles of operant conditioning can be applied to specific targets for the prevention of alcohol abuse.

In summary, then, social learning theory proposes that excessive drinking and alcohol-related problem behavior are to a large extent learned behaviors (P. M. Miller, 1976). It is also generally accepted that the acquisition of appropriate behaviors or the weakening of learned behaviors is most readily accomplished early in life. Although recognizing the importance of an individual's social learning history, the social learning approach focuses on the immediate proximal environment as the primary source of behavioral control in the here-and-now. The social learning viewpoint also encourages a coping skills training approach to prevention that emphasizes learning new habits to increase an individual's ability to exercise appropriate self-control while drinking. Other approaches include self-management techniques, such as self-monitoring of blood alcohol levels, cognitive restructuring techniques, and understanding motivational factors and the stages-of-change model (Prochaska and DiClemente, 1982). These approaches are reviewed briefly below.

The Coping Skills Training Approach

Traditional progressive disease models of alcoholism assume that drinking problems generally intensify inexorably over time as the disease progresses. In contrast, social learning researchers suggest that many individuals can learn to stabilize or even reduce their drinking by acquiring alternative coping skills, changing life-style habits, and learning safe drinking practices. This hypothesis follows from the critical assumption that drinking problems can be aligned along a continuum of severity ranging from moderate drinking to alcohol dependence. Moderation or the controlled use of alcohol may be more acceptable as a goal for primary and secondary prevention programs than as an alternative to abstinence for the treatment of alcohol dependence (Heather and Robertson, 1983; Marlatt, 1984; Marlatt and Gordon, 1985).

Behavioral coping skills training methods can be used to achieve goals of either abstinence or moderate drinking. The skills that are often taught include drink refusal training and how to cope with peer pressures to drink. Such skills are usually taught in group settings in which role playing, direct practice, rehearsal, and corrective feedback can be provided either by the group or by a professional group leader (see Peer resistance training in school-based programs: Flay, 1984; Killen, 1985; Best et al., 1988). Other coping skills (e.g., relaxation training, exercise, anger or assertiveness training) are also taught as alternatives to drinking under the assumption that some individuals drink to manage their moods and interpersonal relations. The goal here is to provide these individuals with "functionally equivalent" substitutes for drinking, which will provide them with a broader repertoire of responses in stressful situations. Behavioral relapse prevention strategies using many of these techniques have been developed as a way to help former alcoholics maintain sobriety (Marlatt and Gordon, 1985).

Although skills programs were originally designed and evaluated for use in adult alcoholism treatment programs (Chaney, O'Leary, and Marlatt, 1978; Monti et al., 1986), such procedures are also being used in primary and secondary prevention programs with children, young adults, and college students (Mills, Pfaffenberger, and McCarty, 1981; McCarty et al., 1983; Schiffman and Wills, 1985; W. R. Miller and Heather, 1986). More research is needed to identify the skills training techniques and methods of dissemination that may be appropriate for different individuals in different settings and to develop ways of adapting these strategies for broad-scale primary prevention interventions.

Self-Management Techniques

Self-management techniques lend themselves to preventive interventions. Clients can be taught the basic principles of habit change, using minimal self-help or media-assisted protocols. The techniques involved in this approach include dealing with problem identification and heightening awareness that a problem exists, setting the stage for change by increasing motivation, teaching the appropriate selection of specific methods of change, and providing technologies to maintain and generalize the change. The targets of change may vary, depending on the priorities and targets of prevention (e.g., excessive drinking, acute drinking-related problem behavior). They will also vary with such individual factors as age, life-span stage, gender, and stage of motivation.

Self-monitoring is a relatively simple procedure that heightens an individual's awareness of the behavior in question and helps to quantify the frequency, severity, and unique patterns of drinking or the associated problematic target behavior. The information gained from self-monitoring can be compared with normative data so that individuals can judge how far their behavior deviates from the norm (e.g., number of times late to work because of a hangover). Self-monitoring increases a person's self-awareness, and sometimes may result in behavior change without any additional intervention. Research on increasing self-awareness can be useful in both primary and secondary prevention programs.

Self-monitoring with feedback can be used to teach individuals how to estimate their blood alcohol levels. A number of public drinking settings now provide instruments that allow people to obtain data to monitor more accurately the severity of their intoxication (Nathan, 1978). The results of studies on blood alcohol level discrimination and feedback training suggest that many normal social drinkers and even some heavy drinkers can be trained to estimate their blood alcohol level accurately. People can then be taught to titrate their blood alcohol level with such methods as spacing drinks over time, interchanging nonalcoholic drinks with alcoholic beverages, and consuming beverages with a lower alcohol content (Hay and Nathan, 1982; Miller and Munoz, 1982).

Cognitive Restructuring

Cognitive restructuring interventions are based on social learning theory models that consider expectancy and self-efficacy to be critical elements in behavior change. In this type of prevention approach, the focus is on the psychological aspects of problem drinking, for example, the thought processes associated with excessive drinking or with drinking-related problem behavior. Interventions using this approach are designed to modify expectancies, beliefs, attributions, and perceived norms about what is culturally appropriate and inappropriate. As noted earlier, persons who take excessive risks or become violent or sexually overactive when intoxicated may be doing so as a result of learned expectations rather than pharmacological effects (Marlatt and Rohsenow, 1980).

One of the more promising avenues for prevention comes from the study of alcohol outcome expectancies. This area has received widespread attention over the past two decades and has resulted in the development of such psychometrically sound assessment instruments as the alcohol expectancy questionnaire (Goldman, Brown, and Christiansen, 1987). For example, young drinkers who show a particularly high-risk expectancy profile (expecting alcohol to act as a mood modifier, producing euphoric states and the alleviation of negative moods, as well as to enhance physical and sexual prowess) are individuals who may be at high risk for developing problematic drinking patterns. Outcome expectancies can develop very early in life and can serve as powerful compelling factors that determine future behavior when intoxicated. Research is needed in this field to examine the potential for modifying expectancies and for determining whether such changes are associated with reductions in actual drinking or in drinking-related problem behavior.

Cognitive-behavioral prevention programs can be targeted to high-risk individuals or groups. The specific content of the program may depend on the target population and the target behaviors within that population.

Motivation and Readiness to Change Behavior

Motivational factors are of prime importance for the cognitive- behavioral mechanisms that mediate behavior change. Individuals who are not aware that problems exist are not going to be receptive to any kind of preventive intervention, whether it be focused on education or skills training. Indeed, motivation is a largely unexplored preven- tion area. A useful conceptual model that was first developed in the areas of mental health and smoking cessation (DiClemente and Prochaska, 1982; Prochaska and DiClemente, 1986) postulates stages of readiness to change. Individuals and even groups or whole organizations can vary along a continuum of readiness to change (Abrams et al., 1986): they may be disinterested in change, in a contemplation phase (considering change but not yet ready), ready for action, or moving into the maintenance and termination of change efforts. Different skills may be appropriate at different stages of readiness. For instance, a person contemplating change may not benefit much from action-oriented skills training because he or she has not yet made a commitment to action. Such individuals display decision-making processes which suggest that, for them, the positive aspects of change have not yet overtaken the negatives; they are not convinced they have a problem that warrants effort to change. Inappropriate pressure toward action could result in a rebellious backlash or increased denial/avoidance of the need for change. The prevention approaches targeted to persons in the contemplation phase would include consciousness raising and supportive efforts to alter the decisional balance. For example, the perceived negative consequences of alcohol abuse may begin to outweigh the perceived benefits of use. Once individuals move from contemplation into readiness for action, the specific prevention strategies change from consciousness raising, support, and education to coping skills training.

Research needs to be undertaken to evaluate the stages-of-change model and to document whether the matching of preventive interventions to specific stages will be of value in the prevention of alcohol- related problems. Research using this model can help identify strategies for accelerating change within individuals, organizations, communities, and society at large. Some individuals within society will be on the forefront of change processes (early adopters); these individuals can serve as role models and agents for the social diffusion of change to others. Once a large enough subgroup within a society begins to change its behavioral practices so that a "critical mass" is achieved, other individuals who have not yet changed (late adopters) may begin to feel that they are not abiding by current cultural norms (Abrams et al., 1986). The processes of diffusion and cultural change can be accelerated to modify individual behavior and to select the behaviors that society deems acceptable for drinking frequency, volume, and comportment (MacAndrew and Edgerton, 1969; Abrams et al., 1986; Abrams and Niaura, 1987).

Research is also needed to facilitate choosing between different interventions that vary in cost, complexity, and degree of impact on the target population. In contrast to universal prevention programs targeted to the whole community or the society, selected preventive interventions could be prioritized on the basis of (a) prior screening or knowledge of individual risk factors; (b) intensity of the intervention (including such factors as cost, degree of individualized skills training, and amount of professional involvement per individual); and (c) their importance (i.e., in terms of the prevalence of the target behaviors to be modified and the degree of individual/societal risk or damage caused by them).

Because the matching process could be very costly, matching subgroups to interventions must first be demonstrated to be superior to universal interventions designed for larger populations. Perhaps optimal prevention using community-based interventions should consist of multilevel, multifaceted universal intervention components with a few, selected individual and small group programs for those who fail to benefit from the more standardized sets of interventions. Thus, individuals or subgroups are "stepped up" to more intensive and costly interventions only when less costly approaches have been attempted and have failed.

The committee recommends controlled trials to test the efficacy of matching versus mismatching or no matching. Suggested questions for testing include the following: Is it necessary to have special programs for adolescent children of alcoholics, or could they benefit as much as other adolescents from general coping skills training programs given to all adolescents as part of a brief, standardized curriculum package? Is it necessary to provide skills training that is directed specifically toward alcohol, or can such training include other drugs and tobacco? To what extent should skills training focus on presumed underlying vulnerabilities (e.g., low self-esteem or poor self-concept) that may mediate the risk of alcohol or drug abuse? Research should be encouraged to identify program components (or combinations of components) that have the largest sustained impact with the least cost and use of human resources.

Life-Style Change

Prevention research should also consider the process of life-style change over time. Naturalistic studies and the methods of anthropology could be useful in this area. It is important to test theories of how changes in life-style are adopted, how they diffuse to others, and how they either become embedded in cultural norms (maintained) or fade away (Abrams et al., 1986; Bandura, 1986). Selected theory-driven questions include these: What specific factors promote diffusion and cultural norm change? How should individual, group, organizational, and community-level theoretical models and principles become integrated into a comprehensive, synergistic blueprint to accelerate the development of healthy life-style norms? How do individuals influence their social network members, and how do these network members reciprocally influence individuals? What factors determine when and how a critical mass is achieved that results in a more permanent normative change in cultural practices (i.e., the maintenance of desired changes because of reciprocal reinforcement) (Rogers and Shoemaker, 1971)?

Recent developments in motivational constructs, such as models of stages of readiness to change and associated processes to accelerate change, should be considered and adapted for alcohol prevention research (Prochaska and DiClemente, 1982, 1985, 1986). The results of life-span developmental research indicating the importance of transition periods should also be integrated into models of the process of change over time. What factors determine resilience, and what mechanisms allow individuals to "grow out of" acute problem behaviors over time?

A variety of specific preventive interventions can be developed and evaluated in controlled trials. The goals of such interventions can vary, ranging from controlled or moderate alcohol use, to modification of cognitive and behavioral factors that might reduce alcohol-related problems, to total abstinence in those populations in which abstinence is indicated (e.g., pregnant women or individuals with chronic alcohol dependence syndrome). Once there is a clear conceptual model that identifies critical mediating mechanisms and accurately measures desired changes in endpoints, effective preventive interventions can be designed based on the principles of individual psychology. Theory-driven research provides the opportunity for testing specific theoretical models and predictions about how and why prevention interventions work or do not work.

The following are opportunities for research based on social learning models:

• There is a need for synthetic efforts among researchers that could explicate the multidetermined and reciprocal interactions among behavioral, cognitive, and environmental processes that bear on the development of alcohol-related problems.
• The role of cognitive-behavioral mediators of drinking and drinking-related behaviors should be explored to better understand the mechanisms that control these behaviors and the interventions required to set processes of change in motion.
• Emphasis should be placed on understanding the role of beliefs and expectations in the acquisition and maintenance of problem drinking practices and behaviors. The relevance of self-efficacy for prevention should also be explored.
• The use of role modeling and vicarious learning factors should be more thoroughly explored in prevention research at both the individual and the community levels (e.g., media influences).
• More effort needs to be directed toward developing and evaluating coping skills training for primary and secondary prevention targets.
• Research should focus more on the motivational factors underlying the processes and stages of readiness to change. How can the process of change be accelerated by considering stages-of-change models? How can immotive and precontemplative individuals be persuaded to want to change their practices?
• More research should be done to examine the matching hypothesis and to gather data to examine the feasibility of cost-effective, stepped-care approaches to prevention. Are screenings for individual differences and tailored (but costly) treatments worthwhile? If so, for which subgroups, at what developmental stages, and in which settings?
• Research should attempt to bridge the gap between individual and sociocultural models and understand how innovations diffuse through society. Studies should focus on advancing theoretical models of diffusion by extending individual change concepts to group, social network, organizational, community, and higher levels of social structure.
• Basic assessments, analogue research, and clinical trials are required that will focus on promising targets for preventive interventions and on understanding their mediating mechanisms-- when and why treatments work and on whom. What mediating mechanisms are crucial for facilitating change? Is timing important? How generalizable are interventions--to what groups, at what time, and in what contexts?

• Research should focus on answering specific questions that test underlying theory rather than on "racehorse" studies that are eclectic in nature. Do different theoretical models apply to different targets or stages of individual change?

GENETIC DETERMINANTS OF RISK

Considerable effort continues to be devoted to identifying those genetic factors that may predispose an individual to alcohol dependence (alcoholism). The types of effort being employed, the relative success of various avenues of research, and future research opportunities are discussed in detail in Causes and Consequences of Alcohol Problems (IOM, 1987:93). Consequently, the committee includes only a short summary below.

Briefly, researchers are looking for chromosomal markers, including restriction fragment-length polymorphisms (RFLPs), and specific genes that predispose an individual to alcohol dependence; they are also pursuing family studies and linkage analysis and searching for physiological indicators of susceptibility (IOM, 1987). This work is promising, and its results may, in the future, enable health care providers to identify specific individuals who are genetically at risk and to provide appropriate counseling. However, these investigations have not yet progressed to the point at which it is possible to recommend that prevention efforts based on them should be undertaken. At present, family history is the single best predictor of severe alcohol problems or dependence. As a group, children of alcoholics are considered to be at high risk, but they are not all equally at risk. Research should continue to allow more specific identification of those individuals among the children of alcoholics who are or are not genetically susceptible.

CONCLUSION

This chapter has focused on factors in the individual that may influence the development of alcohol-related problems. The first concerns individual vulnerabilities from a life-course perspective; the second describes observational theories derived from a social learning perspective that suggest potential interventions for the prevention of alcohol-related problems; and the third briefly notes current work on genetic factors that may predispose an individual to problems. It is clear that each approach offers promising avenues of research that can lead to more effective interventions than are now available. Yet a relatively unexplored issue is how the general principles of social learning can be made more specific to be useful for individuals of varying susceptibility. Future researchers may find the matching of particular patterns of susceptibility vulnerability to specific preventive interventions a very fruitful avenue of investigation.

REFERENCES

Ablon, J. Family structure and behavior in alcoholism: A review of the literature. In B. Kissin and H. Begleiter, eds. The Biology of Alcoholism, vol. 4, Social Aspects of Alcoholism. New York: Plenum, 1976.

Abrams, D. B. Assessment of alcohol-stress interactions: Bridging the gap between laboratory and treatment outcome research. Pp. 61-86 in L. Pohorecky and J. Brick, eds. Stress and Alcohol Use. New York: Elsevier, 1983.

Abrams, D. B., and R. Niaura. Social learning theory of alcohol abuse. Pp. 131-178 in H. T. Blane and K. E. Leonard, eds. Psychological Theories of Drinking and Alcoholism. New York: Guilford Press, 1987.

Abrams, D. B., J. Elder, T. Lasater et al. A comprehensive framework for conceptualizing and planning organizational health promotion programs. In M. Cataldo and T. Coates, eds. Behavioral Medicine in Industry. New York: John Wiley and Sons, 1986.

Alexander, C. N., Jr., and E. Q. Campbell. Peer influences on adolescent drinking. Q. J. Stud. Alcohol 28:444-453, 1967.

Azjen, I., and M. Fishbein. Understanding Attitudes and Predicting Behavior. Englewood Cliffs, NJ: Prentice-Hall, 1980.

Ball, J. C., and C. D. Chambers. The epidemiology of opiate addiction in the United States. Springfield, IL: Charles C. Thomas, 1970.

Baltes, P. B., H. W. Reese, and L. P. Lipsitt. Life-span developmental psychology. Ann. Rev. Psychol. 31:65-110, 1980.

Bandura, A. Principles of Behavior Modification. New York: Holt, Rinehart and Winston, 1969.

Bandura, A. Social Learning Theory. Englewood Cliffs, NJ: Prentice-Hall, 1977.

Bandura, A. Social Foundations of Thought and Action. Englewood Cliffs, NJ: Prentice-Hall, 1986.

Baribeau, J. C., M. Ethier, and C. M. Braun. Neurophysiological assessment of selective attention in males at risk for alcoholism. Electroenceph. Clin. Neurophys. 40:651-656, 1987.

Barnes, G. M., M. P. Farrell, and A. Cairns. Parental socialization factors and adolescent drinking behaviors. J. Marriage Fam. 48:27-36, 1986.

Beardslee, W. R., L. Son, and G. E. Vaillant. Exposure to parental alcoholism during childhood and outcome in adulthood: A prospective longitudinal study. Br. J. Psychiatry 149:584-591, 1986.

Begleiter, H., B. Projesz, B. Bihari, et al. Event-related brain potentials in boys at risk for alcoholism. Science 225:1493-1496, 1984.

Berger, D. E., and J. R. Snortum. A structural model of drinking and driving: Alcohol consumption, social norms, and moral commitments. Criminology 24:139-153, 1986.

Best, J. A., S. J. Thomson, S. M. Santi et al. Preventing cigarette smoking among school children. Pp. 161-201 in L. Breslow, J. E. Fielding, and L. B. Lave, eds. Annual Review of Public Health, vol. 9. Palo Alto, CA: Annual Reviews, 1988.

Biddle, B. J., B. J. Bank, and M. M. Marlin. Social determinants of adolescent drinking. J. Stud. Alcohol 41:215-241, 1980.

Blane, H. T., and K. E. Leonard. Psychological Theories of Alcohol Use and Abuse. New York: Guilford Press, 1987.

Block, J., J. H. Block, and S. Keyes. Longitudinally foretelling drug usage in adolescence: Early childhood personality and environmental precursors. Child Develop. 59:336-355, 1988.

Brooks, J. S., A. S. Gordon, M. Whiteman et al. Dynamics of childhood and adolescent personality traits and adolescent drug use. Dev. Psychol. 22:403-414, 1986.

Burnside, M. A., P. E. Baer, R. J. McLaughlin et al. Alcohol use by adolescents in disrupted families. Alcoholism 10:274-278, 1986.

Cadoret, R. J., E. Troughton, and T. O'Gorman. Genetic and environmental factors in alcohol abuse and antisocial personality. J. Stud. Alcohol 48:1-8, 1987.

Cantwell, D. P. Hyperactivity and antisocial behavior. J. Am. Acad. Child Psychiatry 17:252-262, 1978.

Chaney, E. F., M. R. O'Leary, and G. A. Marlatt. Skill training with alcoholics. J. Consult. Clin. Psychol. 48(3):305-316, 1978.

Christiansen, B. A., M. S. Goldman, and S. A. Brown. The differential development of adolescent alcohol expectancies may predict adult alcoholism. Addict. Behav. 10:299-306, 1985.

Cloninger, C. R. Neurogenetic adaptive mechanisms in alcoholism. Science 236:410-416, 1987.

Cloninger, C. R., M. Bohman, and S. Siguardson. Inheritance of alcohol abuse: Cross-fostering analysis of adopted men. Arch. Gen. Psych. 38:861-868, 1981.

Cohen, M., I. A. Liebson, L. A. Faillace et al. Moderate drinking by chronic alcoholics. J. Nerv. Ment. Dis. 153:434-444, 1971.

Collins, R. L., and G. A. Marlatt. Social modeling as a determinant of drinking behavior: Implications for prevention and treatment. Addict. Behav. 6:233-239, 1981.

Dawkins, M. P. Social correlates of alcohol and other drug-use among youthful blacks in an urban setting. J. Alcohol Drug Educ. 32:15-28, 1986.

DiClemente, C. C., and J. O. Prochaska. Self-change and therapy change of smoking behavior: A comparison of processes of change of cessation and maintenance. Addict. Behav. 7:133-142, 1982.

El-Guebaly, N., and D. R. Offord. The offspring of alcoholics: A critical review. Am. J. Psychiatry 134:357-365, 1977.

Fillmore, K., and L. Midanik. Chronicity of drinking problems among men: A longitudinal study. J. Stud. Alcohol 45:228-236, 1984.

Fillmore, K. M., E. Hartka, B. M. Johnstone et al. Spontaneous remission from alcohol problems: A critical review. Background paper prepared for the Institute of Medicine Committee on Alcohol Treatment. 1988.

Flay, B. R. What we know about the social influences approach to smoking prevention: Review and recommendations. Pp. 67-112 in C. S. Bell and R. Battjes, eds. Prevention Research: Deterring Drug Abuse Among Children and Adolescents. NIDA Research Monograph No. 63. USDHHS Publ. No. (ADM)85-1334. Rockville, MD: NIDA, 1984.

Folsom, A. R., J. R. Hughes, J. F. Buehler et al. Do type A men drink more frequently than type B men? Findings in the multiple risk factor intervention trial (MRFIT). J. Behav. Med. 8:227-235, 1985.

Gaines, L. S., and G. J. Connors. Drinking and personality: Present knowledge and future trends. Pp. 331-346 in Alcohol Consumption Related Problems. NIAAA Research Monograph No. 1. USDHHS Publ. No. (ADM)82-1190. Washington, DC: NIAAA, 1982.

Gibbons, S., M. L. Wylie, L. Echterling et al. Situational factors related to rural adolescent alcohol use. Int. J. Addict. 21:1183-1195, 1986.

Gliksman, L., and B. R. Rush. Alcohol availability, alcohol consumption, and alcohol-related damage. II. The role of sociodemographic factors. J. Stud. Alcohol 47:11-18, 1986.

Goldman, M., S. Brown, and B. Christiansen. Expectancy theory--Thinking about drinking. In H. T. Blane and K. E. Leonard, eds. Psychological Theories of Drinking and Alcoholism. New York: Guilford Press, 1987.

Goodstadt, M. S. Alcohol education research and practice: A logical analysis of the two realities. J. Drug Educ. 16(4):349-365, 1986.

Goodwin, D. W., F. Schulsinger, L. Hermansen et al. Alcohol problems in adoptees raised apart from alcoholic biological parents. Arch. Gen. Psychiatry 28:238-243, 1973.

Goodwin, D. W., F. Schulsinger, N. Moller, et al. Drinking patterns in adopted and nonadopted sons of alcoholics. Arch. Gen. Psychiatry 31:164-169, 1974.

Goodwin, D. W., F. Schulsinger, L. Hermansen et al. Alcoholism and the hyperactive child syndrome. J. Nerv. Ment. Dis. 160:349-353, 1975.

Hagnell, O., P. Isberg, J. Lanke et al. Predictors of alcoholism in the Lundby Study. III. Social risk factors for alcoholism. Eur. Arch. Psychiatry Neurol. Sci. 235:197-199, 1986.

Hay, W. M., and P. E. Nathan, eds. Clinical Case Studies in the Behavioral Treatment of Alcoholism. New York: Plenum, 1982.

Heather, N., and I. Robertson. Controlled Drinking. London: Methuen, 1983.

Heibrun, A. B., J. C. Cassidy, M. Diehl et al. Psychological vulnerability to alcoholism: Studies in internal scanning deficit. Br. J. Med. Psychol. 59:237-244, 1986.

Institute of Medicine. Causes and Consequences of Alcohol Problems: An Agenda for Research. Washington, DC: National Academy Press, 1987.

Jessor, R. Adolescent development and behavioral health. In J. Matarazzo, S. Weiss, J. Herd et al., eds. Behavioral Health: A Handbook of Health Enhancement and Disease Prevention. New York: John Wiley and Sons, 1984.

Jessor, R., and S. L. Jessor. Adolescent development and the onset of drinking: A longitudinal study. J. Stud. Alcohol 36:27-51, 1975.

Jessor, R., and S. L. Jessor. Problem Behavior and Psychosocial Development: A Longitudinal Study of Youth. New York: Academic Press, 1977.

Jones, M. C. Personality correlates and antecedents of drinking patterns in adult males. J. Consult. Clin. Psychol. 32:2-12, 1968.

Jones, M. C. Personality antecedents and correlates of drinking patterns in women. J. Consult. Clin. Psychol. 36:61-69, 1971.

Kandel, D. B. Drugs and drinking behavior among youth. Ann. Rev. Sociology, 6:235-285, 1980.

Kandel, D. B., R. C. Kessler, and R. Z. Margulies. Antecedents of adolescent initiation into stages of drug abuse: A developmental analysis. In D. Kandel, ed. Longitudinal Research on Drug Use: Empirical Findings and Methodological Issues. New York: John Wiley and Sons, 1978.

Kellam, S. G. Developmental epidemiological framework for family research on depression and aggression. In G. R. Patterson, ed. Depression and Aggression: Two Facets of Family Interactions. Englewood Cliffs, NJ: Lawrence Erlbaum Associates, in press.

Kellam, S. G., and L. Werthamer-Larsson. Developmental epidemiology: A basis for prevention. Pp. 154-180 in M. Kessler and S. E. Goldston, eds. A Decade of Progress in Primary Prevention. Hanover, NH: University Press of New England, 1986.

Kellam, S. G., C. H. Brown, and J. P. Fleming. The prevention of teenage substance use: Longitudinal research and strategy. Pp. 171-200 in T. J. Coates, A. C. Petersen, and C. Perry, eds. Promoting Adolescent Health: A Dialogue on Research and Practice. New York: Academic Press, 1982.

Kellam, S. G., M. E. Ensminger, and M. B. Simon. Mental health in first grade and teenage drug, alcohol, and cigarette use. Drug and Alcohol Depend. 5:273-304, 1980.

Kellam, S. G., J. D. Branch, K. C. Agrawal et al. Mental Health and Going to School: The Woodlawn Program of Assessment, Early Intervention, and Evaluation. Chicago: University of Chicago Press, 1975.

Kellam, S. G., C. H. Brown, B. R. Rubin et al. Paths leading to teenage psychiatric symptoms and substance use: Developmental epidemiologic studies in Woodlawn. Pp. 17-51 in S. B. Gure, F. J. Earls, and J. E. Barrett, eds. Childhood Psychopathology and Development. New York: Raven Press, 1983.

Killen, J. D. Prevention of adolescent tobacco smoking: The social pressure resistance training approach. J. Child Psychiatry 26:7-15, 1985.

Knop, J., T. W. Teasdale, F. Schulsinger et al. A prospective study of young men at high risk for alcoholism: School behavior and achievement. J. Stud. Alcohol 46:273-278, 1985.

Labouvie, E. W., and C. R. McGee. Relation of personality to alcohol and drug abuse in adolescence. J. Consult. Clin. Psychol. 54:289-293, 1986.

Linsky, A. S., J. P. Colby, Jr., and M. A. Straus. Drinking norms and alcohol-related problems in the United States. J. Stud. Alcohol 47:384-393, 1986.

MacAndrew, C., and R. Edgerton. Drunken Comportment. Chicago: Aldine Publishing Co., 1969.

MacDonald, D. I., and S. B. Blume. Children of alcoholics. Am. J. Dis. Child. 140:750-754, 1986.

Marlatt, G. A. Alcohol, stress and cognitive control. Pp. 271-296 in J. G. Sarason and C. D. Spielberger, eds. Stress and Anxiety, vol. 1. Washington, DC: Hemisphere Publishing, 1976.

Marlatt, G. A. Alcohol, the magic elixir: Stress, expectancy, and the transformation of emotional states. Paper presented to the Seventh Annual Coatesville Jefferson Conference, V.A. Medical Center, Coatesville, PA, 1984.

Marlatt, G. A., and J. R. Gordon. Relapse Prevention: Maintenance Strategies in the Treatment of Addictive Behaviors. New York: Guilford Press, 1985.

Marlatt, G. A., and D. J. Rohsenow. Cognitive process in alcohol use: Expectancy and the balanced placebo design. In N. K. Mello, ed. Advances in Substance Abuse, vol. 1. Greenwich, CT: JAI Press, 1980.

Marlatt, G. A., J. S. Baer, D. M. Donovan et al. Addictive behaviors: Etiology and treatment. Ann. Rev. Psychol. 39:223-252, 1988.

McCarty, D., M. Poore, K. C. Mills et al. Direct-mail techniques and the prevention of alcohol-related problems among college students. J. Stud. Alcohol 44(1):162-170, 1983.

McCord, J. Alcoholism: Toward understanding genetic and social factors. Psychiatry 51:131-141, 1988a.

McCord, J. Identifying developmental paradigms leading to alcoholism. J. Stud. Alcohol 49:357-362, 1988b.

McCord, W., and J. McCord. Origins of Alcoholism. Stanford, CA: Stanford University Press, 1960.

McCord, W., and J. McCord. A longitudinal study of the personality of alcoholics. Pp. 413-430 in D. F. J. Pittman and C. R. Snyder, eds. Society, Culture and Drinking Patterns. New York: John Wiley and Sons, 1962.

Miller, P. M. Behavioral Treatment of Alcoholism. Oxford: Pergamon Press, 1976.

Miller, W. R. The Addictive Behaviors: Treatment of Alcoholism, Drug Abuse, Smoking, and Obesity. New York: Pergamon Press, 1980.

Miller, W. R., and N. Heather. Treating Addictive Behaviors: Processes of Change. New York: Plenum, 1986.

Miller, W. R., and R. F. Munoz. How to Control Your Drinking. Albuquerque: University of New Mexico Press, 1982.

Mills, K. C., B. Pfaffenberger, and D. McCarty. Guidelines for alcohol abuse prevention on the college campus. J. Higher Educ. 52(4):399-414, 1981.

Monnelly, E. P., E. M. Hartl, and R. Elderkin. Constitutional factors predictive of alcoholism in a follow-up of delinquent boys. J. Stud. Alcohol 44:530-537, 1983.

Monti, P., D. B. Abrams, J. Binkoff et al. The relevance of social skills training for alcohol and drug abuse problems. In C. Hollin and P. Trower, eds. Handbook of Social Skills Training. New York: Pergamon Press, 1986.

Nathan, P. E. Studies in blood alcohol discrimination. Pp. 161-175 in P. E. Nathan, G. A. Marlatt, and T. Loberg, eds. Alcoholism: New Directions in Behavioral Research and Treatment. New York: Plenum, 1978.

Nathan, P. E. Failures in prevention. Am. Psychologist 38:459-467, 1983.

Nathan, P. E., and R. S. Niaura. Prevention of alcohol problems. Pp. 333-354 in W. M. Cox, ed. Treatment and Prevention of Alcohol Problems: A Resource Manual. Orlando, FL: Academic Press, 1987.

Nathan, P. E., and J. S. O'Brien. An experimental analysis of the behavior of alcoholics and nonalcoholics during prolonged experimental drinking behavior therapy. Behav. Ther. 2:455-476, 1971.

Needle, R., H. McCubbin, M. Wilson et al. Interpersonal influences in adolescent drug use: The role of older siblings, parents, and peers. Int. J. Addict. 21:739-766, 1986.

Niaura, R. S., D. J. Rohsenow, J. A. Binkoff et al. Relevance of cue reactivity to understanding alcohol and smoking relapse. J. Abnorm. Psychol. 97(2):133-152, 1988.

O'Leary, K. D., and G. T. Wilson. Behavior Therapy: Application and Outcome, 2nd ed. Englewood Cliffs, NJ: Prentice-Hall, 1988.

Partanen, J., K. Bruun, and T. Markkanen. Inheritance of Drinking Behavior. Helsinki: Finnish Foundation for Alcohol Studies, 1966.

Perry, C. L. Community-wide health promotion and drug abuse prevention. J. School Health 56(9):359-363, 1986.

Pomerleau, O. F., and C. S. Pomerleau. Neuroregulators and the reinforcement of smoking: Towards a biobehavioral explanation. Neuroscience Biobehav. Rev. 8:503-513, 1984.

Prochaska, J. O., and C. C. DiClimente. Transtheoretical therapy: Toward a more integrative model of change. Psychother. 19:276-288, 1982.

Prochaska, J. O., and C. C. DiClimente. Processes and stages of self-change: Coping and competence in smoking behavior change. Pp. 319-343 in S. Shiffman and T. A. Wills, eds. Coping and Substance Use. New York: Academic Press, 1985.

Prochaska, J. O., and C. C. DiClimente. Toward a comprehensive model of change. Pp. 3-27 in W. R. Miller and N. Heather, eds. Treating Addictive Behaviors: Processes of Change. New York: Plenum, 1986.

Robins, L. N. Deviant Children Grown Up. Baltimore, MD: Williams and Wilkins, 1966.

Robins, L. N., W. N. Bates, and P. O'Neal. Adult drinking patterns of former problem children. Pp. 395-412 in D. Pittman and C. R. Snyder, eds. Society, Culture, and Drinking Patterns. New York: John Wiley and Sons, 1962.

Rogers, E. M., and F. F. Shoemaker. Communication of Innovations: A Cross-Cultural Approach. New York: Free Press, 1971.

Selnow, G. W., and W. D. Crano. Formal vs. informal group affiliations: Implications for alcohol and drug use among adolescents. J. Stud. Alcohol 47:48-52, 1986.

Sher, K. J., and R. W. Levenson. Risk for alcoholism and individual differences in the stress-response-dampening effect of alcohol. J. Abnorm. Psychol. 91:350-367, 1982.

Shiffman, S., and T. A. Wills, eds. Coping and Substance Use. New York: Academic Press, 1985.

Smart, R. G. Drinking problems among employed, unemployed, and shift workers. J. Occup. Med. 21:731-736, 1979.

Stephens, R., and E. Cottrell. A follow-up of 200 narcotic addicts committed for treatment under the Narcotic Addiction Act (NARA). Brit. J. Addict. 67:45-53, 1972.

Straus, R., and S. D. Bacon. Drinking in College. New Haven, CT: Yale University Press, 1953.

Tarter, R. E., A. I. Alterman, and K. I. Edwards. Vulnerability to alcoholism in men: A behavior-genetic perspective. J. Stud. Alcohol 46:329-356, 1985.

Temple, M. T., and K. M. Fillmore. The variability of drinking patterns and problems among young men, ages 16-31: A longitudinal study. Int. J. Addictions 20:1595-1620, 1985.

Vaillant, G. E. A twelve-year follow-up of New York narcotic addicts: Some social and psychiatric characteristics. Arch. Gen. Psychiatry 15:599-609, 1966.

Vaillant, G. E. The Natural History of Alcoholism: Causes, Patterns, and Paths to Recovery. Cambridge, MA: Harvard University Press, 1983.

Vaillant, G. E. Cultural factors in the etiology of alcoholism: A prospective study. Ann. N.Y. Acad. Sci. 472:142-148, 1986.

Wilson, G. T. Cognitive process in addiction. Br. J. Addict. 82:343-353, 1987.

Wilson, G. T. Alcohol use and abuse: A social learning analysis. In D. Chaudron and A. Wilkinson, eds. Theories of Alcoholism. Toronto: Addiction Research Foundation, 1988.

Wolin, S. J., and L. A. Bennett. Disrupted family rituals: A factor in the intergenerational transmission of alcoholism. J. Stud. Alcohol 41:199-214, 1980.

Wolin, S. J., L. A. Bennett, and D. L. Noonan. Family rituals and the recurrence of alcoholism over generations. Am. J. Psychiatry 136:589-593, 1979.

Zucker, R. A., and F. H. Barron. Parental behaviors associated with problem drinking and antisocial behavior among adolescent males. In M. E. Chafetz, ed. Research on Alcoholism: Clinical Problems and Special Populations. Proceedings of the First Annual Alcoholism Conference of the National Institute on Alcohol Abuse and Alcoholism. USDHEW Publ. No. (NIH)74-675. Washington, DC: NIAAA, 1973.

Zucker, R. A., and E. S. L. Gomberg. Etiology of alcoholism reconsidered: The case for a biopsychosocial process. Am. Psychol. 41:783-793, 1986.

Zucker, R. A., and R. B. Noll. Precursors and developmental influences on drinking and alcoholism: Etiology from a longitudinal perspective. Pp. 289-327 in Alcohol Consumption Related Problems. NIAAA Research Monograph No. 1. USDHHS Publ. No. (ADM) 82-1190. Washington, DC: NIAAA, 1982.

4

INDIVIDUAL-ENVIRONMENT INTERACTIONS: FOCUS ON THE ENVIRONMENT

This chapter reviews research on a number of the environmental factors that influence the choices individuals make about their use of alcohol. (In its use of the term environment in this case, the committee refers to the drinking setting and the cultural and economic milieu surrounding alcohol use.) Environmental factors can affect many people at a time or only a few. This chapter considers those factors that affect broad populations (e.g., national legislation concerning minimum purchase age requirements, mass media influences), as well as factors that do not have as broad a reach (e.g., the influences of a local bar or restaurant). It will also discuss aspects of the workplace that influence alcohol consumption.

Framing alcohol-related problems from an environmental perspective is part of the public health approach described in Chapter 1 that views behavior as a function of the interaction of individual and agent attributes with factors in the drinking environment. In the past, alcohol abuse and alcohol problems have often been blamed on the "weak will" or irresponsibility of the drinker. Demonstrating that conditions in the environment can affect and alter behavior allows for understanding another part of the behavioral equation relating to alcohol use. Selective modifications of these conditions represent promising approaches to research on the prevention of alcohol-related problems.

ENVIRONMENTAL CONTROLS ON THE AVAILABILITY OF ALCOHOLIC BEVERAGES

The focus of this section is on the mechanisms that influence the availability of alcoholic beverages. The factors considered here include physical availability (e.g., minimum age requirements, geographic density of alcohol outlets), as well as economic availability (the price of alcohol relative to income and other goods).

Although availability and subsequent consumption of alcohol are affected by federal and state restrictions concerning the production and distribution of alcoholic beverages, most of these limits are no longer intended to prevent consumption. State statutes that established alcoholic beverage control (ABC) commissions after the repeal of Prohibition in this country were designed to prevent drunkenness and alcohol misuse. Today, however, state and local control of alcoholic beverages is intended rather to ensure that taxes are collected, that the marketplace is orderly, and that undesirable persons do not secure licenses for retail sales (Rice, 1984).

The study of alcohol availability and its relation to consumption has generally been approached in one of two ways. Researchers have looked at aggregate indices of alcohol availability (e.g., a combination of age restrictions, law enforcement, pricing structures, and other factors thought to be important) and their relationship to the full range of alcohol problems and consumption levels. Alternatively, researchers have studied such specific alcohol availability policies as an increase in the minimum purchase age as it relates to specific types of alcohol problems (e.g., auto crashes).

Studies That Measure the Effect of Multiple Influences on Consumption

Studies of aggregate influences and results frequently show positive associations between aggregate measures of alcohol availability and alcohol consumption. A combined cross-sectional and longitudinal analysis of the consumption of distilled spirits by Hoadley, Fuchs, and Holder (1984) showed that certain laws and restrictions do significantly hold down distilled spirits consumption. In another effort, Rush, Gliksman, and Brook (1986) conducted statistical analyses using linear structural relations applied to a set of county-level data from Ontario, Canada. They found a high positive association among the retail availability of alcohol, alcohol consumption, and alcohol-related morbidity and mortality. These investigators concluded from their analyses that government policies that restrict the availability of alcohol will reduce per capita consumption and indirectly lessen alcohol-related damage.

Another set of studies, however (Popham, Schmidt, and DeLint, 1976; DeLuca, 1981), concluded that state ABC laws and regulations have little or no effect on reducing per capita consumption and alcohol-related problems. Watts and Rabow (1981) claim that interstate tourism, particularly for Nevada, Vermont, New Hampshire, and the District of Columbia, accounts for much of the association between availability and consumption. Their conclusion, however, was based on 1972 state consumption data and on results from a 1977 national survey--a period during which the minimum age for drinking was changed in 29 states. In a study published later, the same research team found positive links between availability and alcohol-related problems in California (Rabow and Watts, 1982). In addition, Colon and colleagues (1981), while controlling for tourism and urban conditions, found a significant association between consumption and two types of composite measures of availability.

Most of the studies noted above used state-level data. Yet it has been argued (Hooper, 1983) that the most appropriate unit of analysis for this type of research is the county because of differences by county in alcoholic beverage regulation. For example, Blose and Holder (1987a) used an interrupted time-series analysis in a quasi-experimental design on alcohol-related crash data in North Carolina following the legalization of liquor by the drink (LBD). They found statistically significant increases in counties that permitted LBD and no changes in matched comparison counties that did not legalize LBD (Blose and Holder, 1987b).

MacDonald and Whitehead (1983) conducted a literature review of U.S. and Canadian studies of the relationship between consumption and the frequency of outlets for alcoholic beverages. As a group, these studies, along with cross-cultural analyses from other countries (see DeLint, 1980; Makela et al., 1981; Single et al., 1981), have provided evidence that environmental restrictions can affect both consumption levels (which are linked to alcohol-related problems) and alcohol abuse. Room (1984, p.310), in reviewing studies from the United States and other countries, concluded, "The evidence is thus by now compelling that alcohol controls can affect the rates of alcohol-related problems, and that they often particularly affect the consumption patterns of high-risk drinkers."

Other researchers have looked into the influence of such factors as statewide alcohol policy changes or the pricing structure of alcoholic beverages as they relate to the level of alcohol consumption. The committee has selected for review three such factors that have received serious study and attention: (1) alcohol prices and taxation, (2) minimum age of purchase, and (3) zoning and conditional-use permits. Certainly, there are other aspects of the drinking environment (e.g., hours of sale, number of outlets, rationing, strikes among brewery workers) that have been investigated and that may provide useful insights into the effects of environmental factors on alcohol-related problems. The committee chose to discuss research on the three topics below as illustrative of the work in this area and as offering particularly rich possibilities for further inquiry.

Studies That Measure the Effects of Specific Factors upon Consumption Alcohol Prices and Taxation

Research has confirmed that alcoholic beverage sales are sensitive to price and that a relationship exists between the price of alcoholic beverages, alcohol consumption, and alcohol-related problems. Alcohol pricing and taxation policy, therefore, is an important consideration in the development of an alcohol problem prevention strategy. Although researchers have not reached a consensus on the exact level of price sensitivity, they agree that alcoholic beverage consumption does respond to changes in price. Cook (1981), Cook and Tauchen (1982), Levy and Sheflin (1983), Ornstein and Hanssens (1983), and Hoadley, Fuchs, and Holder (1984) all confirm a relationship between price and total consumption in the United States. Room (1984) summarized studies in other countries with similar findings. The research of Cook (1981) and Cook and Tauchen (1982) has also shown a strong relationship between cirrhosis mortality (as a surrogate measure of heavy, chronic drinking) and the price of liquor. In addition, Cook (1981) found that increases in liquor taxes tended to reduce auto fatalities.

Researchers differ in their estimates of the price sensitivity of alcoholic beverages. Furthermore, there are likely to be different sensitivity levels for alcoholic beverages by type of beverage and by age of the purchasers (Grossman, Coate, and Arluck, 1987; Saffer and Grossman, 1987a). Young people, for instance, may exhibit a unique alcohol consumption rate as a function of price because their relative inexperience as drinkers also means that they will have less rigid drinking habits (Levy and Sheflin, 1983; Coate and Grossman, 1986). In addition, the marginal cost of alcohol relative to disposable income is greater for young people (Coate and Grossman, 1986).

Grossman, Coate, and Arluck (1987) determined the differential price sensitivity of consumption by young people 16-21 years old. They concluded that youthful consumption is sensitive to price changes in both beer and distilled spirits. They found that a 10-cent increase in the price of beer will result in a 14.8 percent decrease in the number of youthful heavy beer drinkers (defined as three to five drinks of beer per day) and that a 30-cent increase in distilled spirits would result in a 27.3 percent decline in the number of youthful heavy liquor drinkers (three to five drinks of liquor per day).

Saffer and Grossman (1985) examined the association between beer prices and traffic fatalities among young people. Separate analyses were performed for young men and young women in three age groups (15-17, 18-20, and 21-24 years). Minimum purchase age, demographic variables, and driving exposure were controlled. Findings indicated that the states with higher beer prices had lower fatality rates for all of the age groups studied.

Studies of the specific drinking environment have also been undertaken to determine what price-relevant factors in the immediate surroundings might contribute to alcohol-related problems. Babor and his colleagues (1980) found that happy-hour promotions increased consumption in laboratory and barroom settings, but Smart and Adlaf (1986), using aggregate-level data, were unable to detect changes in consumption with the elimination of happy hours in Ontario, Canada. In another study, Geller, Russ, and Altomari (1986) reported that the size of the serving was associated with overall consumption. Those who ordered cups (10 ounces), bottles (12 ounces), or pitchers (40 ounces) of beer drank an average of 10, 15.1, and 35.2 ounces per person, respectively. These differences do not reflect different rates of consumption, however: the pitcher drinkers stayed in the bar approximately three times longer than did the cup drinkers.

Based on the results of price sensitivity research, Cook (1984b), Harris (1984), Levy and Sheflin (1983), Grossman, Coate, and Arluck (1987), Bruun and colleagues (1975), Saffer and Grossman (1987a), and Phelps (in press) have pointed out the policy potential of increasing taxes to reduce or stabilize consumption and to reduce alcohol-related problems. Several observations may be made on this issue, based on current research:

1. Taxes are politically viable as a prevention policy if voters understand that increased prices can reduce alcohol misuse, particularly among the young (Levy and Sheflin, 1983; Mosher and Beauchamp, 1983).
2. Price increases are not regressive because consumption has been shown to increase with income (Cook, 1981; Harris, 1984).
3. Potential reductions in alcohol-related problems as a result of price increases are substantial, even if one allows for overestimates of the reductions in cirrhosis deaths (Cook, 1984a; Harris, 1984).

Minimum Age of Purchase

For the majority of young people, drinking is initiated before they finish their first year of high school, at an average age of 13. By ages 14-15, about 85 percent have drunk alcohol at least once, and 65-70 percent of 14 to 15 year olds drink on at least a monthly basis (NIAAA, 1987).

The early age of onset of drinking and the frequency of alcohol use among young people lead to questions about the role alcohol plays in many social and medical problems that affect teenagers. Alcohol is involved in as many as 50 percent of teen suicides and plays a large role in car crashes, the number one killer of teenagers. There is also concern that the early use of alcohol can lead to later drinking problems and drug use.

Historically, the minimum age of purchase has been used to reduce alcohol consumption by the young and to prevent alcohol-related problems, particularly accidents and injuries, involving young people. The effect of changes in the minimum purchase age on youthful drinking and traffic accidents has been extensively researched. Overall, evidence suggests that a higher minimum purchase age results in lower per capita consumption (Maisto and Rachal, 1980). Longitudinal analyses of aggregate sales, of which young purchasers represent a small part, have shown that beer (and sometimes wine) sales are sensitive to changes in the minimum purchase age (Douglas and Freedman, 1977; Smart and Goodstadt, 1977; Wagenaar, 1983).

An exception to such findings occurred in Massachusetts, where the level of self-reported alcohol consumption by young people did not change following an increase in the minimum drinking age from 18 to 20 years (Hingson et al., 1983; Smith et al., 1984). This exception might be explained by the under-or overreporting of drinking by the young respondents, a lack of compliance with the law, or a lack of enforcement. After the drinking age increase, teenage purchases of alcohol in liquor stores, bars, and restaurants in Massachusetts declined sharply, but the proportion of teens who had other people purchase alcohol for them almost doubled.

In the case of alcohol-related traffic accidents, however, research findings support the conclusion that a higher minimum age of purchase can reduce the number of such accidents. The longest time-series analysis of a state increase in the minimum age was conducted by Wagenaar (1981, 1987) in Michigan. Michigan is a good state for such analyses because the greatest population concentrations are sufficiently far from state borders to reduce the "border effect" whereby underage youths cross to a state with lower minimum-age requirements to purchase alcohol. Wagenaar (1981) found an 18 percent reduction in alcohol-related crashes among young drivers in the first year following a change in the minimum age of purchase from 18 to 21. His follow-up analysis, which was carried out four years after the age change, showed a statistically significant 9 percent reduction over the total five-year period (Wagenaar, 1987). These findings are consistent with those of Filkins and Flora (1981) in an independent analysis also conducted in Michigan.

Other states show similar results. Maxwell (1981) found a statistically significant reduction in alcohol-related accidents in Illinois for 18-to 21-year-old drivers following an increase in the minimum purchase age to 21. These findings were confirmed by a nine-state analysis conducted by Williams and colleagues (1983), who also found decreases in the number of fatal crashes among young drivers following an increase in the minimum alcohol purchase age requirement.

Massachusetts experienced the lowest reduction in fatal crashes following a one-year increase in the minimum purchase age from 18 to 20. No statistically significant changes in fatal crashes in Massachusetts were found by Hingson and coworkers (1983) for the entire 16-to 20-year-old age group and by the same research team (Smith et al., 1984) for the 16-to 17-year-old group. However, a statistically significant reduction in single-vehicle, nighttime fatalities was found in Massachusetts for 18 to 19 year olds over the three years following the increase in the minimum age requirement. These outcomes are consistent with the findings by Williams and colleagues (1983) that Massachusetts had the lowest reduction in fatalities of nine states that raised their minimum purchase age. Other states that appear to have a higher level of enforcement of the minimum purchase age laws and of compliance with the laws have recorded statistically significant reductions in alcohol-related crash involvement among the age groups most affected by the raised minimum ages. A recent study of 26 states by DuMouchel, Williams, and Zador (1987) found similar results.

In an adjoining state, New York, which was used as a comparison state for the Massachusetts study by Hingson and coworkers (1983), a subsequent purchase age change from 18 to 19 yielded statistically significant changes in the auto accident rate. Lillis, Williams, and Williford (1987) reported nearly a 21 percent decrease in fatal and injury crashes and a 46 percent decrease in self-reported drinking and driving for New York young people following the age requirement change. A recent study conducted in Texas also showed that a one-year change in the minimum drinking age affected youthful crashes (Wagenaar and Maybee, 1986).

Taken as a group, such studies of individual states or clusters of states support the conclusion that a higher minimum purchase age requirement has the potential to reduce consumption by youth (particularly of beer, the beverage of choice of the young) and alcohol-related traffic accidents. The potential reduction, like the effects of most restrictions on alcohol availability, appears to be a function of compliance and enforcement. If compliance is poor as a result of the lack of diligence by retail establishments in checking identification or the lack of enforcement by ABC authorities and law enforcement officers, the decline in alcohol-related traffic accidents is reduced.

Three national studies are worthy of note. An analysis by Cook and Tauchen (1982) found a 7 percent increase in the number of youths killed in automobile accidents that was associated with a lowering of the drinking age from 21 to 18. A national comparison by the National Highway Traffic Safety Administration (1982) found that states with higher drinking-age requirements had lower rates of serious injuries.

In a related study, Grossman, Coate, and Arluck (1987) conducted a national evaluation of the sensitivity of youthful consumption of specific alcoholic beverages to minimum-age changes. Based on their projections, they concluded that an increase in the minimum age for the purchase of beer from 20 to 21 would yield a 10 percent drop in the number of youths who drank beer, a 17 percent reduction in those drinking beer two to three times a week, and a 17 percent reduction in the number drinking as many as three to five glasses of beer on a typical drinking day (for a similar analysis, see Saffer and Grossman, 1987b).

A report by the National Highway Traffic Safety Administration (Arnold, 1985) analyzed traffic crash data for drivers up to age 23 in 13 states that had raised their minimum purchase age between 1975 and 1982. The study compared annual figures for drivers in areas affected by minimum age changes who were involved in fatal crashes with those drivers who were involved in fatal crashes in areas not affected by the law change. Pooled data from all states revealed an average reduction of about 13 percent (with a range of 6-19 percent) in fatal accident involvement among the drivers affected by increased minimum-age requirements.

Zoning and Conditional-Use Permits

Recently, decision makers in some municipalities have considered employing local land-use zoning to directly limit the density of alcohol outlets. Another proposal has been to employ conditional-use permits to place specific restrictions on the hours of operation, decor, and perhaps serving practices of any business that plans to serve alcohol (see Wittman, 1986). However, relatively little research has been conducted to date on the topics of zoning and conditional-use permits.

Published research on alcohol zoning practices appears to be limited to a single survey of California cities reported by Wittman and Hilton (1987). The survey's purpose was to describe current zoning practices. It found that approximately 41 percent of the cities did not regulate outlets, 29 percent required conditional-use permits for on-premises sales outlets, and 30 percent required conditional-use permits for both on-and off-premises sales; 26 percent of the cities had incorporated restrictions on alcohol outlets into the local zoning ordinance. It remains unclear what leads cities to adopt these restrictions, although larger urban areas are more likely than smaller areas to adopt zoning regulations of all types.

Although a basic relationship between the overall indicators of alcohol availability and alcohol use and misuse has been demonstrated, research should be focused on the effects of specific changes in the forms and types of restriction on alcohol availability.

The following are some promising opportunities for research on alcohol availability:

• The differential effects of retail price changes for alcohol should be examined in terms of their potential to affect heavy, high-risk drinking. Because age and gender are related to some high-risk consumption behavior, age- and gender-specific studies of price sensitivity for alcoholic beverages are needed to improve our understanding of the economic dimensions of alcohol use and misuse. Current economic models of variables do not differentiate among alcohol-dependent persons, heavy drinkers, and moderate consumers; also, the relative sensitivity of alcoholics and nonalcoholics to price changes is not well delineated.

• Elements of alcohol availability (e.g., happy hour price incentives) have economic and social dimensions that have not been studied. Further investigations in this area could provide direction for the formulation of policy concerning these sales strategies.

• The influence of location, density, and hours of sale of alcohol outlets, as well as the types of outlets that should be permitted and their proximity to major driving locations, is just now being investigated. This research may suggest additional prevention strategies that can be instituted at many different levels of government. Recently, localities have become more involved in the regulation of alcohol availability, a role previously dominated by the state alcoholic beverage control authority.

• As communities become more involved in preventing alcohol problems, new territory will be opened up for studies of the epidemiology of alcohol problems at the community level. An equally important topic for investigation in itself is the use of local community resources for the development of prevention initiatives. For instance, further research could answer questions about (a) the effectiveness of existing local controls on alcohol outlets for reducing alcohol-related problems; (b) the factors that stimulate action by communities to use their own local resources to prevent alcohol problems related to alcohol availability; and (c) the effect of using local proprietors to regulate alcohol availability.

Studies such as these can help to develop knowledge about the potential effectiveness of local planning for alcohol availability and to support policy development. Major questions include the following: Should controls on the distribution of availability remain at the state level, where they have been since the repeal of Prohibition? Should the trend toward de facto allocation of responsibility for control on availability to local authorities continue? How is physical planning for alcohol availability related to other aspects of environmentally based prevention planning (e.g., prices, alcohol advertising, media portrayals of alcohol, age-related aspects of alcohol availability)?

ENVIRONMENTAL INFLUENCES ON INDIVIDUAL DRINKING BEHAVIOR

The environmental influences on an individual's drinking behavior are many and varied, reaching out to encompass a wide range of forces that may affect the development of alcohol problems. The committee discusses several of these influences in the following pages: the normative environment and the mass media, the legal environment, and the effects of drinking context and setting.

The Normative Environment and the Mass Media

The standards set by a community and communicated both explicitly and implicitly play a large role in shaping many different behaviors, including alcohol consumption. Appropriate alcohol-use behavior in one era may not be appropriate in another. Similarly, appropriate drinking behavior may change from setting to setting or from group to group. The normative environment can be rather complex, with one level of norms operating in a local area (e.g., a college campus or even a single dormitory) and a different, perhaps even competing set of norms accepted in the society at large.

The media, especially television, play an increasingly substantive role in communicating information of all kinds to the public, and they are thought to play a significant part in shaping public perceptions and norms about alcohol use. Alcohol-related information is conveyed through at least three media modes: (1) public information campaigns that are designed to educate the public about alcohol (2) advertising by the alcohol industry and (3) fictional television and movie programming that depicts drinkers and drinking situations. The contribution that each is thought to play in shaping the environment in which we operate has been the object of a great deal of research. As one might expect, observations of the impact of commercial advertising and fictional media programming are necessarily different from planning and testing intentional media campaigns as a mode of preventive intervention.

Public Information Campaigns

In the 1970s, several efforts were made to educate the general public about the importance of moderate drinking. A three-year mass media demonstration project in California that promoted responsible drinking showed some increase in citizen awareness but no significant changes in attitudes or behavior (Wallack, 1983). A review of 15 mass media campaigns conducted by Hewitt and Blane (1984) revealed that some campaigns were effective in changing some audience attributes, including knowledge, attitudes, or behavior. In later work, Wallack (1985, 1987) proposed that the mass media can be used as an intentional change agent to alter the social agenda, increase awareness and knowledge, stimulate public discussion, and provide a background of legitimacy for the problems that detract from the health of society. Conclusions from the California campaign and others are that public education may not be sufficient to change behavior, but it could be an important component of a larger prevention effort. There are, however, serious reservations about whether the potential of public education for changing behavior has been adequately tested, especially in the context of a comprehensive program that integrates environmental and regulatory changes with multichannel education.

It is not likely that significant changes in attitudes, behavior, or both, will occur primarily through mass media campaigns (Farquhar, Maccoby, and Wood, 1985). Rather, the evidence from cardiovascular disease prevention programs (Farquhar et al., 1977; Puska et al., 1981) suggests that change may be more likely to occur when a comprehensive campaign involves several change agents in addition to the mass media. At the same time, it is unlikely that a large-scale public health campaign directed at the general public can be successful without mass media involvement.

Existing research indicates that the mass media may be most effective in inducing cognitive (as opposed to behavioral) changes and setting the public agenda about an issue. From reviews of health campaign research compiled in the late 1970s and the 1980s, the most reasonable goals of mass media campaigns in the health area appear to be to increase awareness, information levels, and the salience of specific issues. When the mass media focus on a topic, they create and reinforce public awareness about an issue and contribute to its salience. In addition, continuing emphasis on the issue is likely to increase the absolute level of its perceived importance. Unfortunately, when focus on an issue subsides, so does public attention.

Health issues are brought to public attention in one of two ways: either through selection by the media or through a targeted health education campaign. These two approaches differ greatly because selection by the media is largely uncontrolled, whereas a health organization's efforts generally are purposeful, with specific, measurable goals. Health organizations often initiate efforts to make the public aware of, and informed about, health issues, and these efforts are designed to affect the media agenda. Agencies create films, public service announcements, news releases, photo and interview opportunities, television and radio programs, and so forth, sometimes to stimulate direct public response but more typically to trigger media response as well.

Another goal of mass media campaigns is to provide information in the form of new knowledge, as well as knowledge to replace misinformation and correct myths. The goal is a better informed public, and research indicates that this is a reasonable expectation of a mass media campaign (although target groups are never as well informed as health agency administrators might wish).

If public education campaigns are to be successful in reducing alcohol abuse, there is a need periodically to monitor the target populations, usually through surveys, to accomplish the following:

• assess areas of information and misinformation. (What do people know, and what do they think they know? What should they know that they do not know?);
• determine the public's awareness of alcohol abuse and alcohol problems;
• determine the salience of those problems to the public, both in terms of personal importance and in terms of perceived social importance;
• examine relevant beliefs and attitudes held by the public; and
• identify their alcohol-related behaviors.

This assessment should precede any concerted health campaign because it provides background information for planning such efforts. It should also be the substance for the formative evaluation of media campaign efforts and strategies discussed below. To the extent that campaign themes and strategies are in a developmental phase, they should be pretested through formative research and modified in preparation and design as such evaluation suggests--not when it is too late to make changes. Another element that is critical in developing mass media health messages is to specify the target audience. Specification allows research planners to assess more accurately the knowledge, awareness, salience, and orientation toward alcohol use and abuse that is characteristic of target subgroups. It also permits planners to use each group's message exposure habits to design more effective media campaigns.

Formative research is a necessary tool to create campaign messages for media dissemination and should be carried out in two phases. In the first phase (preproduction), a target group is surveyed to determine members' cognitive knowledge and affective responses to alcohol, their motives for drinking, and their media usage patterns as a way to identify potential areas of "vulnerability" for change. The areas that are so identified are then examined by media, content, and persuasion experts to design messages. Formative research in message design involves informal testing from early tentative versions of a message to the one that is ultimately used. Prototype messages emerging from this process can then be experimentally tested with sample target audience groups in the second (or postproduction) phase to determine whether the campaign's desired goals are being achieved. The results of these tests can serve as the basis for improving the messages. Summative or final evaluation research may follow in the waning days of the campaign or thereafter (Atkin and Freimuth, in press).

Alternative modes of reaching target groups with media messages should also be devised and tested. For example, the radio is a particular favorite of teenagers and could be used for public service announcements directed toward them. In addition, drinking-and-driving messages would appear to be most appropriate if received by radio while driving. Field experiments in selected communities could assess the ability of radio to deliver such messages. Furthermore, there are specialized magazines for virtually all groups that can be appropriately used to deliver alcohol-related messages. Music, in any medium, is another strong influence for young people. The demonstrated attractiveness of some specialized cable channels, such as Music Television (MTV), should be considered as a means to reach this group.

Another major avenue for reaching adolescents is films. For teenagers, moviegoing is a major social experience, often followed by drinking opportunities and incidents. The movie theater is rich in possibilities for intervention: for example, it provides a forum for public service announcements (PSAs) before the movie begins, acts as a venue to mount antidrinking/driving posters, and offers the possibility of print messages on soda and popcorn containers. Another way of reaching adolescents (and others) with alcohol-use messages might be to approach videocassette producers and request the inclusion of PSA messages as trailers on rental or purchase tapes.

A social inoculation approach (i.e., using media messages to "inoculate" individuals against persuasion efforts) has been shown to be effective, not only against persuasion (Lumsdaine and Janis, 1953; McGuire, 1973) but against the effects of counterpersuasive messages. This approach has recently been demonstrated to be effective against social temptation (Killen, 1985) in smoking prevention research. The identification of effective inoculations against some media messages could help to prevent young people from forming unhealthful and dangerous patterns of alcohol use (see the discussion under "Commercial Alcohol Advertising" below).

The following are opportunities for research on public information campaigns and education:

• The formative evaluation process is necessary to identify credible communicators for different groups. The "sources" used to present alcohol-related messages to any particular target audience must be credible. It is as unlikely that there are universally credible sources for different audiences as it is that there is a universal antialcohol message. Questions that require answers include: When are women credible commentators on alcoholism prevention, as well as which women and for whom? Who is a hero to adolescents and, as a hero, an effective spokesperson? A wealth of literature exists on source credibility, little of which is linked to specific content areas. Especially for such contemporary issues as driving after drinking or after using drugs, it may be particularly difficult to predict credible sources accurately. In these cases, pretesting is essential.

• Preproduction research on media campaigns should identify which media are accessible and are used by particular target groups, how often they are used, and when. For example, if a substantial subset of problem drinkers or individuals consists of late-night television fans, that characteristic suggests a time and medium in which to reach them with media messages.

• The coverage of alcohol issues in local newspapers and television programs should be sampled.

Commercial Alcohol Advertising

The majority of the information on alcohol use is presented by the alcoholic beverage industry. About $1 billion is spent annually on alcohol advertising, an amount that greatly exceeds the public education budgets both of federal and state governments and of nonprofit agencies. The messages that are common in alcohol advertising promote drinking as a healthy, attractive, and success-oriented activity (Minkler, Wallack, and Madden, 1987). However, research on the effects of that advertising is conflicting. Smart (1988, p.321) reports that "[n]o study (with one exception) has concluded that alcohol advertising has a substantial effect on alcohol consumption. . . . Current research suggests that advertising is, at best, a weak variable affecting alcohol consumption." Strickland (1983, p.221) concurs, concluding that televised advertising has "meager effects on the level of consumption" by adolescents in school. According to him, television advertising to promote alcohol use is "rarely translated into effects on alcohol problems."

In a notable exception to these studies, Atkin and Bloch (1981) and Atkin, Hocking, and Bloch (1984) concluded that schoolchildren who have seen more television and magazine ads for alcohol generally drink more than those who have seen fewer ads; in addition, among those who do not yet drink, those who have seen more ads report that they are more likely to begin. In his most recent review, Atkin (1988b, p.ii) found the following:

Despite ambiguities about causal direction, the findings indicate that televised beer ads mildly increase beer drinking, magazine liquor ads have a modest positive influence on consumption of spirits, and that the impact of traditional wine advertising is weak.

In reference to the several dozen studies he critiqued in the article, Atkin (1988b, p.iii) concluded,

Although each technique and most specific executions can be attacked, rendering conclusions suggestive and tentative, the preponderance of the evidence from the alcohol advertising literature indicates that ads stimulate higher consumption by both adults and adolescents. . .there is sufficient basis for rejecting the inference of null effects and for rejecting claims that advertising exerts a powerful influence on drinking behavior. It appears that advertising is a contributing factor that increases consumption to a modest extent.

Other researchers agree that advertising may be a contributing factor to increased alcohol use. Farrell (1985, p.27) notes that advertising is "only one element of a complex mix of marketing techniques. . .whose combined impact may well be substantially greater." She also points out that there are no studies that explore the cumulative, long-term effects of advertising on alcohol consumption and alcohol-related problems over the course of a generation, no studies of the impact of a sharp reduction in advertising where it has been pervasive, and no research on the impact of a sharp increase in advertising in cases in which it has been largely unknown (e.g., Third World countries).

Other sections of this report emphasize the importance of a comprehensive or community-wide approach to combating alcohol problems. In that same vein, the most effective use of mass media may be as part of a multimedia effort. The single insertion of a single advertisement is unlikely to produce change in the level of alcohol-related problems or to increase awareness, salience, or knowledge. The proponents of alcohol consumption use all of the mass media; so, too, must the proponents of alcohol problem prevention.

For example, in advertising, there is a need to identify the type and style of advertising content (e.g., life-style appeals versus consumer information, brand imaging) that has the most impact on alcohol consumers. Identification could be followed by theoretically grounded experimental research to determine how inoculating messages might diminish the acceptance and impact of advertising content. Contrary themes could be examined as a potential message strategy. If one theme of commercial alcohol ads is the social benefits of drinking, it is important to determine how alternative messages (e.g., public service advertisements that identify the social deficits of drinking) might be used to counteract the commercial ads. (For a recent review of the research on using alcohol-related advertising as an intentional change agent, see Atkin, 1988a; see also Alcalay, 1983; Hewitt and Blane, 1984; and Wallack, 1985.)

The following are opportunities for research on the effects of commercial advertising on alcohol use:

• Given the association between teenage drinking and driving, targeted examinations are needed to assess the impact of alcohol advertising on those young people currently approaching legal drinking ages, in terms of exposure to advertising and its impact on brand recognition, preference, interest in drinking, and expectations as to the social merits (and demerits, if any) of drinking. Other targeted groups might include light drinkers, women, and ethnic minorities.

• As suggested earlier in the text, studies should explore the cumulative, long-term effects of advertising on alcohol consumption, the impact of a reduction in pervasive advertising, and the impact of increased advertising in situations in which it has not previously been used.

• There is also a need to test the impact of advertising within a specific program context. For example, a study of the short-term effects of beer advertising during a popular sports event covered by the media may provide useful insights.

Fictional Media Content

The focus in this discussion is on the depiction of drinking and drinkers in fictional television programming. Often, the rationale for these studies comes from social learning theory (see Chapter 3), which predicts that learning and behavior change may occur by observing new kinds of behavior (e.g., watching an individual refuse an alcoholic drink and subsequently being rewarded for doing so, seeing attractive persons become ill with drink). In this instance the media can be seen as an object of study rather than as an intentional change agent.

Content analysis clearly demonstrates the prevalence of alcohol on commercial television programs. In 1976-1977, there were 2.2 incidents of alcohol use per hour during prime time and Saturday morning programs (Greenberg et al., 1978); there were 2.7 incidents per hour the following season (Greenberg et al., 1979) and 8.13 incidents per hour in the

10 top-rated prime time shows after the next season (Greenberg, 1981). Similar levels have been identified in afternoon soap operas. No studies have been conducted, however, that directly link the quantity of these portrayals to consumption or attitudes.

It has been suggested by Atkin (1988b) that a group that is particularly vulnerable to such program content would be young adolescents because (1) they watch as much or more television than any other age group; (2) they have limited direct experience with alcohol; and (3) whereas other influential agents such as parents are likely to be uniformly discouraging of alcohol experimentation, the primary message in the TV programs and advertising content they will read, see, or hear is one of positive social consequences. Preteens may be another vulnerable group. In a study by Rychtarik and coworkers (1983), preteens who were exposed to a situation comedy that included multiple drinking scenes were more likely to offer whiskey drinks to potential adult guests than were preteens who did not see the program.

Because media messages may act as formative influences and change agents, content analysis should be used to monitor the portrayal of alcohol use in television programs and films that are most heavily viewed by target groups of interest (e.g., in soap operas, if the target group is adolescent females and nonworking women; in situation comedies featuring minority characters, if the target group is minority). Follow-up research should explore the impact of these alcohol portrayals on their audience, within specified target groups.

In addition, what the national media present to the public about alcohol as news should be regularly monitored and supplemented by a sampling of local coverage in newspapers and on television in communities throughout the country. News media personnel responsible for science writing at the wire services, major newspapers, and television networks should be identified and surveyed about their knowledge of attitudes about alcohol.

The Legal Environment

Alcohol-Impaired Driving

Between 1980 and 1985, the United States experienced an unprecedented emergence of public concern about the problems posed by drunk drivers. More than 400 chapters of local citizens groups such as Mothers Against Drunk Driving (MADD) and Students Against Drunk Driving (SADD) were formed. News media coverage of drunk driving, as measured in numbers of stories, increased 50-fold from 1980 to 1984. A national commission was formed to examine the problem, and more than 500 laws were passed aimed at reducing drunk driving. All of the states now have legal drinking ages of 21. More than 40 states have now adopted laws making it illegal "per se" to drive with a blood alcohol level above 0.10-- the equivalent of four to five drinks for a 150-pound person in an hour on an empty stomach. In addition, half of the states adopted "administrative per se" laws that permit states to hold the licenses of arrested drivers until their court trials. Many other states have recently adopted stiffer penalties for drunk driving, including increased automatic fines, license suspensions, and jail sentences.

These activities have had a profound influence on drinking-and-driving behavior in this country. Serious limitations remain, however, which hamper efforts to evaluate the changes that have occurred.

First, most states do not obtain blood alcohol information on all drivers who are involved in fatal crashes. Accordingly, when a new drunk-driving law is enacted, researchers cannot determine whether there is a change in the number of crashes involving intoxicated drivers as a proportion of all crashes. Because the key dependent variable (blood alcohol level) cannot be precisely observed, researchers have used surrogate measures to study the impact of drunk-driving legislation. However, some researchers have cautioned that such surrogate measures are so imprecise that their use can, on occasion, lead to incorrect conclusions, particularly in short-term studies of small jurisdictions (e.g., Heeran et al., 1985).

A second constraint that prevents researchers from measuring the effectiveness of drunk-driving laws results from the kind of individuals who drive after heavy drinking. They are less likely to wear seat belts, are more likely to drive after using psychoactive drugs, and are more likely to have been arrested for speeding, running red lights, and other moving violations (Hingson and Howland, 1987). Consequently, it may be possible to reduce drunk driving and still not reduce the number of fatal crashes because persons who reduce the amount they drink before driving may still be at high risk for vehicular injury.

Finally, changes in drinking-and-driving laws usually do not occur in isolation. When several related laws are enacted within a short period of time, it is difficult to attribute any effects that might occur to a specific intervention. Numerous confounding variables can influence alcohol-related vehicular crash rates. Such variables as unemployment rates, use of seat belts, and rates of speeding are seldom, if ever, controlled analytically in research evaluating drunk-driving interventions. Previous research also shows that the impact of drunk-driving laws can vary widely among jurisdictions. Thus, findings from one region cannot be generalized to another.

Nonetheless, from 1980 to 1985, when media attention, community organization, and legislative activity peaked nationwide, fatal crashes declined 13 percent from 45,284 to 39,168. Single-vehicle, nighttime fatal crashes--the kind most likely to involve alcohol--declined even more, down 20 percent from 18,277 to 14,603. Among teenage drivers, declines were even steeper: single-vehicle, nighttime fatal crashes declined 34 percent, with 2,497 fewer in 1985 than in 1980 (Hingson, Howland, and Levenson, 1988; Hingson et al., 1988).

These dramatic reductions occurred for many reasons. First, the laws themselves produced positive beneficial effects. As noted earlier, studies of drinking age increases revealed that, although effects were variable from state to state, states that raised their drinking ages typically achieved 10 to 15 percent declines in night-time fatal crashes in targeted age groups relative to states that did not (Hingson et al., 1983; Williams et al., 1983; DuMouchel, Williams, and Zador, 1987; U.S. General Accounting Office, 1987).

An analysis of national traffic data from the period 1978-1985 by the Insurance Institute for Highway Safety (Zador et al., 1988) indicated that states that passed administrative per se laws reduced nighttime fatal crashes on the average of 9 percent relative to states that did not pass such legislation. In addition, states that passed criminal per se laws or imposed increased penalties for drunk driving achieved 6 percent declines in nighttime fatal crashes relative to states that did not pass such laws. Most states have criminal per se laws, but only a few have administrative per se laws; the institute estimated that if all states passed such laws, 2,600 fatal crashes could be avoided annually (Zador et al., 1988). Police enforcement of drunk-driving laws and court conviction rates have also increased in numerous states, developments that may produce further reductions because quasi-experimental community studies have shown that increased drunk-driving enforcement by police is associated with crash declines (Lacey et al., 1986; Voas, Rhodenizer, and Lyon, 1986; Voas and Hause, 1987). An additional finding of interest regarding this topic is that the extensive use of random breath testing in two states of Australia has been shown to substantially reduce alcohol-involved crashes and fatalities (Homel, 1988a,b).

Perhaps equally as important as these formal, legal counter-measures during the early 1980s was the emergence of informal social pressure that discouraged drunk driving. Media attention and political lobbying often preceded new laws. Annual surveys conducted in Massachusetts from 1981 to 1985 revealed that the proportion of drivers who said they would not care at all if their best friends found out that they had been arrested for drunk driving declined from 25 to 12 percent (Hingson et al., 1987). During the same time, the proportion of drivers who reported driving after five or more drinks during the past month also declined, from 18 to 6 percent. Massachusetts' experience in fatal crash declines was comparable to the national trends. Reported drunk-driving and nighttime fatal crash trends began to decline in Massachusetts and in many other states even before major legal changes occurred. Thus, the informal social pressures that stimulated passage of drunk-driving laws may also have produced drunk-driving reductions.

Despite the progress that has been achieved in the United States, however, experience in Great Britain and several other countries indicates that fatal crash declines after the passage of drunk-driving laws may be only temporary if public discussion of the problem diminishes and people become aware that the chances of being caught by the police are really quite low (Ross, 1982). This situation could well occur in the United States. The number of new citizens groups concerned with drunk driving peaked in 1983 (McCarthy, Wolson, and Baker, 1988). News and magazine stories about drunk driving declined sharply after 1984 (Hingson, Howland, and Levenson, 1988). After several years of decline, single-vehicle, nighttime fatal crashes rose 7 percent in 1986; other fatal crashes rose only 3 percent. Parallel estimates of the U.S. Department of Transportation showed an overall increase in alcohol-related fatalities of 6 percent and an increase in such fatalities among teenage drivers of 14 percent in 1986 relative to 1985 (U.S. Department of Transportation, 1988). Compared with 1986, data from 1987 indicate slightly fewer single-vehicle, nighttime fatal crashes among all ages and among teenage drivers; nevertheless, the overall total is still 5 percent higher than in 1985, and the teenage total is still 9 percent higher than in 1985.

Police enforcement of drunk-driving laws may not be sufficient to sustain long-term general deterrence effects of the laws. In a recent study comparing the effects of Maine's 1981 operating-under-the-influence (OUI) law with the 1982 Massachusetts drunk-driving law, only one-quarter of the drivers queried in the surveys in both states believed it likely that drunk drivers would be stopped by police, even though a majority thought arrested drunk drivers would be convicted and receive automatic penalties (both laws had instituted tougher penalties). Their perceptions appear to have had some validity: in Massachusetts in the postlaw period, despite increased police arrests for drunk driving, only one arrest, compared with 2.5 crashes, occurred per 1,000 drunk-driving trips reported by survey respondents (Hingson et al., 1987). Maine's arrest rate was only slightly higher and declined during the third postlaw year.

The study also showed that nighttime fatal crashes in Maine, which had declined 33 percent in the first postlaw year, returned to prelaw levels by the third postlaw year. During the same period, state police speeding arrests also declined by one-third, and the proportion of drivers traveling over 65 miles per hour on five roads posted at 55 miles per hour increased markedly (Hingson et al., 1987). Thirty-eight states raised speed limits on rural interstate highways in 1987. Speeding in general and the return to higher speeds on the highways are an emerging concern; because of poor sensory motor coordination and reaction time, drunk drivers may be particularly vulnerable to crashes at high speeds.

The following are opportunities for research on alcohol-impaired driving:

• The combined effect on actual behavior of social and legal pressures against drinking and driving and the influence of media attention on drinking-and-driving issues should be investigated further. Together, these influences are thought to exert considerable environmental controls on behavior.

• Theoretically, more disposable income is available for alcohol and gasoline purchases in times of strong economic conditions. It would be useful to conduct a study that controls for economic conditions to isolate their effects on automobile crashes.

• Further research is needed to identify the causes of the marked declines in fatal crashes in the early 1980s. We also need to assess whether recent increases in the number of fatal crashes will be temporary or whether other legal interventions, education, or enforcement efforts may be able to sustain long-term declines in the number of fatal crashes.

• The effects of speed limit increases on drunk-driving deaths, new legislation to reduce the blood alcohol levels that are considered to constitute legal intoxication, and the states' adoption of administrative per se laws are all areas for fruitful research. Other topics of interest include the interactive effect of vehicle speed with alcohol use in traffic crashes and the physical characteristics of drinking environments or settings that enhance safer drinking decisions or, alternatively, promote high-risk drinking.

Dram Shop or Server Liability

Server liability refers to the legal responsibility of someone who serves alcohol (usually for profit in a retail establishment). Server liability includes civil responsibility for damage and injury caused by a patron who is served while obviously intoxicated and later causes damage or injury to him- or herself or to others (e.g., in an auto accident). The term also encompasses criminal liability for service to an underage person. Before and after Prohibition, server liability laws (also called dram shop laws) were often enacted as an element of public prevention policy; most recently, such statutes have been used as the basis for individual litigation to obtain damages.

During the past several years, Mosher (1984a,b) and others have called for the use of server liability as part of a comprehensive approach to prevention called server intervention. According to Mosher, server intervention has three components: (1) legal, (2) training, and (3) environment. The legal component is discussed below; server training and the serving environment are discussed later under "Server Intervention."

The legal component of the server intervention approach includes state and local ABC statutes and regulations, criminal statutes, and dram shop liability. The dram shop liability element in particular has been explored by Mosher, who developed the Model Alcoholic Beverage Retail Licensee Liability Act of 1985 (Mosher, 1985). In its full form, this approach is designed to be incorporated into existing state ABC statutes and emphasizes the preventive potential of the legal approach. The statute would provide both deterrents and incentives. Dram shop liability could be considered the "stick," that is, the threat of financial (and possibly criminal) liability of the server or retail establishment that makes alcohol available either illegally or irresponsibly. The "carrot," or reward, would be the availability of the statute as a defense by a licensed beverage outlet that engages in responsible serving practices and can prove that it did so on a specific occasion. The preventive approach embodied in the statute would also reduce liability insurance premiums.

A parallel issue that warrants additional research is social host liability. As noted earlier in this chapter, many teenagers under the legal age of purchase obtain alcohol by having persons over the legal age purchase it for them (Hingson et al., 1983). Whether such persons should be held liable for the actions of those teenagers while under the influence of the liquor purchased for them is being debated. The effects of such liability on behavior should be explored.

Context and Setting as Environmental Influences

Drinking contexts and settings are studied by researchers in the alcohol field to determine how drinking behavior varies across different situations and to investigate whether certain strategies can be applied to different situations to reduce alcohol-related problems. One such strategy is server intervention training, which is discussed below. The context or setting in which drinking occurs may also influence alcohol consumption. Context includes such elements as the time of day, the occasion, and drinking companions. A setting is generally characterized by place (e.g., workplace, home, school) or by elements in the physical environment (e.g., lighting, size of tables).

Server Intervention

The most recent research to examine drinking settings arises from an interest in server intervention as a prevention strategy. The goal of server intervention is to reduce a customer's likelihood of intoxication or of driving while intoxicated through a combination of revised management and serving practices, server training, and changes in the physical environment. One of the first evaluations of server intervention (to determine its impact on customer consumption) was reported by Saltz (1987), who studied a Navy enlisted persons' club that had implemented a comprehensive server intervention program. The program itself involved extensive consultation with the club manager, which produced several changes in club policies and practices and an 18-hour training course for all staff.

The policy changes included promoting nonalcoholic beverages and food, overtly delaying service of an alcoholic beverage if it would put the patron at or above the legal limit for intoxication, and the discontinuance of beer sales in pitchers. Where before, food service had been separated from the bar area, a food service station was now installed in the barroom, and money incentives were provided to servers and cooks to promote food sales. In addition, servers had been free to roam anywhere in the building to serve customers; under the new program, servers were assigned to specific sections of optimal size to monitor customers' consumption. The food and beverage menus were expanded, and drink prices were marginally raised to cover the program's costs.

For two months before and after the program was in place, randomly selected customers were interviewed on Thursday, Friday, and Saturday evenings at both the study site and a comparable Navy club at which no program was implemented. Data from the interviews were used to estimate customer consumption and blood alcohol concentration (BAC). Results showed that the program led to a 50 percent drop in the likelihood of intoxication.

Although the Saltz study included changes in both bar practices and server training, other evaluations have been conducted on server training alone. Russ and Geller (1987) employed research assistants who posed as patrons who attempted to drink beyond the limits of intoxication at two bars at which approximately half of the staff had been trained. By recording the frequency and type of interventions used by the servers, they were able to show that the trained servers intervened in some way significantly more often than did untrained servers. Furthermore, when the pseudopatron's BAC was measured after leaving the bar, those who had been served by trained servers had lower BACs than those who had been served by the untrained personnel.

Another evaluation of server training is currently being prepared for the National Highway Traffic Safety Administration (NHTSA) by James A. McKnight. This study also employs pseudopatrons who in this case affect intoxication to see if servers who have been trained are less likely to serve them alcoholic beverages. The results from this study are not yet available.

Server intervention and server training studies suggest that environments can influence consumption and that these environments can be altered to lower the risk of alcohol-related problem outcomes. At the current stage of development of this strategy, however, the serving policies or training topics are most effective in bringing about these changes cannot yet be identified.

Drinking Establishments

The bar and restaurant are public settings in which alcohol typically makes up a large portion of the total revenue earned by the establishment. There are several good observational studies of bars and restaurants that examine the influence of the drinking group and its impact on consumption.

Several researchers have found that the size of drinking groups is correlated with the duration of drinking and thus with the total amount of alcohol consumed, although not necessarily with the rate of consumption (Somer, 1965; Foy and Simon, 1978; Rosenbluth, Nathan, and Lawson, 1978; Graves et al., 1981; Storm and Cutler, 1981; Harford et al., 1983; Geller, Russ, and Altomari, 1986). An additional influence on the drinking done by members of the group has to do with social modeling: it appears that faster drinking companions have more influence over the group than do slower drinkers (Caudill and Marlatt, 1975; DeRicco and Garlington, 1977; DeRicco, 1978; Reid, 1978; Skog, 1979; DeRicco and Niemann, 1980).

Other studies have suggested that bars with entertainment (e.g., live music, dancing, television, games) prolong the duration of a customer's stay and presumably increase overall consumption (Bach and Schaeffer, 1979; Ratcliffe et al., 1980); however, no one has directly observed whether individuals who actually engage in those activities are likely to drink more.

Naturalistic studies of drinking contexts are a helpful tool for framing research questions and generating research hypotheses. Unfortunately, they cannot tell us about causal influences on consumption and intoxication or about adverse consequences. By their nature, most observational studies have been unable to assess the interaction between characteristics of the individual and facets of the drinking environment. Indeed, to date, most experimental research in drinking behavior has focused on interpersonal influences rather than contextual ones (for a discussion of the need to integrate these influences, see Harford, 1979).

The following are opportunities for research on the drinking context:

• The contribution of the context of drinking to the development or inhibition of alcohol-related problems is a major factor that is not yet fully documented or understood. For example, we know that a majority of driving-while-intoxicated (DWI) offenders do most of their drinking in on-premises alcohol outlets (see the review by O'Donnell, 1985), but we do not know if this is a personal preference only of high-risk drinkers or whether the drinking site contributes to the development of the problem outcome.
• Measures of drinking contexts also need to be developed, especially because they are likely to involve structured observations of public drinking, a form of data collection that has not developed as rapidly as survey sampling and instrumentation. Measures of drinking environments need to be developed, refined, and assessed for reliability. Research into environmental influences is also likely to require integrating several forms and modes of data collection (survey, observation, archival) to maximize the reliability of measurement.

The Workplace as a Drinking Setting

Problem drinking exacts high costs for any work organization. Trice and Roman (1978) point out three direct costs: (1) the worker's on-the-job behavior (e.g., lower production, reductions in quality); (2) the impact of the drinker on other employees; and (3) the costs associated with treating problem drinking once it has been identified. A fourth cost that is not mentioned by Trice and Roman is the generally direct association between problem drinking and absenteeism. Although a dollar value can be attached to these costs, the subtle and indirect costs of problem drinking--in terms of loss of morale, erosion of supervisory authority, and errors in decision making--can only be estimated roughly. When only directly identifiable costs are considered, it has been estimated that a problem drinker costs the employer at least twice as much as an employee who is not a problem drinker in terms of the need for treatment, the increased utilization of medical facilities and benefits, the expenses associated with disciplinary measures, and below-average job performance (Winslow et al., 1966; Trice and Roman, 1978). Because of the demonstrable extent of the physical, social, psychological, and economic costs of problem drinking to the individual and to the employer, a great deal of research has focused on the workplace setting as it relates to alcohol use by employees.

In general, the literature on occupational drinking does not make a clear distinction between on-the-job, job-related, and non-job-related drinking. The assumption seems to be that because drinking behavior is an element of a person's entire social life and because work is a significant component of a person's existence, workplace factors are as important as nonworkplace factors in understanding patterns of drinking. Essentially, the problem with this research is one of failing to distinguish among the varying role domains through which people move in their day-to-day lives and thus failing to specify the linkages and overlaps between them. Drinking at work, drinking after work, drinking at home, and drinking at a bar on weekends with neighbors are all important phenomena to consider. In each social arena, the role, contexts, and meanings of drinking are likely to be unique.

As noted in Chapter 3, one way of conceptualizing a person's environment is as a series of domains. Hannerz (1982) also employs this concept to emphasize that urban life is a composite of roles that individuals play in different social arenas or role domains. Several significant domains may be identified: work, leisure, family, neighborhood, kin, and community. For some individuals, particularly those in well-established, ethnically based communities, the people who occupy roles in these distinct domains are relatively few; that is, coworkers are neighbors, may be kin, are certainly friends, and are those with whom one spends leisure time. Such networks--often termed "close-knit" (Bott, 1957)--are significant insofar as they are able to exert social control on network members (Mitchell, 1969). In these communities there will clearly be a spillover effect of work-related drinking into the family, neighborhood, and leisure domains.

Conversely, in very loose-knit networks, which are often the result of social and geographic mobility, the people an individual knows in the work domain are rarely met in roles outside that domain. Coworkers may be friendly at work, but there is often no significant social interaction outside that setting. The same may be said of the community and leisure domains. In loose-knit networks the social control exerted on the network member is weak overall (although possibly significant within some contexts) and is not consistent across the role domains. In these cases, workers may drink together on the job, at the union hall, or at an after-work softball game, but the style of drinking the individual does in such settings may not carry over into other domains. In the case of loose-knit networks, it may be important to specify clearly the differences, similarities, and overlaps between the work and nonwork worlds in terms of drinking behavior (Janes and Ames, 1986).

Until now, research has focused primarily on two aspects of occupational drinking: (1) occupational characteristics of clinical populations and the use of mortality statistics to identify "high-risk" jobs; and (2) examination of the relationship between subjective perceptions of work structure, satisfaction, or stress and drinking behavior or problems. The results of these studies generally indicate that alcohol problems are unevenly distributed across occupations and industries and that the determinants of this distribution stem either from the self-selection of deviant drinkers into certain occupations or from workplace conditions that foster problematic drinking in susceptible individuals (Cosper, 1979; Fillmore and Caetano, 1982; Parker and Brody, 1982).

There is a clear and unresolved discrepancy in the available literature between investigations that locate the source of drinking problems in the environment and those that specify individual, psychosocial attributes. The specific occupational risk factors that have been identified (Archer, 1977; Trice and Roman, 1978; Cosper, 1979; Fennel, Rodin, and Kantor, 1981; Parker and Brody, 1982) include

  • lack of visibility (e.g., nonexplicit production goals, flexible work schedules, lack of supervision);
  • stress factors stemming from the absence of a structured work environment, including work addition, occupational obsolescence, novel job roles;
  • stress factors stemming from overstructured work (low job complexity, time pressure, little control over work);
  • the absence of social controls; and
  • the high social availability of alcohol in work or work-related contexts, including occupational subcultures in which heavy drinking is normative.

Although the majority of findings point to the possible importance of certain kinds of work roles or occupational characteristics in the development of alcohol-related problems in the workplace, no single job-based risk factor emerges consistently across studies. The difficulty with much of this work is that it relies primarily on survey methods that combine individuals from many different industries into occupational categories that are defined a priori. Thus, it fails to consider the unique social and cultural contexts that characterize different workplace environments. Given the tremendous variety of work settings within a single industry, it seems superficial to focus on individual workers without considering the impact of environmental and sociocultural factors.

Although seldom addressed explicitly, conceptual models used in the occupational field frequently do not consider the relationship between environmental and individual factors in explaining alcohol-related behavior. Nowhere is this more evident than in the apparent dichotomy between the "subculture" and "social control" models. The subculture model, developed most extensively by Cosper (1979), argues for the normative underpinnings of alcohol use in specific occupational groups or settings. Heavy drinking by group members is thus "normal" and may even be functional in enhancing social solidarity in work groups, developing a coherent identity for group members, expressing masculinity, and other such effects.

Conversely, Roman and Trice (1970) have developed a "social control" model that posits deviant drinking as an outcome of ineffective or absent social controls (loose supervision and low work visibility) in the workplace. Related to this supposition of deviance is that those individuals who are deviant may in fact select themselves (or may be placed) in environments in which they can express such deviance. Although on their face these are contradictory explanations, both models address different explanatory levels of reality. For example, occupational drinking, although deviant from a management perspective, may in fact be adaptive under certain conditions: it may relieve the stress, tension, or boredom that characterize many jobs.

The point to be emphasized here is that the values suggested by attributions of "normative" or "deviant" labels to describe worker drinking unnecessarily distract attention from the real issue: individual heavy drinking may be considered a cultural artifact (the individual is following normative guidelines), a group response to work conditions, or a consequence of individual proclivities to join drinking groups. The real research concern should be with whether, how, why, and to what purpose occupational drinking groups evolve, and the determinants of an individual's affiliation with such groups.

The tendency to treat subcultural and deviant drinking models as opposing explanations points up the unwillingness of scholars to consider the intersection of individual and environmental factors. Understanding this intersection is vital for considering the relationship between quality or kind of work and alcohol-related behavior. Some work obviously is stressful; much work is boring; and few jobs offer a great deal of flexibility. Why do some people react to such conditions by drinking, and how does drinking as a social behavior develop out of individual responses to stress? Do poor working conditions have alternative effects? This question has often been posed in stress research in which the assumption is made that stress leads to a general susceptibility to one or more of a range of possible adverse health outcomes: heart disease, anxiety, depression, suicide, drinking, drug abuse, ulcers, and so forth (Cassel, 1976).

The following are opportunities for research on the workplace as a drinking setting:

• Conceptual models should be developed in which drinking may be considered as an outcome of a complex set of interrelationships among the work environment, the social organization of work, the evolution of informal work groups, other social spheres of the worker's life, and specific characteristics of the worker. Such a conceptual model demands a research strategy that can attend to different levels of analysis with some rigor.

• Research should be undertaken to identify those observable aspects of work (e.g., the structural organization of work, job stress, job complexity) that may explain differential rates of drinking practices and problems in the workplace.

• Studies should be conducted to determine the effects of formal and informal workplace alcohol policies, levels of supervision, and relative visibility of workers and job performance on alcohol consumption and alcohol-related problems.

• Research is needed to determine the level of alcohol availability in the workplace and the characteristics of workplace social networks or subcultures in relation to alcohol use.

FACTORS THAT AFFECT THE RISK OR SEVERITY OF THE NEGATIVE CONSEQUENCES OF DRINKING

There is another area of prevention in the alcohol field that is not specifically targeted at reducing alcohol consumption per se but that aims to reduce the risk or severity of subsequent alcohol-related problems. These measures tend to be problem specific and include such strategies as reducing deaths and injuries from alcohol-impaired driving by promoting the use of safety belts; reducing drownings through mandatory life preserver laws or the redesign of boats to make capsizing or falling overboard less likely; or reducing loss from fires (often alcohol related) through the manufacture of cigarettes that extinguish themselves quickly when unattended. Measures to reduce the violence that may attend heavy drinking are also a part of this area of prevention and have been the subject of recent research. For example, a study in Vancouver, British Columbia, looked at the physical characteristics of bars and taverns to discover which characteristics most influence the level of aggression associated with drinking (Graham, 1985). Other useful work in the area of alcohol-related violence has been carried out by Coleman and Strauss (1983) and Collins and Schlenger (1988). Also of interest in this area is the book edited by J. J. Collins (1981) entitled Drinking and Crime: Perspectives on the Relationships Between Alcohol Consumption and Criminal Behavior.

One prevention measure of this type that specifically targets youthful drinking is the adoption of a nighttime curfew, which can be a component of a comprehensive prevention policy. Curfews are meant to reduce crash risks by preventing the young from driving during late-night and early-morning hours, the greatest crash-risk periods. Curfews also tend to limit nighttime access of the young to alcohol and the opportunity to drive while drinking at night. As of May 1984, 12 states had curfew laws. These laws vary with respect to the ages of the drivers covered, the curfew hours, and the exceptions permitted (Williams, Lund, and Preusser, 1984).

In a study of 4 of the 12 curfew states, Preusser and colleagues (1984) found that crashes of 16 year olds were reduced 25 to 69 percent during restricted hours. In interviews with young people in New York and Louisiana, which are both curfew states, Williams, Lund, and Preusser (1984) found that most high school students generally know about the curfew law in their state and conform to the restrictions to a considerable extent. The research team also found that, although the students believe the police do not enforce the curfew law, many parents believe they do.

In considering opportunities for research in the area of reducing the risk or severity of the negative consequences of drinking, one must recognize the considerable gap in knowledge about the circumstances surrounding alcohol-related assaults, homicides, and suicides. The availability of handguns and other weapons may be a significant intervening factor in the high rate of alcohol involvement in these acts. A need exists to integrate alcohol prevention strategies with current research related to the use of firearms.

REFERENCES

Alcalay, R. Impact of mass communication campaigns in the health field. Soc. Sci. Med. 17:87, 1983.

Archer, J. Occupational alcoholism: A review of issues and a guide to the literature. Pp. 2-28 in C. J. Schramm, ed. Alcoholism and Its Treatment in Industry. Baltimore, MD: Johns Hopkins University Press, 1977.

Arnold, R. D. Effect of Raising the Legal Drinking Age on Driver Involvement in Fatal Crashes: The Experience in Thirteen States. Washington, DC: National Highway Traffic Safety Administration, 1985.

Atkin, C. K. Advertising and Marketing. Report of the Surgeon General's Workshop on Drunk Driving, Washington, 1988a.

Atkin, C. K., A Critical Review of Media Effects on Alcohol Consumption Patterns. Report prepared for the Alcoholic Beverage Medical Research Foundation, Baltimore, MD, 1988b.

Atkin, C. K., and M. Block. Content and Effects of Alcohol Advertising. Prepared for the Bureau of Alcohol, Tobacco and Firearms. Report No. Pb82-123142. Springfield, VA: National Technical Information Service, 1981.

Atkin, C., and V. Freimuth. Formative evaluation research in campaign development. In R. Rice and C. Atkin, eds. Public Communication Campaigns. Beverly Hills, CA: Sage, in press.

Atkin, C., J. Hocking, and M. Block. Teenage drinking: Does advertising make a difference? J. Communications 34:157-167, 1984.

Babor, T. F., J. H. Mendelson, I. Greenberg et al. Drinking patterns in experimental and barroom settings. J. Stud. Alcohol 41(7):635-651, 1980.

Bach, P. J., and J. M. Schaeffer. The tempo of country music and the rate of drinking in bars. J. Stud. Alcohol 41(7):635-651, 1979.

Blose, J. O., and H. D. Holder. Liquor-by-the-drink and alcohol related traffic crashes: A natural experiment using time-series analysis. J. Stud. Alcohol 48:52-60, 1987a.

Blose, J. O., and H. D. Holder. The public availability of distilled spirits: Structural and reported consumption changes associated with liquor-by-the-drink. J. Stud. Alcohol 48(4):371-379, 1987b.

Bott, E. Family and Social Networks. London: Travistock Publishers, 1957.

Bruun, K., G. Edwards, M. Lumio et al. Alcohol control policies in public health perspective. Helsinki: Finnish Foundation for Alcohol Studies, 1975.

Cassel, J. C. The contribution of the social environment to host resistance. Am. J. Epidemiology 104:107-123, 1976.

Caudill, B. D., and G. A. Marlatt. Modelling influences in social drinking: An experimental analogue. J. Consult. Clin. Psychol. 43(3):405-415, 1975.

Coate, D., and M. Grossman. Effects of Alcoholic Beverage Prices and Legal Drinking Ages on Youth Alcohol Use. Cambridge, MA: National Bureau of Economic Research, 1986.

Coleman, D. H., and M. A. Strauss. Alcohol abuse and family violence. Pp. 104-124 in E. Gottheil et al., eds. Alcohol, Drug Abuse and Aggression. Springfield, IL: Charles C. Thomas, 1983.

Collins, J. I., and W. E. Schlenger. Acute and chronic effects of alcohol use on violence. J. Stud. Alcohol 49(6):516-521, 1988.

Collins, J. J., Jr., ed. Drinking and Crime: Perspectives on the Relationships Between Alcohol Consumption and Criminal Behavior. New York: The Guilford Press, 1981.

Colon, I., H.S. Cutter, and W.C. Jones. Alcohol control policies, alcohol consumption, and alcoholism. Am. J. Drug Alcohol Abuse 8:347-362, 1981.

Cook, P. J. The effect of liquor taxes on drinking, cirrhosis, and auto accidents. Pp. 255-285 in M. H. Moore and D. R. Gerstein, eds. Alcohol and Public Policy: Beyond the Shadow of Prohibition. Washington, DC: National Academy Press, 1981.

Cook, P. J. The economics of alcohol consumption and abuse. Pp. 56-77 in L. J. West, ed. Alcoholism and Related Problems: Issues for the American Public. Englewood Cliffs, NJ: Prentice-Hall, 1984a.

Cook, P. J. Increasing the federal alcohol excise tax. Pp. 24-33 in D. R. Gerstein, ed. Toward the Prevention of Alcohol Problems. Washington, DC: National Academy Press, 1984b.

Cook, P. J., and G. Tauchen. The effect of liquor taxes on heavy drinking. Bell J. Econ. 13(2):379-390, 1982.

Cosper, R. Drinking as conformity: A critique of sociological literature on occupational differences in drinking. J. Stud. Alcohol 40:868-891, 1979.

DeLint, J. E. Alcohol control policy as a strategy of prevention. J. Public Health Policy 1:41-49, 1980.

DeLuca, J. R., ed. Fourth Special Report to the U.S. Congress on Alcohol and Health. U.S. Department of Health and Human Services. USDHHS Publ. No. (ADM)81-1080. Washington, DC: Government Printing Office, 1981.

DeRicco, D. A. Effects of peer majority on drinking rate. Addictive Behaviors 3:29-34, 1978.

DeRicco, D. A., and W. K. Garlington. The effect of modeling and disclosure of experimenter's intent on drinking rate of college students. Addictive Behaviors 2:135-139, 1977.

DeRicco, D. A., and J. E. Niemann. In vivo effects of peer modeling on drinking rate. J. Appl. Behav. Anal. 13(1):149-152, 1980.

Douglas, R. L., and J. A. Freedman. Alcohol-Related Casualties and Alcohol Beverage Market Response to Beverage Alcohol Availability Policies in Michigan. Ann Arbor: University of Michigan, Highway Safety Research Institute, 1977.

DuMouchel, W., A. Williams, and P. Zador. Raising the alcohol purchase age: Its effects on fatal motor vehicle crashes in 26 states. J. Legal Stud. 16:249-266, 1987.

Farquhar, J., N. Maccoby, and P. Wood. Education and communication strategies. Pp. 207-221 in W. Holland, R. Detels, and G. Knox, eds. Oxford Textbook of Public Health, vol. 3. London: Oxford University Press, 1985.

Farquhar, J., N. Maccoby, P. Wood et al. Community education for cardiovascular health. Lancet 1:1192-1195, 1977.

Farrell, S. Review of National Policy Measures to Prevent Alcohol-Related Problems. Geneva: World Health Organization, 1985.

Fennel, M.L., M. Rodin, and G.K. Kantor. Problems in work settings, drinking, and reasons for drinking. Social Forces 60:114-132, 1981.

Filkins, C. D., and J. D. Flora. Alcohol-related accidents and D.U.I. arrests in Michigan: 1978-1979. Ann Arbor: University of Michigan, Highway Safety Research Institute, 1981.

Fillmore, K. M., and R. Caetano. Epidemiology of alcohol abuse and alcoholism in occupations. Pp. 21-88 in Occupational Alcoholism: A Review of Research Issues. NIAAA Research Monograph No. 8. USDHHS Publ. No. (ADM)82-1184. Washington, DC: Government Printing Office, 1982.

Foy, D. W., and S. J. Simon. Alcoholic drinking topography as a function of solitary versus social context. Addict. Behav. 3:39-41, 1978.

Geller, E. S., N. W. Russ, and M. G. Altomari. Naturalistic observations of beer drinking among college students. J. Applied Behavior Analysis 19:391-396, 1986.

Graham, K. Determinants of heavy drinking and drinking problems: The contribution of the bar environment. In E. Single and T. Storm, eds. Public Drinking and Public Policy. Toronto: Addiction Research Foundation, 1985.

Graves, T., N. Graves, V. Semu et al. The social context of drinking and violence in New Zealand's multi-ethnic pub settings. In T. Harford and L. Faines, eds. Social Drinking Contexts: Proceedings of a Workshop, September 17-19, 1979. NIAAA Research Monograph No. 7. Washington, DC: NIAAA, 1981.

Greenberg, B. Smoking, drinking and drugging in top-rated TV series. J. Drug Educ. 11:227-233, 1981.

Greenberg, B., C. Collado, C. Atkin et al. Sexual intimacy and drug use in TV series. J. Communications 28:30-37, 1978.

Greenberg, B., C. Collado, D. Graef et al. Trends in use of alcohol and other substances on television. J. Drug Educ. 9:243-253, 1979.

Grossman, M., D. Coate, and G. M. Arluck. Price sensitivity of alcoholic beverages in the United States: Youth alcohol consumption. Pp. 169-198 in H. D. Holder, ed. Control Issues in Alcohol Abuse Prevention: Strategies for States and Communities. Greenwich, CT: JAI Press, 1987.

Hannerz, U. Tales of the City: Inquiries Toward an Urban Anthropology. New York: Columbia University Press, 1982.

Harford, T. Ecological factors in drinking. In H. T. Blane and M. E. Chafetz, eds. Youth, Alcohol and Social Policy. New York: Plenum Press, 1979.

Harford, T., S. Feinhandler, J. O'Leary et al. Drinking in bars: An observational study of companion status and drinking behavior. International Journal of the Addictions 18(7):937-950, 1983.

Harris, J. E. More data on tax policy. Pp. 33-38 in D. R. Gerstein, ed. Toward the Prevention of Alcohol Problems. Washington, DC: National Academy Press, 1984.

Heeran, T. R., S. Smith, S. Morelock et al. Surrogate measures of alcohol involvement in fatal crashes: Are conventional measures adequate? J. Safety Res. 16:127-134, 1985.

Hewitt, L. E., and H. T. Blane. Prevention through mass media communication. Pp. 281-323 in P. M. Miller and T. D. Nirenberg, eds. Prevention of Alcohol Abuse. New York: Plenum Press, 1984.

Hingson, R., and J. Howland. Alcohol as a risk factor for injury or death resulting from accidental falls: A review of the literature. J. Stud. Alcohol 48:212-219, 1987.

Hingson, R., J. Howland, and S. Levenson. Effects of legislative reform to reduce drunken driving and alcohol related fatalities. Public Health Reports 103:659-667, 1988.

Hingson, R., N. Scotch, T. Mangione et al. Impact of legislation raising the legal drinking age in Massachusetts from 18-20. Am. J. Public Health 73:163-170, 1983.

Hingson, R., T. Heeran, S. Smith et al. Effects of Maine's 1981 and Massachusetts' 1987 driving under the influence legislation. Am. J. Public Health 77:593-597, 1987.

Hingson, R., J. Howland, T. Heeran, et al. Effects of legal penalty changes and laws to increase drunken driving convictions on fatal traffic crashes. Bull. N.Y. Acad. Med. 64:662-677, 1988.

Hoadley, J. F., B. C. Fuchs, and H. D. Holder. The effect of alcohol beverage restrictions on consumption: A 25-year longitudinal analysis. Am. J. Drug Alcohol Abuse 10:375-401, 1984.

Holder, H. D., and J. O. Blose. Impact of changes in distilled spirits availability on apparent consumption: A time-series analysis of liquor-by-the-drink. Br. J. Addictions 82:623-631, 1987.

Homel, R. Drunk-driving countermeasures in Australia. Alcohol, Drugs, and Driving 4(2):113-144, 1988a.

Homel, R. Policing and Punishing the Drinking Driver: A Study of General and Specific Deterrence. New York: Springer-Verlag, 1988b.

Hooper, F. J. The relationship between alcohol control policies and cirrhosis mortality in United States counties. Paper presented at meetings of the American Public Health Association, Dallas, November 16, 1983.

Janes, C. R., and G. M. Ames. Men, Blue Collar Work and Drinking: Alcohol Use and Misuse in an Industrial Subculture. Berkeley, CA: Prevention Research Center, 1986.

Killen, J. D. Prevention of adolescent tobacco smoking: The social pressure resistance training approach. J. Child Psychiatry 26:7-15, 1985.

Lacey, J. H., L. Stewart, L. Marchette et al. Enforcement and Public Information Strategies for DWI General Deterrence: Arrest Drunk Driving--The Clearwater and Largo, Fla., Experience. Doc. DOT HS 807 066. Washington, DC: U.S. Department of Transportation, 1986.

Levy, D., and N. Scheflin. New evidence on controlling alcohol use through price. J. Stud. Alcohol 44(6):929-937, 1983.

Lillis, R. P., T. P. Williams, and W. R. Williford. The impact of the 19-year-old drinking age in New York. Pp. 133-146 in H. D. Holder, ed. Control Issues in Alcohol Abuse Prevention: Strategies for States and Communities. Greenwich, CT: JAI Press, 1987.

Lumsdaine, A. A., and Janis, I. L. Resistance to counter propaganda produced by one-sided and two-sided propaganda. Public Opinion Quarterly 17:311-318, 1953.

MacDonald, S., and P. C. Whitehead. Availability of outlets and consumption of alcoholic beverages. J. Drug Issues, Fall: 477-486, 1983.

Maisto, S. A., and J. V. Rachal. Indication of the relationships among adolescent drinking practices, and drinking-age laws. Pp. 155-176 in H. Webster, ed. Minimum-Drinking-Age Laws. Lexington, MA: D.C. Heath, 1980.

Makela, K., R. Room, E. Single et al. Drink in Finland: Increasing alcohol availability in a monopoly state. Pp. 31-60 in Alcohol and the State. II. A Social History of Control Policies in Seven Countries. Toronto: Addiction Research Foundation, 1981.

Maxwell, D. M. Impact Analysis of the Raised Legal Drinking Age in Illinois. Washington, DC: National Highway Traffic Safety Administration, 1981.

McCarthy, J., M. Wolson, and D. Baker. The founding of local citizens groups opposing drunken driving. In G. R. Caroll, ed. Ecological Models of Organizations. Cambridge, MA: Cambridge Press, 1988.

McGuire, W. J. Persuasion, resistance and attitude change. In I. Pool, W. Schramm, F. W. Fray, N. Maccoby, and E. B. Parker, eds. Handbook of Communications. Chicago, IL: Rand McNally College Pub. Co., 1973.

Minkler, M., L. Wallack, and P. Madden. Alcohol and cigarette advertising in Ms. Magazine. J. Public Health Policy 8(2):164-179, 1987.

Mitchell, J. C. The concept and use of social networks. In J. C. Mitchell, ed. Social Networks in Urban Situations. Manchester, U.K.: Manchester University Press, 1969.

Mosher, J. F. The impact of legal provisions on barroom behavior: Toward an alcohol problems prevention policy. J. Stud. Alcohol 1:205-211, 1984a.

Mosher, J. F. Legal liabilities of licensed alcoholic beverage establishments: Recent developments and policy implications. Paper presented at the Conference on Public Drinking and Public Policy: A Symposium on Observational Studies, April 26-28, Banff, Alberta, Canada, 1984b.

Mosher, J. F. The Model Alcoholic Beverage Retail License Liability Act of 1985. Western States Law Review 12(2):443-517, 1985.

Mosher, J. F., and D. Beauchamp. Justifying alcohol taxes to public officials. J. Public Health Policy 4:422-439, 1983.

National Highway Traffic Safety Administration. Evaluation of Minimum Drinking Age Laws Using the National Electronic Injury Surveillance System. Washington, DC: National NHTSA, 1982.

National Institute on Alcohol Abuse and Alcoholism. Sixth Special Report to the U.S. Congress on Alcohol And Health. USDHHS Publ. No. (ADM)87-1519. Rockville, MD: NIAAA, 1987.

O'Donnell, M. Research on drinking locations of alcohol-impaired drivers: Implications for prevention policies. J. Public Health Policy 6:510-525, 1985.

Ornstein, S. K., and D. M. Hanssens. Alcohol control laws and the consumption of distilled spirits and beer. Working paper, Research Program in Competition and Business Policy, Graduate School of Management, University of California at Los Angeles, 1983.

Parker, D. A., and J. A. Brody. Risk factors for alcoholism and alcohol problems among employed women and men. In Occupational Alcoholism: A Review of Research Issues. NIAAA Research Monograph No. 8. USDHHS Publ. No. (ADM)82-1184. Washington, DC: Government Printing Office, 1982.

Pearl, D., L. Bouthilet, and J. Lazar, eds. Television and Behavior, vol. 2. Washington, DC: National Institute of Mental Health, 1982.

Phelps, C. E. Death and taxes: An opportunity for substitution. J. Health Econ., in press.

Popham, R. E., W. Schmidt, and J. DeLint. The effects of legal restraint on drinking. Pp. 579-625 in B. Kissin and H. Begleiter, eds. Social Aspects of Alcoholism: The Biology of Alcoholism, vol. 4. New York: Plenum Press, 1976.

Preusser, D. F., A. F. Williams, P. L. Zador et al. The effect of curfew laws on motor vehicle crashes. Law and Policy 6:115-128, 1984.

Puska, P., J. Tuomilehto, J. Salonen et al. The North Karelia Project: Evaluation of a comprehensive community programme for control of cardiovascular diseases in 1972-77 in North Karelia, Finland. Public Health in Europe, WHO/EURO Monograph Series. Copenhagen: World Health Organization, 1981.

Rabow, J., and R. K. Watts. Alcohol availability, alcoholic beverage sales, and alcohol-related problems. J. Stud. Alcohol 44:767-801, 1982.

Ratcliffe, W. D., R. W. Nutter, D. Hewitt et al. Amenities and drinking behaviors in beverage rooms. Research report. Edmonton, Alberta: Alberta Alcoholism and Drug Abuse Commission, 1980.

Reid, J. Study of drinking in natural settings. In G. Marlatt and P. Nathan, eds. Behavioral Approaches to Alcoholism. New Brunswick, NJ: Rutgers Center of Alcohol Studies, 1978.

Rice, B. The role of state alcoholic beverage control in alcohol abuse prevention. Pp. 23-26 in H. D. Holder and J. B. Hallan, eds. Control Issues in Alcohol Abuse Prevention: Local, State and National Designs for the 80's. Columbia, SC: South Carolina Commission on Alcohol and Drug Abuse, 1984.

Roman, P. M., and Trice, H. M. The development of deviant drinking behavior: Occupational risk factors. Arch. Environ. Health 20:424-435, 1970.

Room, R. Alcohol control and public health. Annual Rev. Public Health 5:293-317, 1984.

Rosenbluth, J., P. E. Nathan, and D. M. Lawson. Environmental influences on drinking by college students in a college pub: Behavioral observation in the natural environment. Addict. Behav. 3:117-121, 1978.

Ross, H. L. Deterring the Drinking Driver: Legal Policy and Social Control. Lexington, MA: Lexington Books, 1982.

Rush, B., L. Gliksman, and R. Brook. Alcohol availability, alcohol consumption and alcohol-related damage. I. The distribution of consumption model. J. Stud. Alcohol 47:1-10, 1986.

Russ, N. W., and E. S. Geller. Training bar personnel to prevent drunken driving: A field evaluation. Am. J. Public Health 77(8):952-954, 1987.

Rychtarik, R. G., J. A. Fairbank, C. M. Allen et al. Alcohol use in television programming: Effects on children's behavior. Addict. Behav. 8:19-22, 1983.

Saffer, H., and M. Grossman. Effects of Beer Prices and Legal Drinking Ages on Youth Motor Vehicle Fatalities. New York: National Bureau of Economic Research, 1985.

Saffer, H., and M. Grossman. Beer taxes, the legal drinking age, and youth motor vehicle fatalities. J. Legal Stud. 16:351-374, 1987a.

Saffer, H., and M. Grossman. Drinking age laws and highway mortality rates: Causes and effect. Economic Inquiry 25:403-418, 1987b.

Saltz, R. The role of bars and restaurants in preventing alcohol- impaired driving: An evaluation of server intervention. Evaluation and the Health Professions 10(1):5-27, 1987.

Single, E., et al. Alcohol, Society and the State: A Social History of Control Policy in Seven Countries. Toronto: Addiction Research Foundation, 1981.

Skog, O. Drinking behavior in small groups: The relationship between group size and consumption level. Oslo: Statens Institutt for Alkoholforskning, 1979.

Smart, R. G. Does alcohol advertising affect overall consumption? A review of empirical studies. J. Stud. Alcohol 49:314-323, 1988.

Smart, R. G., and E. M. Adlaf. Banning happy hours: The impact on drinking and impaired-driving charges in Ontario, Canada. J. Stud. Alcohol 47(3):256-258, 1986.

Smart, R. G., and M. S. Goodstadt. Effects of reducing the legal alcohol purchasing age on drinking and drinking problems: A review of empirical studies. J. Stud. Alcohol 38:1313-1323, 1977.

Smith, R. A., R. W. Hingson, S. Morelock et al. Legislation raising the legal drinking age in Massachusetts from 18-20: Effect on 16 and 17 year-olds. J. Stud. Alcohol 45:534-539, 1984.

Somer, R. The isolated drinker in the Edmonton beer parlor. Q. J. Stud. Alcohol 46(6):459-466, 1965.

Storm, T., and R. Cutler. Observations of drinking in natural settings: Vancouver beer parlors and cocktail lounges. J. Stud. Alcohol 42(11):972-997, 1981.

Strickland, D. E. Advertising exposure, alcohol consumption and misuse of alcohol. Pp. 201-222 in M. Grant, M. Plant, and A. Williams, eds. Economics and Alcohol: Consumption and Controls. New York:Gardner Press, 1983.

Trice, H. M., and Roman, P. M. Spirits and Demons at Work: Alcohol and Other Drugs On the Job. New York: New York State School of Industrial and Labor Relations, Cornell University, 1978.

U.S. Department of Transportation. Fatal Accident Reporting System 1986. DOT HS 807 245. Washington, DC: National Highway Traffic Safety Administration, 1988.

U.S. General Accounting Office. Drinking Age Laws: An Evaluation and Synthesis of Their Impact on Highway Safety. Doc. GAO/PEMD 87-10. Washington, DC: U.S. Government Accounting Office, 1987.

Voas, R., and J. Hause. Deterring the drinking driver: The Stockton experience. Accident Analysis and Prevention 19:81-90, 1987.

Voas, R., A. E. Rhodenizer, and C. Lyon. Evaluation of a Charlottesville checkpoint operation: Final report to the National Highway Traffic Safety Administration. Charlottesville, VA, April 1986.

Wagenaar, A. C. Effects of an increase in the legal minimum drinking age. J. Public Health Policy 2:206-225, 1981.

Wagenaar, A. C. Alcohol, Young Drivers, and Traffic Accidents. Lexington, MA: D.C. Heath, 1983.

Wagenaar, A. C. Effects of minimum drinking age on alcohol-related traffic crashes: The Michigan experience five years later. Pp. 119-131 in H. D. Holder, ed. Control Issues in Alcohol Abuse Prevention: Stategies for States and Communities. Greenwich, CT: JAI Press, 1987.

Wagenaar, A. C., and R. Maybee. The legal minimum drinking age in Texas: Effects of an increase from 18 to 19. J. Safety Research 17:165-176, 1986.

Wallack, L. Alcohol advertising reassessed: The public health perspective. Pp. 243-248 in M. Grant, M. Plant, and A. Williams, eds. Economics and Alcohol: Consumption and Controls. New York: Gardner Press, 1983.

Wallack, L. The prevention of alcohol-related problems: Health educators and the "new generation" of strategies. Inter. J. Health Educ. 4(2):23-30, 1985.

Wallack, L. Mass media and health promotion: Ideological and practical foundations. School of Public Health, University of California, Berkeley, 1987.

Wallack, L., W. Breed, and J. Cruz. Alcohol on prime-time television. J. Stud. Alcohol 48:33-38, 1987.

Watts, R. K., and J. Rabow. The role of tourism in measures of alcohol consumption, alcohol availability and alcoholism. J. Stud. Alcohol, 42:797-801, 1981.

Williams, A. F., A. K. Lund, and D. F. Preusser. Night driving curfew in New York and Louisiana: Results of a questionnaire survey. Accident Analysis and Prevention 17:461-466, 1984.

Williams, A. F., P. L. Zador, S. S. Harris et al. The effect of raising the legal minimum drinking age on involvement in fatal crashes. J. Legal Stud. 12:169-179, 1983.

Winslow, W.W., K. Hayes, L. Prentice, et al. Some economic estimates of job disruption from an industrial mental health project. Archives of Environmental Health, 13:213-219, 1966.

Wittman, F. Community planning for alcohol availability. Bull. Alcohol Policy, 5(1):9-10, 1986.

Wittman, F., and M. Hilton. Local regulation of alcohol availability: Uses of planning and zoning ordinances to regulate alcohol outlets in California cities. In H. Holder, ed. Control Issues in Alcohol Abuse Prevention: Strategies for States and Communities. Greenwich, CT: JAI Press, 1987.

Zador, P., A. Lund, M. Fields et al. Fatal Crash Involvement and Laws Against Alcohol Impaired Driving. Washington, DC: Insurance Institute for Highway Safety, 1988.

Wittman, F., and M. Hilton. Local regulation of alcohol availability: Uses of planning and zoning ordinances to regulate alcohol outlets in California cities. In H. Holder, ed. Control Issues in Alcohol Abuse Prevention: Strategies for States and Communities. Greenwich, CT: JAI Press, 1987.

Zador, P., A. Lund, M. Fields et al. Fatal Crash Involvement and Laws Against Alcohol Impaired Driving. Washington, DC: Insurance Institute for Highway Safety, 1988.

5

COMMUNITY APPROACHES AND PERSPECTIVES FROM
OTHER HEALTH FIELDS

Major advances in the prevention of health-related problems have been made recently in several public health fields through the development and application of theory, the careful documentation of implementation processes, and the application of formative and summative evaluation methods. As a result of several well-planned, community-wide prevention programs based on sound experimental research designs, significant changes have been effected in the health behaviors of Americans, and declines in the risk of morbidity and premature mortality have been achieved. These systematic efforts to reduce cigarette consumption, control high blood pressure, lower accident rates, and modify unhealthy eating habits have resulted in sustained, community-wide health risk reductions that can be linked to a lowered incidence of disease and early death. The use of controlled experimentation to test prevention theory in programs such as these provides research findings that can guide the design of alcohol prevention approaches and permit the evolution of sound program designs and methods. This chapter reviews current perspectives on alcohol-related prevention and identifies applicable findings from prevention efforts in other public health fields.

Published reports of research on alcohol using comprehensive approaches at the community level are limited in number. Wallack (1984-1985) reports on one case study, and Geisbrecht, Douglas, and McKenzie (1981) are evaluating a three-community demonstration project in Canada. There have also been several other studies, but they have not involved the total "community" and have not been evaluated. Consequently, they are not reported here.

The Midwestern Prevention Project (MPP), also referred to as Project STAR, is an example of the community-wide approach to alcohol problem prevention. It is an as yet incomplete federally funded demonstration project under way in the states of Kansas, Missouri, and Indiana. The STAR project is a multilevel program addressing individual, social, and environmental factors that are thought to influence adolescent drinking. The project staff developed a school-based curriculum and supplements classroom studies with media messages, vendor education, police patrols, and alternative activities. The project has reported significant reduction in the use of three drugs (tobacco, marijuana, and alcohol) in a two-year follow-up of 15 communities near Kansas City, Missouri (Pentz et al., 1989). A full report is not expected until around 1991, following a two-year trial in communities in Indiana, which serve as controls for the Kansas City phase of the project. Probably the most ambitious and comprehensive existing program with an alcohol-use prevention component, MPP will contribute many insights relevant to the prevention of alcohol-related problems even though it is restricted to adolescents.

Comprehensive approaches need not be limited to cities or counties. Kraft (1984) and Mills and associates (1983) described comprehensive programs for college campuses that employed media, discussion groups, and experimental workshops. Community organizational planning was used to modify campus regulations. The programs appeared to be successful in modifying knowledge and attitudes regarding alcohol but not behavior. Although not as yet fully evaluated, a similar project targeted at high school youth, has demonstrated changes in knowledge, attitudes, and behaviors of teachers and peer leaders

5

(Mecca, 1984).

Other examples of community-based prevention are the actions taken by local, grass-roots movements to reduce such specific alcohol-related problems as drunk driving on prom night. A descriptive case study of parent groups sponsored by the National Institute on Drug Abuse (NIDA), found wide differences in activity, organization, and perceived efficacy (Moskowitz, 1985; Klitzner et al., 1987). Preliminary results of a study by NIAAA of Students Against Drunk Driving (SADD) programs have not detected measurable effects at two high schools (M. Klitzner, Pacific Institute for Research and Evaluation, personal communication). Another study (Ungerleider et al., 1986) used questionnaires sent to members of Mothers Against Drunk Driving (MADD) chapters to gather data for a descriptive study; no data are yet available.

LIMITATIONS OF ALCOHOL PREVENTION RESEARCH

Prevention research in the alcohol field--in general and at the community level--has been limited by problems in program design and evaluation. Project designs have relied heavily on the acceptance of prevention strategies based on the face validity of the intervention. For example, innovative means of education and policy changes such as warning signs at the point of purchase and bans on the sale of beer or wine at gas stations have been widely adopted without sufficient evidence of their effectiveness.

Other design weaknesses include focusing on a single strategy for change rather than using multiple and mutually reinforcing strategies. Another problem has been a tendency among policymakers to ignore complementary policy change strategies and legislative measures, such as local zoning ordinances. Surprisingly, these problems persist despite the well-accepted principle that successful health promotion and disease prevention programs maximize program effects through the integration of several components (Green and McAlister, 1984; Farquhar et al., 1985). Room (1984) also contends that alcohol problem prevention efforts should be designed as a system rather than conceived of as isolated components. Because limited controls on alcohol consumption do not appear likely to have a significant effect, Room calls for the concurrent use of several strategies that can result in synergistic effects.

The measurement of outcomes has also posed difficulties in research on the prevention of alcohol-related problems. Tax receipts from the sale of alcoholic beverages have been used successfully as a quantitative measure for some studies that have furnished considerable empirical data on interventions designed to control consumption. Yet most studies have only used such measures as the number of participants in a program or have relied entirely on changes in knowledge or self-reports of behavior change. Only a few have measured such outcome variables as blood alcohol levels of individual participants or changes in community rates of injuries or arrests for driving under the influence.

The sections that follow first present a case study of two cardiovascular disease (CVD) prevention programs in California. An in-depth look at these programs illuminates some of the major lessons learned from more than 15 years of effort to achieve measurable risk reduction for cardiovascular disease. Next, selected examples from other primary prevention efforts are reviewed, both to report on successes and to identify principles for possible application to alcohol abuse prevention.

COMMUNITY-BASED CARDIOVASCULAR DISEASE PREVENTION STUDIES

The Stanford Three-Community Study (TCS) conducted during the 1970s provided evidence that community-wide health education involving the mass media and supplemental face-to-face instruction can be quite effective in changing knowledge, attitudes, and behavior and, consequently, in reducing CVD risk factors (Farquhar et al., 1977). The results of the TCS demonstrated the potential for community-wide risk reduction using a three-year program of education. The TCS was carried out in one town largely through the mass media (including electronic media, newspapers, and printed self-help booklets) and in another town through the mass media supplemented by a face-to-face program of intensive instruction. A third town served as a reference community.

In contrast to prior projects in health education, the TCS project staff relied heavily on formative evaluation to develop educational strategies. The results strongly suggest that health status at the community level can be improved significantly through a well-designed educational program using both mediated and interpersonal channels.

Results of the TCS educational components were assessed over time, by using a multiple logistic function of CVD risk that incorporated age, sex, plasma cholesterol, systolic blood pressure, relative weight, and smoking. Several techniques were used to collect these data, including periodic field surveys of knowledge, behavior, and physiological testing in representative samples of the general population.

During a two-year period of community education, a statistically significant reduction was achieved in the composite risk score for cardiovascular disease as a result of significant declines in blood pressure, smoking, and cholesterol levels. This risk score decreased approximately 25 percent for the media-only community and 30 percent for the community in which media were supplemented by face-to-face instruction (Farquhar et al., 1977). This outcome suggests that considerable success was achieved when mass media programs were supplemented with intensive instruction but that adequate exposure to mass media alone was often successful without the supplemental education (Maccoby et al., 1977).

The Stanford Five-City Project (FCP), an ongoing, 13-year study that began in 1978, is an outgrowth of the TCS. It involves 350,000 people and employs multiple methods of education and community organization. The primary goal of the FCP is to reduce the risk of cardiovascular disease; however, subsidiary goals of the program also have important public health implications. These goals include cost-effectiveness analysis, development of educational and community organization methods, transfer of control to community organizations, and measurement of morbidity and mortality end points through a new, low-cost community surveillance method (Farquhar et al., 1985). The FCP represents an ambitious new endeavor in experimental epidemiology of potential relevance to field applications of noncommunicable disease control methods. It also offers a significant opportunity for testing generalizable and cost-effective community organization and health education methods.

Interim results from the FCP show that the risk factor reduction that has been achieved through this program is quite promising. Smoking rates have declined significantly in both treatment and reference communities, with a 2.5 percent per year greater drop in the proportion of smokers occurring in the treatment communities than in those locales in which no intervention occurred. The interventions also produced significant improvements in such health status indicators as blood pressure, blood cholesterol, and physical activity.

The multiple logistic of CVD risk for total mortality and for coronary heart disease events was reduced significantly in treatment communities by amounts ranging from 7 to 29 percent measured during four time periods from 2 to 5-1/3 years after education began (Farquhar et al., 1988).

Promising results have also been achieved in meeting other program goals. For example, preliminary results support the feasibility of transferring responsibility for program maintenance to local organizations. In addition to the overall community effect, the FCP provided evidence for individual or combined effects on various groups (in school and work site settings) of environmental or regulatory changes when coupled with mediated or face-to-face educational programs. Other data have shown that, although all three components were effective and have a place in a comprehensive prevention program, low-cost self-help booklets for smoking cessation are more cost-effective than either classes or contests (Altman et al., 1987).

Lessons from the Three-Community Study and the Five-City Project

The successful reduction of risk factors for cardiovascular disease through a primary prevention approach has been very encouraging. The results are promising because they suggest that it is possible to change the health habits of entire communities and to mobilize existing community resources to achieve those changes. The next step, however, is to learn how to replicate these results. Although there have been successes in other fields of primary prevention, the results of the CVD efforts have been much better documented. Therefore, the two CVD prevention programs in California may serve as models (Farquhar et al., 1977; Maccoby et al., 1977; Farquhar, 1978; Farquhar, Maccoby, and Wood, 1985). Several "lessons" or "keys to success" that were used repeatedly by these projects to ensure that the program was well-planned, well-implemented, and well-evaluated are described below.

Theory should be used as a basis for program planning, implementation, and evaluation. To provide a foundation for planning, implementing, and evaluating a large-scale community intervention to reduce the risk of heart disease, the Stanford group drew from several disciplines to develop a theoretical framework for individual behavior change. Relying on theory-based planning was essential for interpreting the results of evaluations and hypothesis testing. Without a theory or a model for change, outcome evaluation results would have been difficult to explain; without a previously determined hypothesis, it would have been nearly impossible to determine which strategies were effective and which were ineffective.

Theories and models that have been used in community CVD prevention include the communication-behavior change model, the social marketing framework, and the community organization model (Farquhar, Maccoby, and Wood, 1985). The communication-behavior change model draws on Bandura's social learning theory, McGuire's communication-persuasion model, and Rogers' diffusion theory (Farquhar et al., 1985) to identify a series of sequential steps for behavior change: (1) creating awareness of the need for behavior change; (2) producing a change in attitude toward the behavior; (3) increasing the motivation to change; (4) learning skills for change; and (5) learning maintenance and relapse prevention skills.

The Stanford group used social marketing theory to develop health messages for communities. Kotler and Zaltman (1971) define social marketing as "the design, implementation and control of programs seeking to increase the acceptability of a social idea or cause in a target group or groups." Based on its consumer orientation, social marketing dictates that the product--in this case, either a health information product such as a public service announcement (PSA) or a behavior--be developed and promoted to meet the needs of the consumer.

The community organization model is founded on the notion that the process of organization within the community is required to create a mechanism for collaborative action that leads to the adoption of programs, a step needed to ensure both cost-effectiveness and program maintenance.

A comprehensive, integrated program is needed. Primary prevention approaches used in effective programs have sought to address the entire population rather than high-risk individuals only. Because complex health problems involve individual and institutional behavior, social norms, and family modeling influences, a comprehensive, integrated program is required for program success. The "comprehensive" feature embraces the notion of Room's "system," an approach that he advocated for the prevention of alcohol-related problems (Room, 1984). The "integrated" feature implies that the components of the system, which may be inadequate when initiated singly, are more effective when they are integrated and when they are delivered in the right sequence. Comprehensive health promotion programs are those that actively involve all of the following elements:

• Multiple channels of communication (e.g., media, face-to-face contacts). Regulatory change and environmental change are additional "channels" of influence.
• Multiple target audiences (e.g., youth, families, health professionals, adults). For example, high-risk individuals or families, "hard-to-reach" individuals, highly motivated "early adopters," and less knowledgeable adults are common subgroups. Groups or organizations such as schools or work sites may also be the target.
• Multiple outcome objectives (e.g, knowledge gain, behavior change, policy change, physical environmental change, media promotion). These different outcome objectives reflect the use of different intervention strategies--for example, the use of advocacy activities to change organizational or community policy.
• Multiple levels of evaluation, including formative, process, and summative evaluation, applied to individuals, groups, organizations, and communities.

An integrated program ensures that each program component reinforces and strengthens other program components. For example, a smoking cessation program may rely primarily on self-help booklets and classes, but it will also reinforce its message through a campaign at local work sites, publicize itself in the local media, and collaborate with other local agencies on such events as a "quit-smoking" contest or legislation to restrict smoking in public areas. An integrated program must also be transferable to institutions within the community so that it can be maintained over time.

Formative and process evaluation is needed for success. Three general categories of formative evaluation were employed in the Stanford risk reduction programs: (1) needs analysis, (2) pretesting of educational programs, and (3) analysis of the implementation process following the introduction of the educational programs into the field. These three categories of formative research are based on social marketing theory by Kotler and are analogous to methods used in product marketing (Kotler and Zaltman, 1971).

In the California programs, an audience needs analysis was used to discover the interests, educational needs, media use, and other characteristics of the different subsections of the community. This type of formative research helped determine the proper name, location, and time for educational activities, as well as the cost and comprehensibility of any educational materials developed. Prototypes of educational programs were developed and tested to determine the appropriate content and method of delivery of the message. The pretest data were then used to revise the message or program prior to implementation to ensure effectiveness.

Process evaluations, or analyses of educational programs following their introduction into the community, were also employed to revise programs and examine content issues. Process evaluation identified some of the factors that influenced attendance, dictated how much was learned, and determined whether an event or program actually affected behavior.

Extensive evaluation of outcomes is essential. Cardiovascular disease prevention programs in the United States and other countries have invested considerable resources in evaluating the effects of their projects. For example, the FCP involved two intervention and three control communities. Periodic independent and cohort surveys were conducted in these communities throughout the life span of the project, and epidemiological data on CVD morbidity and mortality were also collected.

In addition to collecting outcome measures during the entire five years of the multicomponent intervention, specific risk reduction strategies (e.g., smoking cessation, dietary counseling) were evaluated to determine their effects on individual knowledge, attitudes, and behavior. For example, the effects of one quit-smoking contest with 500 participants were evaluated through several outcome measures: a mail survey of contest finishers; a telephone survey of selected nonrespondents; a carbon monoxide (CO) assessment of contestants who quit; and a one-year follow-up CO test of those same contestants (King et al., 1987). Data from this study allowed program planners to see both the successes and the shortcomings of the contest. The findings showed that the quit rate for contestants was twice as high as the rate in the general adult population in the control communities, and the cost of the program--including its evaluation--was lower than that of traditional classes or groups. Program planners concluded that the contest could be strengthened by adding a relapse prevention element (in this case, extending the length of the program) and by the use of incentives to maintain abstinence.

Because the TCS and FCP attempted to change both individual and organizational behavior, many levels of analysis were used to measure these changes. Change occurring at the individual level was perhaps the most studied outcome in these two projects and had the strongest basis in theory. Individual change strategies included the use of booklets, self-help kits, correspondence courses, contests, and classes. Limiting analysis to the individual, however, makes an artificial distinction between the individual and the environment. Therefore, change in organizations, including social service agencies, restaurants, grocery stores, hospitals, and work sites, was examined in a second level of the intervention analysis. Community change--for example, changes in laws, regulations, and taxation--was considered in a third analytical tier.

Each of these levels of change was conceptualized differently and required different intervention strategies and somewhat different evaluation methods. Throughout the TCS and FCP, component testing was the critical first step in designing strategies that had positive, short-term effects. Once these program components were tested, those that were found to be successful were incorporated into a larger multicomponent program. For example, school-based, peer resistance programs to prevent the adoption of cigarette smoking in seventh-grade students was one of the first components tested (McAlister, Perry, and Maccoby, 1979). Analogous studies have recently been extended to older adolescents in a broad nutrition, exercise, and weight control project (Killen et al., 1988). School-based and work site studies are prime examples of "components" that, once developed, may be used together with an expectation of synergistic effects.

Results from Other Comprehensive CVD Prevention Programs

A growing number of community-based studies in CVD prevention have been reported or are under way. The status of some 10 projects initiated between 1972 and 1982 was reviewed by Farquhar, Maccoby, and Wood (1985). The best known of such projects outside of the United States is the Finnish North Karelia Project, which began in 1972 (Puska et al., 1981). The successes in cholesterol reduction, blood pressure control, and smoking cessation after two and three years of education in the Stanford TCS were comparable to those achieved after the first five years of education in the North Karelia Project. The Finnish study was extended for a total of 10 years to allow scrutiny of its impact on CVD morbidity and mortality. The favorable effects of the interventions mounted by the project were reported in comparison not only with the adjoining county but also with respect to trends in the remaining parts of Finland (Tuomilehto et al., 1986).

The results of four other community-based studies that used methods similar to those of the TCS and the North Karelia Project have been published. Only one of them, which took place in three small, rural South African towns, reported significant changes in cholesterol levels and blood pressure control as well as in smoking cessation (Rossouw et al., 1981). Another study, which was undertaken in four Swiss towns (Gutzwiller, Nater, and Martin, 1985), and a three-town study in Australia (Egger et al., 1983) reported significant decreases of 6 and 9 percent, respectively, in smoking rates. In the fourth project, which was carried out at work sites in two Pennsylvania counties, favorable body weight and dietary habit effects were reported (Felix et al., 1985; Stunkard, Felix, and Cohen, 1985).

At this point, the analogous results achieved in replications of the two Stanford programs, along with the comparable results of the North Karelia Project, support the notion that this extensive type of community approach may be reasonably generalizable, at least to cardiovascular disease and quite possibly to the prevention of alcohol-related problems as well. An important caveat is that trials of extensions of these methods to alcohol-related problems should first be carried out in a research format.

Two additional ambitious and well-evaluated studies are now in progress in the United States: the Minnesota Heart Health Study, involving six communities with a total population of 356,000 (Blackburn et al., 1984), and the Pawtucket Heart Health Study, involving two cities in Rhode Island with a total population of 173,000 (Lasater et al., 1984). Results from these two studies will add additional information about the feasibility of carrying out such research and will help identify effective methods that can be used in community recruiting and implementation and in institutionalization of the projects to maintain effects. One exciting finding to date in the Minnesota study is that food labeling, nutrition education, and environmental changes at the "point of purchase" in grocery stores and restaurants have been shown to be effective (Mullis et al., 1987; Glanz and Mullis, 1988; Mullis and Pirie, 1988). This finding is another example of "component development," which may occur prior to the use of a component in a more comprehensive community campaign. The result of this research is that now the three studies (the Stanford FCP and the Pawtucket and Minnesota studies) all use point-of-purchase components in their overall programs.

RESULTS FROM PRIMARY PREVENTION PROGRAMS
IN OTHER HEALTH FIELDS

Although cardiovascular disease prevention has a relatively long and well-documented history, success stories from many other public health fields provide evidence that prevention in matters involving life styles is possible. Lessons from these programs shed new light on how specific health risk behaviors can be prevented and offer guidance on program planning and evaluation. Although there are as yet no examples of comprehensive community-wide programs in fields other than cardiovascular disease, there are many successful illustrations of potential components of broad programs: studies in work sites, examples of the use of regulatory change, the use of the national mass media, or education and environmental change at the point of purchase of tobacco. From the extensive published literature on prevention, several successful programs that have particular relevance to alcohol problem prevention are highlighted below.

Promoting Seat Belt Use

Because injuries are a leading cause of morbidity and mortality in the United States, many public health programs address this problem. Promoting seat belt use as a means of preventing injuries from car crashes is one example of the successful use of statewide legislation and work site-based incentives and education in prevention. Strategies to promote seat belt use can be mandated by legislation or encouraged through public education campaigns. Both of these approaches have been used and evaluated, and a comparison of the results of two studies offers insight into these very different means of achieving a preventive health behavior change. Fortunately, a reduction in automobile fatalities has also been noted as a consequence of increased seat belt use, although enforcement procedures that allow random inspection have also been found to be a necessary step to ensure continued compliance with new seat belt laws (Campbell, 1988; Williams and Lund, 1988). Nevertheless, questions remain on the relative roles of regulations, education, and incentives and on the role of work site programs in achieving change in seat belt use.

Michigan's mandatory seat belt law serves as an example of using legislation for prevention purposes. To study its effects, random samples of drivers were observed in various locations in the state before passage of the law, immediately after implementation, and five months later. Results revealed a dramatic increase in use immediately after the change in the law and a slight decrease five months later. Still, Wagenaar and Wiviott (1986) observed an increase of 117 percent over the prelaw use rates.

Two lessons relevant to the prevention of alcohol-related problems can be extracted from the results of the Michigan study. First, legislation can promote behavior change, at least with respect to seat belt use. Because the results raised some questions about whether the public would maintain the behavior, it appears that legislation combined with periodic campaigns to remind the public to use seat belts may be a more effective strategy than legislation alone. The second lesson applicable to the prevention of alcohol-related problems and to all programs that intend to measure behavior change is the value of an extended data collection effort. Assessing change after five months gave researchers a more accurate picture of how adoption rates fluctuated over time than would have been possible with a more limited period.

In a review of 28 voluntary seat belt use campaigns at work sites, Geller and his colleagues (1987) found that all programs effectively increased use, although at varying rates. Programs were compared on the basis of motivational messages and the use of incentives to encourage seat belt use. Although some programs offered such incentives as meal coupons, cash awards, and prizes, those that emphasized an awareness of, and commitment to, seat belt use but offered no incentives were by far the most effective. The net gain in use from intervention to follow-up several months later varied from 15 to 62 percent in incentive-based programs; it was 152 percent in awareness/commitment programs (Geller et al., 1987).

Geller's conclusions counter previous assumptions about the use of incentives in health behavior change programs. For example, such incentives as free trips and cash prizes have been used successfully in community-wide smoking cessation programs and are an integral part of health promotion strategies based on social marketing (King et al., 1987). Other studies show that incentives increase effectiveness when they are added to campaigns that include components to enhance awareness, knowledge, and behavior change skills (Brownell et al., 1984; Sallis et al., 1986). Because the studies reviewed by Geller were not symmetrical with respect to their educational components, the independent effect of providing incentives is difficult to ascertain.

Cancer Prevention Through Mass Media Advertising

From the long history of education and screening programs to prevent cancer, only the dietary education campaign to promote a low-fat, high-fiber diet will be discussed. The National Cancer Institute (NCI) Cancer Prevention Awareness Program, now in its fourth year, is a nationwide program that seeks to change individuals' knowledge, attitudes, and behavior to prevent cancer. NCI hopes to achieve these goals through the launching of a mass media campaign on cancer prevention, the production and distribution of print materials for the general public, and the education of health professionals about cancer prevention. After the start of these efforts, a campaign intended especially for black Americans was initiated in an effort to reduce the relatively high incidence of cancer in the black population (NCI, 1986).

An evaluation of one component of the NCI program revealed dramatic behavior changes in diet. NCI collaborated with Kellogg Company to publicize a message promoting a low-fat, high-fiber diet in the national media and to promote Kellogg's new bran cereal. A two-year cereal advertising campaign that publicized NCI's diet message and telephone number in television ads and on the back of cereal boxes produced more than 20,000 telephone calls and 30,000 written inquiries to NCI. Furthermore, a study of cereal sales in the greater Washington, D.C., area revealed that sales of all high-fiber cereals, not merely Kellogg's brand, increased (Freimuth, Hammond, and Stein, 1988).

This publicity campaign demonstrates the powerful role that private industry can play in health promotion: NCI was able to reach an audience of millions as a result of the cooperation and extensive financial backing of Kellogg's cereal company. This lesson has important ramifications for the alcohol problem prevention field, because there are many potential allies in the food and nonalcoholic beverage industries that could promote their products as healthful alternatives to alcoholic beverages. However, cooperation between health promotion agencies and the private sector must be carefully considered because the alcoholic beverage industry is not likely to assist in any attempt to reduce sales. Some large companies have integrated the production, distribution, and sales of food, nonalcoholic beverages, and alcoholic beverages. As a result, alcohol abuse prevention efforts will not serve the corporate objectives of such organizations.

A second lesson that can be derived from the NCI program is that consumers were able to generalize the health message promoted by Kellogg's to the purchase of all types of high-fiber cereals. For the alcohol field, this finding may mean that the promotion of one particular nonalcoholic beverage may translate into an increase in consumption of many types of nonalcoholic beverages. Further research on consumer behavior is necessary before any conclusions can be drawn.

Smoking Prevention and Cessation

Smoking prevention and cessation programs are components of prevention programs in several fields of public health because smoking is a risk factor both for cardiovascular disease and for certain types of cancers. The terms prevention and cessation refer to different techniques and different target audiences. Smoking prevention programs are designed to prevent the onset of smoking among adolescents; smoking cessation programs are designed to help smokers quit. From the large body of research on both of these topics, only a few examples have been selected for review here.

Although evidence is still needed to establish long-term effectiveness, smoking prevention programs in schools have been successful in delaying the onset of smoking among early teens. Among such programs, the most effective method appears to be what Killen has called the social pressure resistance training approach (Flay, 1985; Killen, 1985; Best et al., 1988). The resistance training approach alerts young people to the various pressures that may encourage them to smoke and teaches specific skills to use in resisting those pressures. Generally, these programs are evaluated through follow-up surveys conducted several months after the intervention and through the use of carbon monoxide tests to detect recent smoking. Results show that the rate of smoking is significantly lower in treatment populations than in control groups (McAlister, Perry, and Macoby, 1979; Botvin, 1982; Telch et al., 1982; Luepker et al., 1983; Flay, 1985; Killen, 1985; Hansen et al., 1988; Telch, Miller, and Killen, in press).

Best and colleagues (1988) draw the following conclusions and make recommendations for future research based on the adolescent smoking/peer resistance training experience: (1) social influence peer resistance curricula are effective, but more needs to be learned about individual participant, provider, and setting factors that mediate effectiveness; (2) research must continue with renewed vigor and a focus on lessons learned from the previous decade's work (in the area of program development, for example, it is suggested that research focus on those individuals who seem able to "resist" the current smoking prevention curricula); and (3) research must focus not only on program development issues but also on how to achieve widespread diffusion. There are five factors to address in diffusion research: (1) how best to plan diffusion, (2) program packaging, (3) provider training, (4) implementation monitoring and corrective feedback, and (5) determination of costs, efficacy, and cost-effectiveness.

Finally, it is unclear how generalizable the findings from adolescent smoking prevention are to the area of alcohol abuse and especially to the domain of alcohol-related problem behaviors. Some of the targets for behavior change with respect to alcohol (e.g., violence, drunk driving, vandalism) are very different from the targets for adolescent smoking. Research must focus on the commonalities and differences in conceptual models and the clustering (or lack thereof) of problem behaviors and substances of abuse.

Another research question is whether drug abuse programs should focus on single or multiple drugs and which type of program is the more cost-effective. It is of interest that self-reported decreases in both marijuana and alcohol were reported in two separate studies on adolescent smoking prevention by the Stanford group, even though intervention was directed solely toward tobacco (McAlister Perry, and Macoby, 1979; Telch et al., 1982; Telch, Miller, and Killen, in press). Furthermore, a school project in Los Angeles, Project SMART, which used analogous peer resistance training on substance abuse, has also shown reductions in tobacco, marijuana, and alcohol use (Hansen et al., 1988).

A recent study by Altman and coworkers (Altman et al., 1989) has shown that a very low-cost mobilization of political action, volunteer community worker efforts, and the mass media succeeded in reducing retail outlets' illegal sales of cigarettes to minors. As in the seat belt example, the Altman results suggest that community-wide environmental change strategies could interact with education to increase overall effectiveness.

An even larger volume of research has been conducted on smoking cessation, mostly in adults, and essentially all since the 1964 Surgeon General's Report on Smoking and Health. There is a surprising consensus on the use of group or classroom methods as successful approaches to smoking cessation (Glasgow, 1986), but less has been done in large-scale community efforts beyond those included as components of the Stanford studies and other CVD community prevention programs.

In Flay's (1987) review of 40 smoking cessation programs designed for adults, he finds that mass media-only or media with print material campaigns were somewhat successful in changing knowledge and attitudes about smoking but that mass media combined with support groups produced significant changes in behavior and actually affected the quit rate of participants (Flay, 1987). This conclusion lends credence to the argument that combined prevention strategies reinforce each other and suggests that a combination strategy should be adapted to other fields of health promotion, including alcohol problem prevention.

Research on smoking cessation programs also demonstrates that program costs can be reduced by using methods other than the six class sessions that are usually offered (Altman et al., 1987). A cost-effectiveness study of a community-wide smoking cessation program in the Stanford Five-City Project found that, although instructor-led classes produced the highest quit rate, this prevention strategy was three times as expensive as an intervention using a manual (a six-step approach to quitting) and about twice as expensive as a strategy using minimal personal contact (a smoking cessation contest).

Preventing Adolescent Pregnancy Through School-Based Clinics

Among the adolescent population in the United States, the problem of unplanned pregnancy has nearly reached epidemic proportions. Because teenage pregnancies result in long-term medical, economic, and social consequences for the teenage parents and their children, prevention programs have sought to bring about lower rates of unplanned pregnancies in this age group. Few of these prevention programs have been evaluated to determine whether teenagers who participate in prevention programs have a lower incidence of unplanned pregnancy. The most systematic of the available evaluations showed little change in knowledge and no change at all in attitudes or behaviors resulting from one such program (Scales and Kirby, 1981).

Some success has been reported in reducing teenage pregnancy through the use of school-based clinics (Zabin et al., 1986). Zabin and colleagues argue, however, that it may be impossible to assess the full impact of school-based clinics on teenage pregnancy owing to the difficulty of following students over a period of several years after graduation, dropping out, or moving. They overcame this problem with a methodology that has potential application to alcohol problem prevention: another variable--the amount of time between first intercourse and first contraceptive use (i.e., the first clinic visit)--was used as a valid and feasible substitute for the real variable of interest, the incidence of pregnancy (Zabin et al., 1986). This proxy variable was derived from the findings of an earlier study, which revealed that half of all initial teenage pregnancies occurred within the first six months of intercourse (Zabin, Kantner, and Zelnik, 1979). Dr. Zabin and her colleagues are currently measuring this and other variables as part of their evaluation of two school-based clinics in Baltimore. In lieu of data on the incidence of pregnancy among teenagers, these researchers track the proxy variable; then, if the time between first intercourse and the first clinic visit decreases, they can conclude that the risk of an unplanned pregnancy has been effectively reduced.

Developing valid measures based on epidemiological data is especially useful for programs that address early indicators of problem behaviors that have delayed consequences, as in the case of pregnancy. A similar method could be developed to measure the delayed consequences of drinking behavior. This development would promote epidemiological research into the antecedents of alcohol-related problems and would allow for the development of more innovative and revealing evaluations.

SUMMARY OF LESSONS LEARNED FROM OTHER FIELDS

From this examination of comprehensive, integrated, community-based programs in preventing cardiovascular disease and of certain more limited studies (potential components of comprehensive programs), eight lessons may be derived:

1. As previously stated, theories of change are an important part of any successful intervention. Theory should guide not only the development of the intervention and its evaluation but also the interpretation of the intervention's effects. Studies vary in their use of theory. In general, programs oriented toward changing the behavior of individuals by direct education are more theory driven than environmental change efforts or efforts to change organizations. This difference may reflect what has been only a recent initiation of scientific investigations on environmental change programs as solutions to health problems.

2. Establishing multiple outcome objectives and matching those outcome objectives to the level of intervention is important to increase our understanding of change. For example, few work site programs measure organizational change along with individual change. Yet most investigators agree that organizational characteristics determine much of the success of such interventions. In addition, comprehensive programs should create a hierarchical, ordered set of outcome objectives. For individuals, these objectives should include awareness, knowledge, and behavior change. For organizations, programs should seek evidence of commitment, adoption, policy change, regulatory change, environmental change, implementation, and maintenance of policies and programs.

3. Extensive formative, process, and outcome evaluations are needed for the development of the program, for monitoring the implementation process, and for determining program effects over time.

4. Programs should attend to the special needs of the target population. Teen clinics illustrate the successful effects of making information and health resources accessible to young adolescents, of providing support for change at the place at which change is needed (i.e., norm changes within the school and community), and of actively providing resources to a particular target audience during a phase in personal development when only certain types of outreach may succeed.

5. There is a potentially beneficial synergistic effect that may be achieved by combining approaches across different levels of intervention. In the case of seat belt use, combining legislation with education serves to inform the public of the benefits of use and the hazards of nonuse and to keep the issue on the public agenda.

6. Primary prevention strategies are particularly important for adolescents. Prevention strategies that include delaying the onset of a particular behavior, minimizing the use of harmful substances, or preventing entirely the initiation of a behavior are important components to any population-wide strategy for prevention. Attention to high-risk subsets of adolescents is particularly important in selecting prevention strategies.

7. The generalization of principles from previous efforts should be a carefully planned endeavor involving formative evaluation, pilot testing, behavioral analysis, and the critical review of research. Table 5-1 presents a matrix of studies conducted in various health fields that cover such components as work sites, schools, and regulatory change. Decisions on studies that may be analogous to alcohol-related problem prevention and on needed replications should stem from surveys of existing data to reveal any important gaps. Table 5-1 lists by author and year studies that are described in this chapter. A further breakdown of each study into the relative importance of different intervention strategies can also be done to identify additional research necessary. Moreover, a judgment as to the strength, validity, and cost-effectiveness of intervention strategies is needed to create a prospective master plan for research in the prevention of alcohol-related problems. Table 5-1 is therefore presented only as an example of an early step in displaying what has been accomplished to date.

8. Objective data should be collected to assess the specific impact of interventions on targeted behaviors. Issues of validity must be considered.

IMPLICATIONS FOR ALCOHOL PROBLEM PREVENTION

Each of the lessons derived from these varied prevention programs has challenging implications for the prevention of alcohol-related problems. The first, and perhaps most important, is that community-level prevention is possible. Beyond that, applying each lesson to alcohol problem prevention raises additional challenging questions:

• What theories have been used in alcohol problem prevention planning, and how thoroughly have they been tested?
• Is it possible to integrate a variety of seemingly unrelated prevention strategies into a single effective program to prevent alcohol-related problems?
• How can such social marketing techniques as audience needs analysis be used in prevention efforts?
• What role do these lessons play in designing alcohol-related policy changes?

The techniques from a program designed to prevent one public health problem will never fit exactly the needs and goals of another prevention effort. Nonetheless, it would be

Table 5-1. Matrix of Successful Primary Prevention Interventions in Six Health Areas

Health Area	School-based Education	Worksite Education	County or State Regulatory Change	National Mass Media	Comprehensive, Integrated Community Studies
Cardiovascular disease	Killen et al. (1988)	Brownell et al. (1984 Felix et al. (1985) Sallis et al. (1986)			Farquhar et al. (1977, 1985) Roussow et al. (1981) Egger et al. (1983) Gutzwiller, Nater, and Martin (1985) Puska et al. (1981)
Injuries		Geller et al. (1987)	Wagenaar and Wiviott (1986)		
Smoking	McAlister, Perry, and Maccoby (1979) Botvin (1982) Luepker et al. (1983) Killen (1985) Best et al. (1988) Hansen et al. (1988)		Flay (1987) Altman et al. (1989)		King et al. (1987)
Cancer				Freimuth, Hammond, and Stein (1988)	
Teenage pregnancy	Zabin et al. (1986)				
Adolescent alcohol and drug use	McAlister, Perry, and Maccoby (1979) Telch (1982) Hansen (1988) Telch, Miller, and Killen (in press)				Pentz et al. (in press)

imprudent to disregard the years of experience in CVD prevention and the lessons to be learned from the failures and successes of other community-level primary prevention programs. This discussion of the possible applications of these lessons to the prevention of alcohol-related problems will begin with the use of theory as a basis for program planning.

Behavior change theory has important implications for the prevention of alcohol-related problems at the level of the individual. For example, it can be used as a model to test the teaching of resistance skills to youth and the promotion of moderate, low-risk drinking among adults. If, as suggested by the theory, either abstinence or awareness of the problem is the first step in the change process, there is much more work to be done in educating the public about the scope and severity of alcohol problems before contemplating any move to the next step of changing attitudes and behavior.

Social marketing theory also offers practical guidance to alcohol problem prevention. Applying its principles requires an investigation into the orientation of "consumers" of prevention efforts rather than merely focusing on the prevention strategy. To use this theory for preventing alcohol problems, one must begin by asking: How do such preventive behaviors as moderate drinking or such prevention "products" as special zoning ordinances for alcohol outlets meet the needs of the consumer? How does the repeal of prohibition laws affect the public's perception of prevention programs, and how can this perception be used to design effective education programs?

Studies of the effects of legislation to promote positive health behaviors are especially relevant to the prevention of alcohol problems because many of these prevention strategies (e.g., legislating server responsibility, zoning ordinances) are based on policy change. Results from studies of mandatory seat belt use suggest that legislation can have some effect on health behaviors, but more study is needed before conclusions can be drawn about the effects of the policy changes that have been proposed for alcohol problem prevention. Nonetheless, the expectation is that the marginal impact of a single intervention will be compounded when used in concert with other interventions.

Finally, prevention programs directed toward adolescents offer some interesting directions to programs that seek to reduce alcohol problems among youth. The use of resistance skills training in program design and employing epidemiological data to identify periods of intensified risk for adolescents (see Chapter 3) are two possible routes.

In considering the evidence for success that has been obtained in areas other than alcohol-related problems, certain generalizations emerge about community-level approaches to prevention. It appears that life-style issues of cigarette smoking, diet, and physical activity can be influenced in both young and old through complementary change strategies directed at individuals, groups, organizations, and communities. The health habits that have been altered are all influenced by social norms, peers, and environmental and regulatory factors. Alcohol use shares many of the same predictors and precursors as the health habits that have been successfully changed by prevention programs in other health fields. Given the growing evidence of success in these other areas, it seems clear that the prevention of some alcohol-related problems can be achieved through the use of analogous methods.

REFERENCES

Altman, D., J. Flora, S. Fortmann et al. The cost-effectiveness of three smoking cessation programs. Am. J. Public Health 77(2):162-165, 1987.

Altman, D., V. Foster, L. Rosenick-Douss et al. Reducing illegal sales of cigarettes to minors. J. Am. Med. Assoc. 261:80, 1989.

Best, J. A. , S. J. Thomson, S. M. Santi et al. Cigarette smoking among school children. Ann. Rev. Public Health 9:161-201, 1988.

Blackburn, H., R. Luepker, F. Kline et al. The Minnesota Heart Health Program: A research and demonstration project in cardiovascular disease prevention. Pp. 1171-1178 in J. D. Matarazzo, N. E. Miller, S. M. Weiss et al., eds. Behavioral Health: A Handbook of Health Enhancement and Disease Prevention. New York: John Wiley and Sons, 1984.

Botvin, G. Broadening the focus of smoking prevention strategies. Pp. 137-148 in T. J. Coates, A. R. Peterson, and C. Perry, eds. Promoting Adolescent Health: A Dialogue on Research and Practice. New York: Academic Press, 1982.

Brownell, K. D., R. Y. Cohen, A. J. Stunkard et al. Weight loss competitions at the work site: Impact on weight, morale, and cost-effectiveness. Am. J. Public Health 74:1283-1285, 1984.

Campbell, B. J. Casualty reduction and belt use associated with occupant restraint. In J. Graham, ed. Preventing Automobile Injuries. Dover, MA: Auburn Publishing, 1988.

Egger, G., W. Fitzgerald, G. Frape et al. Results of a large scale media antismoking campaign: North Coast "Quit For Life" Programme. Br. Med. J. 296:1125, 1983.

Farquhar, J. The community-based model of lifestyle intervention trials. Am. J. Epidemiology 108:103-111, 1978.

Farquhar, J., N. Maccoby, and P. Wood. Education and communication strategies. Pp. 207-221 in W. Holland, R. Detels, and G. Knox, eds. Oxford Textbook of Public Health, vol. 3. London: Oxford University Press, 1985.

Farquhar, J., N. Maccoby, P. Wood et al. Community education for cardiovascular health. Lancet 1:1192-1195, 1977.

Farquhar, J., J. Flora, L. Good et al. Integrated comprehensive health promotion programs. Unpublished monograph prepared for the Kaiser Family Foundation, Menlo Park, CA, March 13, 1985.

Farquhar, J., S. Fortmann, J. Flora et al. The Stanford Five-City Project: Results after 5 1/3 years of education. Abstract presented at the 28th Annual Conference on Cardiovascular Disease Epidemiology, Santa Fe, New Mexico, March 17-19, 1988.

Felix, M. R. J., A. J. Stunkard, R. Y. Cohen et al. Health promotion at the worksite. 1. A process for establishing programs. Prev. Med. 14:99-108, 1985.

Flay, B. R. What we know about the social influences approach to smoking prevention: Review and recommendations. In Prevention Research: Deterring Drug Abuse Among Children and Adolescents. Research Monograph Series No. 63. USDHHS Publ. No. (ADM)85-1334. Washington, DC: National Institute on Drug Abuse, 1985.

Flay, B. Mass media and smoking cessation: A critical review. Am. J. Public Health 77(2):153-160, 1987.

Freimuth, V., S. Hammond, and J. Stein. Health advertising: Prevention for profit. Am. J. Public Health 78(5):557-561, 1988.

Geisbrecht, N., R. Douglas, and D. McKenzie. A proposal to test the flexibility of the distribution and consumption of alcohol via a secondary prevention program. Paper presented at the 27th International Institute on Prevention and Treatment of Alcoholism, Vienna, Austria. Toronto: Addiction Research Foundation, 1981.

Geller, S., J. Rudd, M. Kalsher et al. Employer-based programs to motivate safety belt use: A review of short term and long term effects. J. Safety Res. 18:1-7, 1987.

Glanz, K., and R. M. Mullis. Environmental interventions to promote healthy eating: A review of models, programs, and evidence. Health Educ. Q. 15(4):1-21, 1988.

Glasgow, R. E. Smoking. Pp. 91-126 in K. Holroyd and T. Creer, eds. Self-Management of Chronic Disease: Handbook of Clinical Interventions and Research. New York: Academic Press, 1986.

Green, L., and A. McAlister. Macro-intervention to support health behavior: Some theoretical perspectives and practical reflections. Health Educ. Q. 11(3):322-339, 1984.

Gutzwiller, F., B. Nater, and J. Martin. Community-based primary prevention of cardiovascular disease in Switzerland: Methods and results of the National Research Program (NRP 1A). Prev. Med. 14:482-491, 1985.

Hansen, W. B. C. A. Johnson, B. R. Flay et al. Affective and social influences approaches to the prevention of multiple substance abuse among seventh grade students: Results from Project SMART. Prev. Med. 17:135-154, 1988.

Killen, J. Prevention of adolescent tobacco smoking: The social pressure resistance training approach. J. Child Psychol. Psych. 26:7-15, 1985.

Killen, J. D., M. J. Telch, T. Robinson et al. Cardiovascular disease risk reduction for tenth graders: A multiple-factor school-based approach. J. Am. Med. Assoc. 260(12):1728-1733, 1988.

King, A. C., J. A. Flora, S. P. Fortmann et al. Smokers' challenge: Immediate and long-term findings of a community smoking cessation contest. Am. J. Public Health 77:1340-1341, 1987.

Klitzner, M., P. J. Gruenewald, E. Bamberger et al. Students Against Driving Drunk: A national study--final report. Vienna, VA: Center for Advanced Health Studies, Pacific Institute for Research and Evaluation, 1987.

Kotler, P., and G. Zaltman. Social marketing: An approach to planned social change. Journal of Marketing 35:3-12, 1971.

Kraft, D. A comprehensive program for college students. Pp. 327-370 in P. Miller and T. Nirenberg, eds. Prevention of Alcohol Abuse. New York: Plenum Press, 1984.

Lasater, T., D. Abrams, L. Artz et al. Lay volunteer delivery of a community-based cardiovascular risk factor change program: The Pawtucket Experiment. Pp. 1166-1170 in J. D. Matarazzo, N. E. Miller, S. M. Weiss et al., eds. Behavioral Health: A Handbook of Health Enhancement and Disease Prevention. New York: John Wiley and Sons, 1984.

Luepker, R., C. Johnson, D. Murray et al. Prevention of cigarette smoking: Three year follow-up of an education program for youth. J. Behav. Med. 6:53-62, 1983.

Maccoby, N., J. Farquhar, P. Wood et al. Reducing the risk of cardiovascular disease: Effects of a community-based campaign on knowledge and behavior. J. Community Health 23:100-114, 1977.

McAlister, A., C. Perry, and N. Maccoby. Adolescent smoking: Onset and prevention. Pediatrics 63:650-658, 1979.

Mecca, A., ed. Comprehensive drug abuse and alcohol prevention strategies. California Health Research Foundation, San Rafael, 1984.

Mills, K., D. McCarty, J. Ward et al. A residence hall tavern as a collegiate alcohol abuse prevention activity. Addict. Behav. 8:105-108, 1983.

Moskowitz, J. M. Evaluating the effects of parent groups on the correlates of adolescent substance abuse. J. Psychoactive Drugs 17(3):173-178, 1985.

Mullis, R. M., and P. Pirie. Lean meats make the grade: A collaborative nutrition intervention program. J. Am. Dietetic Assoc. 88:191-195, 1988.

Mullis, R. M., M. K. Hunt, M. Foster et al. The "Shop Smart for Your Heart" grocery program. J. Nutr. Educ. 19:225-228, 1987.

National Cancer Institute. Technical Report: Cancer Awareness Survey, Wave II. Bethesda, MD: Office of Cancer Communications, 1986.

Pentz, M. A., J. H. Dwyer, D. P. MacKinnon et al. A multi-community trial for primary prevention of adolescent drug abuse: Effects on drug use prevalence. J. Am. Med. Assoc. 261(22):3259-3266, 1989.

Puska, P., J. Tuomilehto, J. Salonen et al. The North Karelia Project: Evaluation of a comprehensive community programme for control of cardiovascular diseases in 1972-77 in North Karelia, Finland. In Public Health in Europe. WHO/EURO Monograph Series. Copenhagen: World Health Organization, 1981.

Room, R. Alcohol control and public health. Pp. 293-317 in L. Breskow, J. E. Fielding, and L. B. Lave, eds. Annual Review of Public Health, vol. 5. Palo Alto, CA: Annual Reviews, Inc., 1984.

Rossouw, J. E., P. L. Jooste, J. P. Kotze et al. The control of hypertension in two communities: An interim evaluation. S. Afr. Med. J. 60:208, 1981.

Sallis, J. F., R. D. Hill, S. P. Fortmann et al. Health behavior change at the worksite: Cardiovascular risk reduction. Prog. Behav. Modification 20:161-197, 1986.

Scales, P., and D. Kirby. A review of exemplary sex education programs for teenagers offered by nonschool organizations. Family Relations 30:238-245, 1981.

Stunkard, A. J., M. R. J. Felix, and R. Y. Cohen. Mobilizing a community to promote health: The Pennsylvania County Health Improvement Program (CHIP). In J. C. Rosen and L. J. Solomon, eds. Prevention in Health Psychology. Hanover, NH: Hanover University Press of New England, 1985.

Telch, M., I. Miller, and J. Killen. Social pressures resistance training for smoking prevention: The effects of a videotape delivery with and without same age peer leader participation. Addictive Behav., in press.

Telch, M. J., J. D. Killen, A. L. McAlister et al. Long-term follow-up of a pilot project on smoking prevention with adolescents. J. Behav. Med. 5:1-8, 1982.

Tuomilehto, J., J. Geboers, J. T. Salonen et al. Decline in cardiovascular mortality in North Karelia and other parts of Finland. Br. Med. J. 293:1068-1071, 1986.

Ungerleider, S., S. A. Bloch, R. F. Connor et al. The Drunk Driving Prevention Project. Eugene, OR: Integrated Research Services, 1986.

Wagenaar, A., and M. Wiviott. Effects of mandating seatbelt use: A series of surveys on compliance in Michigan. Public Health Reports 101(5):505-513, 1986.

Wallack, L. A community approach to the prevention of alcohol related problems: The San Francisco experience. International Quarterly of Community Health Education 5:82-102, 1984-1985.

Williams, A., and A. Lund. Mandatory seat belt laws and occupant crash protection in the United States. In J. Graham, ed. Preventing Automobile Injuries. Dover, MA: Auburn Publishing, 1988.

Zabin, L., J. Kantner, and M. Zelnik. The risk of adolescent pregnancy in the first months of intercourse. Family Planning Perspectives 11(4):215-222, 1979.

Zabin, L., M. Hirsch, E. Smith et al. Adolescent pregnancy prevention program: A model for research and evaluation. J. Adolescent Health Care 7(2):77-88, 1986.

6

METHODOLOGICAL ISSUES IN ALCOHOL PREVENTION RESEARCH: CONCLUSIONS AND RECOMMENDATIONS

No single set of research designs or analytical strategies has characterized research on the prevention of alcohol problems. A variety of approaches can be used depending on the goals of the research, the setting or opportunity afforded, the amount and type of variation one wishes to control or explain, and the generalizability of the findings. One of the difficulties in prevention research--particularly the kind of research that is most relevant to public policy deliberations--is the need to conduct such research outside the laboratory setting. "Real-world" research, however, is difficult to undertake, often expensive to conduct, and difficult to analyze. It is less precise than laboratory work because researchers do not have the opportunity to manipulate variables as they would in laboratory experimentation. It also raises questions of ascertainment and of the validity of self-reports and other measures that are commonly used to assess the efficacy of a preventive intervention. On the other hand, because of the controlled or "hothouse" conditions used in laboratory settings, the extent to which prevention research undertaken in the laboratory can be generalized to the real world is not known.

In recent years, alcohol prevention research has made use of a variety of qualitative and quantitative methods. For example, ethnographic methods and the observation of behavior in natural settings have been employed. Ethnographers gather data through semistructured interviews and through traditional participant-observer techniques. Examples of ethnographic/observational studies in prevention include studies of blue-collar workers and family drinking (Ames and Janes, 1987), of public drinking and drinking contexts (Rosenbluth, Nathan, and Lawson, 1978; Storm and Cutler, 1981; Harford et al., 1983; Single and Storm, 1985; Geller, Russ, and Altomari, 1986), and of the work site (Ames, 1987).

In many respects, the social and health problems that are associated with alcohol need to be viewed in a historical context. Historical analysis, by using both U.S. and international data sources, offers promising opportunities for prevention research. For example, it has been reported that between 1830 and 1850 there was a dramatic decline in per capita consumption in the United States (Rorabaugh, 1976) and that the temperance movement and government policies contributed to this decline and to a concomitant decrease in alcohol problems (Popham, 1978; Moore and Gerstein, 1981; Pendergast, 1987). Historical analysis could provide a method to discover potential "lessons" that might be useful in the modern alcohol problem prevention arena.

Community, school, and work site prevention trials have begun to reflect the use of combinations of several relevant theories (learning, organization, communication, behavior change, health education, and social marketing) in their design. Interest in such designs has been stimulated by the success in health promotion programs to reduce heart disease that are discussed in Chapter 5 (Farquhar et al., 1984; Puska et al., 1985). These approaches have been used in studies of community interventions for alcohol problems at schools (see the review by Moskowitz, 1989), local availability of alcohol (Wittman and Hilton, 1987), and the influence of the mass media (Hewitt and Blane, 1984). Because of the difficulty of random assignment in field studies, quasi-experimental designs have been used (Cook and Campbell, 1979). These designs are often employed in the policy analysis of "natural" experiments, such as changes in alcohol availability. One useful statistical tool is the interrupted time-series analysis (Box and Tiao, 1975; Box and Jenkins, 1976), which has more power than conventional least-squares regression to deal with problems of autoregression, seasonality, and trending (Skog, 1986; Wagenaar, 1986; Blose and Holder, 1987; Holder and Blose, 1987a).

Quasi-experimental designs are also used to address problems related to nonequivalent control conditions or groups (Cook and Campbell, 1979). These designs frequently employ multivariate analysis techniques to increase statistical power. Examples include evaluations of server intervention (Saltz, 1987), happy-hour bans (Smart and Adlaf, 1986), college prevention programs (Mills et al., 1983), cross-cultural drinking behavior (Moskowitz, 1989), alcohol taxes (Cook and Tauchen, 1982), and changes in driving-under-the-influence sanctions and enforcement in Maine (Hingson et al., 1987).

The multifaceted and dynamic nature of the social, cultural, and economic systems in which prevention occurs requires techniques that can deal with such complexity. One approach that has been used is computer modeling. This tool is used in astronomy, physics, and business and economic research and has particular utility for prevention research because it provides the ability to predict potential outcomes prior to expensive field implementation (Katzper, Ryback, and Hertzman, 1976; Holder and Blose, 1987b). For example, complex statistical modeling has been used to examine the sensitivity of drinking and alcohol problems to changes in price levels. Examples include studies by Grossman, Coate, and Arluck (1987) and by Levy and Sheflin (1983).

RESEARCH DESIGN FOR FUTURE ALCOHOL PREVENTION RESEARCH PROGRAMS

There are several primary issues relevant to the design of prevention research in the alcohol field. Three of these issues are discussed below: (1) the importance of using theory as a basis for design, (2) the need for both laboratory and field research, and (3) the practical as well as the statistical significance of research findings.

The Importance of Theory

A truly comprehensive theory for prevention research must encompass complex and dynamically changing biobehavioral mechanisms, individual and group behaviors, organizational influences, and cultural patterns. It is particularly important to incorporate the dimension of time into theoretical models in order to take account of life-span or developmental milestones. Theory is required to establish priorities, to develop and test hypotheses about mediating mechanisms, and to develop or select appropriate interventions, program evaluation, and intermediate and longer term outcome measures. When used for these purposes, theory can help prevention researchers identify the active ingredients in prevention programs and anticipate and account for intervention effects. Theory-driven programmatic research could then be undertaken by using combinations of methodologies including laboratory-based randomized trials, analogue studies, ethnographic and other naturalistic data collection methods, and complex model building. Such research can be undertaken within and between different levels of the social structure ranging from the individual to the community.

In other public health efforts that have utilized community, school, or work site as the base in prevention trials, combinations of several relevant theories (learning, organizational, communication, behavior change, health education, media, social marketing) have been used to guide intervention and evaluation (Flay, 1984; Farquhar et al., 1985; Abrams et al., 1986). This diversity in approach is illustrated by the Stanford, Minnesota, and Pawtucket heart disease prevention trials discussed in the preceding chapter (Maccoby et al., 1977; Blackburn et al., 1984; Lasater et al., 1984; Farquhar et al., 1985). Crucial to developing effective and adequate strategies of prevention intervention is the use of formative research, program evaluation, process tracking, and assessment of program impact and potential problems.

A variety of research approaches can be used in which the design of programs results from an interactive process, combining theoretical and scientific input with practical input from the community and individual consumers. These approaches include ethnographic methods derived from anthropology, unobtrusive or naturalistic observation, the use of focus groups, random-digit rapid telephone surveys, and the use of small-scale randomized designs in the field or laboratory. Such evaluation methods are crucial for developing effective interventions, for making early or midcourse corrections in a program, and for evaluating whether, in fact, the manipulation of independent variables did occur at a sufficiently strong level (dosage) and with the intended impact on the target variables, mediating mechanisms, or processes.

In community prevention programs, interactive and synergistic effects sometimes occur or are intentionally encouraged, making it necessary to consider the question of contamination and to measure impact in areas other than the direct intervention targets. For example, do single-focus, school-based smoking prevention programs actually reduce (or increase) alcohol and other drug use? Are multifocus programs more or less effective? Unlike traditional research in which one variable is manipulated whereas all other factors are controlled, the use of multiple criteria (including factors such as cost-effectiveness) may be more appropriate in program evaluation or prevention research (e.g., Warner and Luce, 1982; Altman et al., 1987). In some cases, the spillover effects that result from such multifocused, synergistic processes as changing social norms and social network interactions in a school, work site, or other system are regarded as beneficial. They are viewed as an intentional part of the intervention and evaluation process rather than "contamination." However, it is crucial to decide what is acceptable synergism and what is contamination, especially with respect to the unit of analysis, the questions being asked, and the comparison groups and settings being used.

Need for Both Laboratory and Field Prevention Research

The term laboratory research is used here to mean research conducted under conditions that permit the direct manipulation of the variables under investigation. Studies conducted within a controlled environment to allow the manipulation of variables have the advantage of providing better opportunities to assign subjects randomly to treatment and no-treatment conditions. Laboratory studies permit the examination of particular variables and the determination of whether specific experimental factors may play a role in a prevention program or policy. For example, the potential role of retail price in alcohol use can be demonstrated in a laboratory experiment that simulates an actual retail drinking situation in which the subjects' drinking is measured as the price of alcohol is manipulated. Such analogue studies can demonstrate (or fail to demonstrate) that retail price (or the economic accessibility of alcohol) affects drinking behavior. Such studies cannot tell, however, whether price is actually a significant variable in the natural setting, given the number of other factors at work.

Prevention research also requires studies that are conducted in the field or in naturalistic environments in which physical manipulation of the situation may be difficult or impossible. Such studies can be more generalizable, but they lack the convenience or appropriateness of random assignment for controlling variance in extraneous factors; however, multivariate statistical tools are available as the means for control. Both laboratory and field studies are needed in prevention research because they have complementary strengths. In particular, the validity of conclusions is strengthened when consistency is demonstrated between the two approaches.

In recent years, empirically minded social scientists have become increasingly concerned with the problem of inferring individual-level behavior from aggregate data (Lanbein and Lichtman, 1978). (The term ecological fallacy has been used to describe an incorrect inference about individual behavior based on group data.) By far the most obvious intervening variable in need of disaggregation is the consumption history of the drinker. Many authors who have written about the policy implications of economic variables have lamented the fact that current models have been unable to differentiate among alcohol-dependent persons, heavy drinkers, and moderate consumers.

Although there has never been a systematic program of experimental research designed to investigate the interaction between environmental variables and alcohol consumption, a number of studies have been conducted to investigate the important policy questions raised by economic and epidemiological studies. For example, several studies have investigated the relative impact of economic variables on the behavior of alcohol abusers (Mello, 1968; Cohen et al., 1971; Bigelow and Liebson, 1972; Engle and Williams, 1972; Marlatt, Demming, and Reid, 1973). The findings in these studies suggest that the strengths of both experimental and quasi-experimental research designs can be combined in complementary studies that move from laboratory analogues to more complicated natural settings.

One question of interest in prevention research concerns whether persons with alcohol problems differ from persons without alcohol problems in their responsiveness to economic incentives for drinking or abstinence. Babor and colleagues (1978) demonstrated that heavy drinkers were as responsive as casual drinkers to the afternoon price manipulation known as the happy hour. Indeed, one of the most encouraging findings of the happy-hour studies was the extent to which the discount drink policy was associated with similar alterations in drinking behavior in both laboratory and natural settings (Babor et al., 1980).

Laboratory analogue research was also combined with naturalistic observation in the studies of Langenbucher and Nathan (1983). Three experiments were used to test the ability of social drinkers, bartenders, and police officers to estimate sobriety. This study has important implications for public policy regarding alcohol sale or use and the legal penalties for purveyors who knowingly or unknowingly serve alcohol to intoxicated persons.

Naturalistic studies have the advantage of being heuristic, realistic, and relevant to important social problems when they include three important dimensions: natural behavior (e.g., drinking), natural settings (e.g., a tavern or bar), and natural treatment (e.g., price variations).

In addition to the concern that no false conclusions be drawn from data, the prevention researcher must also consider the practical significance of any finding. A statistical change may be too small to justify the operational costs of a prevention strategy. Alternatively, the level of statistical significance may be set so high by the researcher, or the variable selected for measurement may occur so infrequently, that a finding of practical significance is overlooked. In selecting a research design, the variables to be studied, and the statistical approach, researchers should be aware that prevention research must accommodate both substantive and statistical significance.

DIRECTION AND DESIGN OF FUTURE ALCOHOL PREVENTION RESEARCH PROGRAMS: CONCLUSIONS AND RECOMMENDATIONS

The conclusions discussed below constitute the committee's recommendations for future directions in research designed to reduce alcohol-related problems.

- Attempts should be made to integrate findings from biomedical research (e.g., biobehavioral vulnerability) with theories on individual, social, educational, and economic variables that influence alcohol use and abuse. Integrated models can then be used to guide the development of prevention interventions and the matching of at-risk subgroups with appropriate intervention strategies.
- It is important to ensure that theory drives the research, which can be achieved by borrowing theory-based analogues from studies in other health fields. Although such theories as social learning approaches have helped in understanding behavior change in individuals, there is little assurance that an adequate theoretical framework is available for the fields of community organization, regulatory and policy-based interventions, environmental change strategies, and interventions that depend on changing the organizations themselves.
- Life-span considerations and developmental factors over time should be incorporated into comprehensive theories. If it can be anticipated that a specific interaction between individual characteristics (e.g., social skills deficits) and environmental/cultural demands (e.g., peer pressure to conform during early puberty) is likely to produce a large at-risk group, then such predictions can be used to plan both individual and community prevention programs. In this manner, findings from biological, psychological, and cultural areas can be used to plan prevention strategies for use during an earlier developmental phase so as to "inoculate" a vulnerable population prior to exposure. Research should also be undertaken to shed light on the determinants of social norms regarding alcohol use. Such research should include creative methods to determine the effects of corporate policies, advertising, and the popular mass media on the nation's attitudes regarding the use of alcohol.
- Multidisciplinary collaboration in theory development should be encouraged from such diverse fields as the biomedical sciences, econometrics, education, psychology, sociology, clinical epidemiology, anthropology, and other relevant disciplines. The development of theories that examine the interactions among variables derived from different levels of analysis or different disciplines should be particularly encouraged, especially if the theories can be used to guide the selection of intervention components and evaluation approaches. The use of new methodologies for formal theory development and model building should also be encouraged. Such methods as structural modeling and path-analytic procedures, computer simulation, and other multivariate approaches to causal analyses appear promising.

• Program planning and implementation should be integrated with evaluation. The use of formative research, one of the main components of social marketing, should be increased to ensure success in pilot studies of untested components of programs. Researchers are often unable to obtain sufficient funding to implement programs they may want to evaluate, and program personnel often do not have the funds to support a full evaluation of their programs. The result is that major prevention programs are "evaluated" after the fact and only in a descriptive or cursory manner. A mechanism needs to be found to facilitate a coherent demonstration evaluation plan whereby program and research designs are fully integrated. Until then, program evaluations, particularly at the community level, will remain piecemeal, inconsistent, and generally inadequate. (One of the great barriers to community prevention research is the enormous cost of collecting the data necessary for measuring whether an intervention has had an effect. NIAAA may want to consider ways to encourage local and county agencies to develop information management systems that can serve as existing data bases for measuring changes within the community. As local agencies begin to see the value of such data bases, they would undoubtedly expand their range to incorporate community and environmental variables that at first may seem remote to their needs. Ideally, such a system might include regular spot surveys of the alcohol-related concerns, knowledge, consumption, and problems of the community.)

• Community trials of prevention strategies should be instituted. One essential prevention research finding derived from heart disease and cancer prevention studies is the value of long-term community trials, such as those reported in Chapter 5. Such approaches have rarely been undertaken in efforts to prevent or reduce alcohol problems or to conduct alcohol problem prevention research. Tested research components should be combined into comprehensive, integrated, and reasonably long-term community-based projects to test the hypothesis that synergistic effects occur and that significant reductions in alcohol-related problems may be demonstrated. Effective community trials are long-term investments in the health and well-being of community members. They represent an opportunity to carefully monitor changes or the absence of change in targeted behaviors and situations. Prevention efforts to reduce alcohol problems have matured to a stage at which cost-effective longitudinal research projects could be undertaken. Such community prevention research trials will require (a) a long-term funding commitment for project development, implementation, and evaluation; (b) an effective partnership between prevention program specialists and prevention researchers; and (c) application of the latest research findings to identify behaviors and situations that can be effectively targeted for change.

• Prevention research should be used in policy development. The interests of researchers, prevention policymakers, and program planners are similar but not identical. Policymakers and planners are interested not merely in understanding the general effects of a particular strategy or documenting its past impact but also in anticipating its future impact in a specific situation. Conventional research and evaluation studies do not by themselves provide the types of "prospective" information that policymakers require. Although traditional research methods are often the most effective approach for examining a small number of variables in isolation from other factors, the policymaker must deal with the considerable "messiness" of detail contained in the real world. Tools are needed to assist policymakers and planners in making the best use of available resources, which would enable them to bring empirical and theoretical knowledge to bear on (a) understanding the complex network of factors that surround a set of alcohol problems and (b) estimating the likely impact of interventions in specific situations. Prevention research must develop the methods and techniques needed to assist prevention planners in estimating potential effects based on the best available research. One potentially valuable area of research is computer simulation, which permits perturbation ("what if") experiments to be undertaken to examine changes in a complex system. In such research, the computer is programmed to act like the system under study and changes are made to represent the analogous changes expected with a planned prevention policy or program. This type of computer-based experiment is intended to provide policymakers and researchers with data about likely or possible long-term results or outcomes of a set of potential prevention actions.

• Cost factors must be considered in prevention research. Much of prevention research is still in a formative stage and thus basic in nature. However, some areas of prevention research have developed beyond this stage to a point at which public policy and programs to prevent or reduce alcohol problems have already been based on such research. In these cases, both program costs and effects should be part of the evaluation; that is, what does it cost to undertake this program or policy given its effect in comparison with other strategies? As has been learned in other public health prevention efforts, cost/effect considerations aid in the selection of the best mix of programs and policies for reducing problems. All prevention approaches do not have similar costs or similar effects. To date, most prevention research has addressed contributory and risk factors and the potential effects of specific prevention strategies. Such research has not addressed the cost to implement or create programs based on research findings. Prevention research should include cost as a part of the outcome measures when such research has moved beyond the formative and developmental stages to a point at which programs can be based on this research.

Together, these recommendations present an ambitious program for the coming years. Considerable financial resources and a commitment from researchers in the field will be required to realize the progress called for in this report. Yet the benefits to be gained from reductions in the human and economic tolls of alcohol-related problems will most certainly justify the needed investments of money and intellectual energy.

REFERENCES

Abrams, D. B., J. Elder, T. Lasater et al. A comprehensive framework for conceptualizing and planning organizational health promotion programs. In M. Cataldo and T. Coates, eds. Behavioral Medicine in Industry. New York: John Wiley and Sons, 1986.

Altman, D., T. Flora, S. Fortmann et al. The cost effectiveness of three smoking cessation programs. Am. J. Public Health 77(2):162-165, 1987.

Ames, G. Environmental factors can create a drinking culture at worksite. Business and Health 5:44-45, 1987.

Ames, G., and C. R. Janes. Heavy and problem drinking in an American blue collar population: Implications for prevention. Soc. Sci. Med. 25:949-960, 1987.

Babor, T., J. Mendelson, I. Greenberg et al. Experimental analysis of the happy hour: Effects of purchase price on alcohol consumption. Psychopharmacology 58:35-41, 1978.

Babor, T., J. Mendelson, I. Greenberg et al. Drinking patterns in experimental and barroom settings. J. Stud. Alcohol 41(7):635-651, 1980.

Bigelow, G., and I. Liebson. Cost factors controlling alcohol drinking. Psychol. Rec. 22:305-314, 1972.

Blackburn, H., R. Luepker, F. Kline et al. The Minnesota Heart Health Program: A research and demonstration project in cardiovascular disease prevention. Pp. 1171-1178 in J. D. Matarazzo, N. E. Miller, S. M. Weiss et al., eds. Behavioral Health: A Handbook of Health Enhancement and Disease Prevention. New York: John Wiley and Sons, 1984.

Blose, J. O., and H. Holder. Liquor-by-the-drink and alcohol-related traffic crashes: A natural experiment using time-series analysis. J. Stud. Alcohol 48:52-60, 1987.

Box, G. E., and G. M. Jenkins. Time Series Analysis: Forecasting and Control. San Francisco: Holden-Day, 1976.

Box, G. E., and G. C. Tiao. Intervention analysis with applications to economic and environmental problems. J. Am. Statist. Assoc. 70:70-79, 1975.

Cohen, M., I. A. Liebson, L. A. Faillace et al. Alcoholism: Controlled drinking and incentives for abstinence. Psychol. Reports 28:575-580, 1971.

Cook, P. J., and G. Tauchen. The effect of liquor taxes on heavy drinking. Bell J. Economics 13(2):379-390, 1982.

Cook, T. D., and D. T. Campbell. Quasi-Experimentation: Design and Analysis Issues for Field Settings. Boston: Houghton-Mifflin, 1979.

Engle, K. B., and T. K. Williams. Effects of an ounce of vodka on alcoholics' desire for alcohol. Q. J. Stud. Alcohol 33:1099-1105, 1972.

Farquhar, J., S. Fortmann, N. Maccoby et al. The Stanford Five City Project: An overview. Pp. 1154-1165 in J. D. Matarazzo, N. E. Miller, S. M. Weiss et al., eds. Behavioral Health: A Handbook of Health Enhancement and Disease Prevention. New York: John Wiley and Sons, 1984.

Farquhar, J., S. Fortmann, J. Flora et al. The Stanford Five City Project: Designs and methods. Am. J. Epidemiol. 122:323-343, 1985.

Flay, B. R. What do we know about the social influences approach to smoking prevention? Review and recommendations. Pp. 67-112 in C. S. Bell and R. Battjes, eds. Prevention Research: Deterring Drug Abuse Among Children and Adolescents. NIDA Research Monograph No. 63. USDHHS Publ. No. (ADM)85-1334. Rockville, MD: National Institute on Drug Abluse, 1984.

Geller, E. S., N. W. Russ, and M. G. Altomari. Naturalistic observations of beer drinking among college students. J. Appl. Behav. Anal. 19:391-396, 1986.

Grossman, M., D. Coate, and G. M. Arluck. Price sensitivity of alcoholic beverages in the United States: Youth alcohol consumption. Pp. 169-198 in H. D. Holder, ed. Control Issues in Alcohol Abuse Prevention: Strategies for States and Communities. Greenwich, CT: JAI Press, 1987.

Harford, T., S. Feinhandler, J. O'Leary et al. Drinking in bars: An observational study of companion status and drinking behavior. Inter. J. Addict. 18:937-950, 1983.

Hewitt, L. W., and H. T. Blane. Prevention through mass media communication. Pp. 281-323 in P. M. Miller and T. D. Nirenberg, eds. Prevention of Alcohol Abuse. New York: Plenum Press, 1984.

Hingson, R., T. Heeren, D. Kovenock et al. Effects of Maine's 1981 and Massachusetts' 1982 D.U.I. legislation. Am. J. Public Health 77:593-597, 1987.

Holder, H., and J. Blose. Impact of changes in distilled spirits availability on apparent consumption: A time series analysis of liquor-by-the-glass. Br. J. Addict. 82:623-631, 1987a.

Holder, H., and J. Blose. The reduction of community alcohol problems: Computer simulation experiments in three counties. J. Stud. Alcohol 48(2):124-135, 1987b.

Katzper, M., R. Ryback, and M. Hertzman. Preliminary Aspects of Modeling and Simulation for Understanding Alcohol Utilization and the Effects of Regulatory Policies. Report submitted to the National Institute on Alcoholism, September 1976.

Kellam, S., C. Brown, B. Rubin et al. Paths leading to teenage psychiatric symptoms and substance use: Developmental epidemiological studies in Woodlawn. Pp. 17-51 in S. Guze, F. Earls, and J. Barrett, eds. Childhood Psychopathology and Development. New York: Raven Press, 1983.

Lanbein, L. J., and A. J. Lichtman. Ecological Inference. London: Sage Publications, 1978.

Langenbucher, J. W., and P. E. Nathan. Psychology, public policy and the evidence for alcohol intoxication. Am. Psychologist 383(10):1070-1077, 1983.

Lasater, T., D. Abrams, L. Artz et al. Lay volunteers of a community- based cardiovascular risk factor change program: The Pawtucket Experiment. Pp. 1171-1178 in J. D. Matarazzo, N. E. Miller, S. M. Weiss et al., eds. Behavioral Health: A Handbook of Health Enhancement and Disease Prevention. New York: John Wiley and Sons, 1984.

Levy, D., and N. Sheflin. New evidence on controlling alcohol through price. J. Stud. Alcohol 44:929-937, 1983.

Maccoby, N., J. Farquhar, P. Wood et al. Reducing the risk of cardiovascular disease: Effects of a community-based campaign on knowledge and behavior. J. Community Health 23:100-114, 1977.

Marlatt, G. A., B. Demming, and J. B. Reid. Loss of control drinking in alcoholics: An experimental analog. J. Abnormal Psychol. 81:223-241, 1973.

Mello, N. K. Some aspects of the behavioral pharmacology of alcohol. Pp. 787-809 in D. H. Efrow, ed. Psychopharmacology: A Review of Progress, 1957-1967. Public Health Service Publ. No. 1836. Washington, DC: Government Printing Office, 1968.

Mills, K., D. McCarty, J. Ward et al. A residence hall tavern as a collegiate alcohol abuse prevention activity. Addict. Behav. 8:105-108, 1983.

Moore, M. H., and D. R. Gerstein. Alcohol and Public Policy: Beyond the Shadow of Prohibition. Washington, DC: National Academy Press, 1981.

Moskowitz, J. M. The primary prevention of alcohol problems: A critical review of the research literature. J. Stud. Alcohol, 50(1):54-88, 1989.

Pendergast, M. L. A history of alcohol problem prevention efforts in the United States. Pp. 25-52 in H. Holder, ed. Advances in Substance Abuse, vol. 1, Control Issues in Alcohol Abuse Prevention: Strategies for States and Communities. Greenwich, CT: JAI Press, 1987.

Popham, R. The social history of the tavern. Pp. 225-302 in Y. Israel et al., eds. Research Advances in Alcohol and Drug Problems, vol. 4. New York: Plenum Press, 1978.

Puska, P., A. Nissinen, J. Tuomilehto et al. The community-based strategy to prevent coronary heart disease: Conclusions from the ten years of the North Karelia Project. Ann. Rev. Public Health 6:147-193, 1985.

Rorabaugh, W. Estimated U.S. alcoholic beverage consumption, 1790 - 1860. J. Stud. Alcohol 37:357-364, 1976.

Rosenbluth, J., P. E. Nathan, and D. M. Lawson. Environmental influences on drinking by college students in a college pub: Behavioral observation in the natural setting environment. Addict. Behav. 3:117-121, 1978.

Saltz, R. The role of bars and restaurants in preventing alcohol- impaired driving: An evaluation of server intervention. Evaluation and the Health Professions 10:5-27, 1987.

Single, E., and T. Storm, eds. Public drinking and public policy. Proceedings of a Symposium on Observation Studies held at Banff, Alberta, Canada, April 26-28, 1984. Toronto: Addiction Research Foundation, 1985.

Skog, O. Trends in alcohol consumption and violent deaths. Br. J. Addict. 81:365-379, 1986.

Smart, R. G., and E. M. Adlaf. Banning happy hours: The impact on drinking and impaired-driving charges in Ontario, Canada. J. Stud. Alcohol, 46(3):256-258, 1986.

Storm, T., and R. Cutler. Observations of drinking in natural settings: Vancouver beer parlors and cocktail lounges. J. Stud. Alcohol 42:972-997, 1981.

Wagenaar, A. Preventing highway crashes by raising the legal minimum age for drinking: The Michigan experience six years later. J. Safety Res. 17:101-109, 1986.

Warner, K. E., and B. R. Luce. Cost Benefit and Cost Effectiveness Analysis in Health Care: Principles, Practice and Potential. Ann Arbor, MI: Health Administration Press, 1982.

Wittman, F., and M. Hilton. Local regulation of alcohol availability: Uses of planning and zoning ordinances to regulate alcohol outlets in California cities. In H. Holder, ed. Control Issues in Alcohol Abuse Prevention: Strategies for States and Communities. Greenwich, CT: JAI Press, 1987.

II

RESEARCH OPPORTUNITIES IN THE TREATMENT OF ALCOHOL-RELATED PROBLEMS

INTRODUCTION

Within the framework of universal, selected, and indicated interventions noted in Chapter 1 of this report, treatment can be said to be an indicated intervention; its focus is on persons with already evident problems rather than on the preventions of problems in unaffected individuals. Given the heterogeneity of persons with alcohol problems-- and the wide range of such problems--reflected in the concept espoused by the committee of a continuum of severity, it should be no surprise to find that a variety of treatment methods and modalities have arisen in response. These numerous approaches testify to the vigorous interest of treatment providers and researchers and offer numerous opportunities for continued development and research on treatment efficacy and effectiveness.

In response to its charge, the committee conducted an extensive review of recent treatment research with a view toward identifying promising avenues of inquiry for future studies. Chapters 7 though 14 summarize its findings, necessarily presenting illustrative as opposed to comprehensive considerations of the various topics. Chapter 7 describes the social and historical context of alcohol treatment research, noting the past extent of federal support as well as emerging trends in service delivery and demographics that may affect future funding and research interests. Chapter 8 deals with issues of assessment, methodology, and research design. It describes some of the notable achievements in treatment evaluation in recent years (e.g., conceptual advances, new measurement techniques) and discusses a number of the major unresolved research issues. Many of the available treatment approaches have not been systematically or rigorously evaluated. Nevertheless, Chapter 9 surveys outcome evaluation research since 1980 on several treatment modalities (e.g., pharmacotherapies, psychotherapy and counseling, mutual help groups) and also considers recent process evaluation research.

Chapters 10 and 11 discuss research on two recent trends that appear to offer promise for impairing treatment outcome--namely, early identification of persons with alcohol problems and patient-treatment matching. Both of these areas hold promise for improving treatment outcome. Chapter 12 highlights selected findings from treatment studies of other psychoactive substance-use disorders that may be applicable to research on the treatment of alcohol problems; Chapter 13 discusses treatment of health consequences of heavy alcohol use or dependence; and Chapter 14 considers recent research on some of the public policy implications of alcohol treatment, particularly those related to costs and efficiency. In all of these chapters, the committee reviews research directions that have already been pursued and highlights potentially fruitful opportunities for further progress in identifying effective treatment approaches for alcohol problems.

7

THE SOCIAL AND HISTORICAL CONTEXT OF
ALCOHOL TREATMENT RESEARCH

A variety of factors, many of them outside the academic scientific community, have influenced the course of alcohol treatment research during the past few years. These historical factors and trends need to be understood before considering new research directions because they will continue to influence future research efforts. Some of the factors that affect treatment research priorities include (a) changing federal involvement in alcohol treatment; (b) emerging trends in the size, financing, and public/private ownership of alcohol treatment services; (c) demographic trends in the general population; and (d) popular movements in treatment and referral.

FEDERAL INVOLVEMENT IN ALCOHOL TREATMENT

The foundation of a federal alcoholism effort was laid during the late 1960s through a series of policy studies, court decisions, and congressional initiatives (Lewis, 1982). The 1967 and 1969 amendments to the Economic Opportunity Act created the first federally funded alcoholism treatment programs. In 1970, amendments to the Community Mental Health Centers Act authorized direct grants for special alcohol treatment projects. Around this time, separate treatment systems were also established at the federal level within the Veterans Administration (VA) and the military. Despite these initiatives, however, alcohol treatment services in the United States were administered primarily through state, local, and voluntary efforts.

This situation changed dramatically with the enactment of the Hughes Act in late 1971. Officially known as the Comprehensive Alcohol Abuse and Alcoholism Prevention, Treatment, and Rehabilitation Act, this legislation created the National Institute on Alcohol Abuse and Alcoholism from a section of the National Institute of Mental Health and charged the new agency with responsibility for education, training, research, and planning in the areas of alcohol treatment and prevention. One year after its inception, NIAAA inherited nearly 200 alcohol treatment programs from the Office of Economic Opportunity. Under the leadership of Morris Chafetz, its first director, NIAAA launched a major effort to alter the public's perception of alcoholism and encourage people to see it as a treatable disorder (Chafetz, 1975). During this time, high priority was given to the development of a comprehensive system of treatment services at the state and community levels, primarily through the mechanism of formula grants (NIAAA, 1977).

By 1981, NIAAA had distributed $654.4 million in project grants and contracts and $468.3 million in formula grants to the states (Lewis, 1982). In choosing grant recipients the agency placed special emphasis on the development of innovative treatment services, especially those that were accessible to underserved populations such as women, racial and ethnic minorities, the disabled, the elderly, young persons, and the families of alcoholics (NIAAA, 1980). In contrast to its role in the development of treatment services, however, only a small portion of NIAAA's total budget was spent to support research and training.

During this period, the agency initiated several innovative programs in the areas of treatment evaluation and reimbursement policy. In 1977, NIAAA contracted for a study of the barriers to third-party reimbursement for alcohol treatment and initiated a National Alcoholism Program Information System (NAPIS). By monitoring categorical community treatment programs in terms of client characteristics, services provided, and treatment outcomes, NIAAA created a valuable data base for the influential Rand Corporation study, the first comprehensive evaluation of treatment effectiveness (Armor, Polich, and Stambul, 1978). During this period, NIAAA also initiated special cost and utilization studies of various federally and state-mandated programs to provide health insurance coverage for alcohol treatment (NIAAA, 1980, 1985; Plotnick et al., 1982).

In addition to its direct support of treatment services and program evaluation research, the agency promoted early intervention activities directed at high-risk groups. NIAAA gave impetus to the development of occupational alcohol programs, drinking driver education programs, the federal employees alcohol program, and criminal justice programs, as well as efforts to educate pregnant women about the risks of excessive alcohol consumption (NIAAA, 1977, 1980).

In the early 1980s, NIAAA's pivotal role in the dramatic expansion of treatment services came to an end. Direct service grants were curtailed as third-party insurance expanded to cover the costs of alcohol treatment services. Congress then eliminated project formula grants, and funds were henceforth distributed directly to the states as part of the block grant mechanism. This action coincided with a shift in NIAAA's priorities away from treatment services to the support of biomedical and psychosocial research and the development of a basic science infrastructure through the agency's intramural research program, investigator-initiated grants, and the National Research Centers Program. Despite its recognized expertise in the area of alcohol treatment and the continued support of NIAAA by influential constituency groups, NIAAA's treatment efforts were rapidly eclipsed by other initiatives, creating a leadership vacuum that has been filled only recently through the agency's renewed commitment to treatment research. This renewed interest has been signaled by the creation of the new Division of Clinical and Prevention Research within the institute and by the congressional appropriation of funds specifically to support treatment research.

EMERGING TRENDS IN TREATMENT SERVICES

Coincident with the shift in NIAAA's role from treatment provider to research institute, changes have occurred in the organization and ownership of alcohol treatment services in the United States (Lowman, 1983; U. S. Department of Health and Human Services, 1983; Korcor, 1985). Alterations in reimbursement policy for treatment of alcohol problems, the expansion of inpatient treatment, an increase in the number of for-profit treatment providers, the growth of Alcoholics Anonymous (AA) (Robertson, 1988), and the emergence of nontraditional sources of recruitment into treatment (e.g., media advertising, employee assistance programs, drinking driver programs) have all been part of these changes.

According to a survey by the federal government, in 1984 there were 6,963 alcoholism units providing treatment services to more than a half-million patients (Reed and Sanchez, 1986). (Compared with 1982, 6,963 units is an increase of 64 percent in the number of service units.) Of the 540,231 patients in treatment on the date of the survey, 82.9 percent were being treated as active outpatients, whereas smaller proportions were receiving treatment in inpatient (7.6 percent) or residential (9.6 percent) settings. Almost half of the alcoholism treatment units were freestanding facilities; 21 percent were based in community mental health centers; and 19 percent were allocated to general, specialized, or VA hospitals. Compared with previous surveys, this study showed a large increase in the number of proprietary programs, especially in the proportion being run on a profit-making basis. For-profit units had increased almost 200 percent from 1982 and constituted 12 percent of all alcoholism treatment units. Another more recent study has documented the emergence of two separate treatment systems within the United States: one is privately owned and serving middle- and upper-income clients, while the other is publically owned and serving uninsured lower-income patients (Yahr, 1988).

Within both of these treatment systems, there has been a marked trend toward diversification and specialization. Early counseling or referral to specialized treatment is becoming increasingly prevalent in employment settings and health maintenance organizations (HMOs). Both inpatient and outpatient programs are directing their services toward special population groups (e.g., the military, adolescents, children of alcoholics, employee groups, professionals, women, homosexuals, and drunk drivers). Media advertising is being used to promote program utilization in many parts of the country (Korcor, 1985).

Alongside the tremendous increases in the availability and scope of alcohol treatment services, there has also been a trend to organize therapeutic approaches around a single inpatient rehabilitation model consisting of detoxification, alcohol education, group confrontational therapy, AA meetings, and disulfiram therapy (Miller and Hester, 1986). This treatment package is typically delivered to all types of patients in the course of a standard three- to four-week residential program. What is surprising about this trend is the relative lack of empirical data that could serve as a rational basis for the selection of these or other treatment components or to justify the duration of intensive care (Saxe, 1983; Miller and Hester, 1986).

The trend toward rapid expansion, standardization, and integration of alcohol treatment services creates special challenges and opportunities for research. The emergence of a complete continuum of services from detoxification to aftercare makes it imperative to investigate how best to assign a patient to the least expensive, yet therapeutically appropriate, alternative. The broad range of available services makes it possible to study the relative efficacy of different therapeutic modalities and treatment programs. For example, "social model" detoxification and rehabilitation programs were developed in California during the 1970s (Borkman, 1986). They feature community-based facilities, variable lengths of stay, and treatment of clients by nonprofessional staff. These programs apparently treat clients at a fraction of the cost of standard, medical-model private programs. A fundamental and as yet unanswered research question concerns the relative effectiveness of these programs for similar types of clients.

DEMOGRAPHY, EPIDEMIOLOGY, AND THE DELIVERY OF TREATMENT SERVICES

Recent demographic trends in the American population, coupled with changing patterns of alcohol and drug abuse, may have important implications for the demand for alcohol-related health services in the future. These trends may also affect the need for more carefully evaluated treatment interventions that go beyond the specialized treatment systems that have developed in recent years. National and regional surveys of the adult U.S. population

(Regier et al., 1984) have indicated that alcohol abuse and dependence are among the most prevalent psychiatric conditions. Survey data and hospital records have consistently shown that alcohol dependence reaches its peak prevalence among persons 35 to 45 years old (Hilton, 1987). The maturing of the postwar baby boom population, which encompasses the 1945-1960 birth cohorts, means that an increasingly larger proportion of the population is passing through this period of greatest risk for alcohol-related consequences (Williams et al., 1987). Other demographic trends that have the potential to influence the nature and availability of treatment services are increases in the Hispanic population, changes in the configuration of the nuclear family, increases in the number of homeless persons, the aging of the population, and the deinstitutionalization of psychiatric patients.

Epidemiological data point to a broad diversity of alcohol-related problems, only some of which overlap with the continuum of alcohol dependence symptoms. For example, a 1979 survey estimated that there were 10 million adult men and women who consumed four or more drinks per day, a common criterion for heavy drinking (U. S. Department of Health and Human Services, 1981). Although heavy or frequent drinking is not necessarily indicative of alcoholism, it is an important risk factor and can lead to health problems even in the absence of alcohol dependence (Babor, Kranzler, and Lauerman, 1987). The findings of a 1982 study showed that the prevalence of alcohol-related problems and heavy drinking in patients seeking treatment for other health problems in general hospital settings ranged from 15 to 20 percent of male patients and from 4 to 10 percent of female patients (MacIntosh, 1982).

Epidemiological surveys indicate that the baby boom cohorts of younger heavy drinkers are also frequent users of other psychoactive substances (e.g., marihuana, cocaine) and are more likely than primary alcoholics to have other psychiatric comorbidities (especially depression or antisocial personality disorder). These trends toward multiple substance-use patterns, greater numbers of individuals at risk, and the pervasiveness of alcohol-related problems in general medical patients not only should be taken into consideration in the planning of health services but also should guide the design of health services research. For example, the high prevalence of heavy drinking and alcohol abuse among general medical patients suggests that attempts should be made to integrate the identification and management of alcohol abuse into general medical practice and to evaluate the impact of this practice change on the health of the primary care population. Similarly, the high concordance of tobacco dependence, alcohol dependence, and dependence on other psychoactive substances means that alcohol-specific treatments may have to be broadened to include the remediation of multiple substance-use disorders.

Finally, the projected increase in the absolute numbers of persons at risk, as well as the anticipated changes in patterns of substance abuse, argues for the development of a more empirically based approach to estimations of the need for treatment services. These estimation techniques should rely on current social indicators, census data, or other readily available information sources. They may also rely on extrapolation or "synthetic" estimates drawn from well-executed population surveys such as the Epidemiologic Catchment Area Study (Regier et al., 1984) or the National Health Interview Survey. These techniques must be sensitive to variations in those demographic variables (e.g.,age, sex, ethnicity, education, socioeconomic status) that are related to the prevalence of alcohol problems and to the conditions that promote efficacious treatment. The development of these techniques may involve research on uniformly coded data bases to help reduce the variability of current social indicator data. It may also involve the comparative evaluation of these techniques in a variety of field settings.

The assessment of a community's need for alcohol treatment services consists of an accurate estimate of three factors: (1) the actual need for treatment in the community; (2) the total treatment resources available to the community at all levels of care; and (3) the demand for those resources from the community. Once these components are known, they can be analyzed to see how need, resources, and utilization compare; where the gaps of unmet need are located; what types of resources are required; and where the new resources ought to be placed.

Although considerable progress has been made since the 1950s in assessing the need for treatment services, more work should be done to refine the needs assessment methods that are currently used. These methods are vital to local, state, and national planners who are attempting to allocate limited resources in the most efficient way.

POPULAR TRENDS IN TREATMENT AND REFERRAL

Popular trends in treatment and referral may have a profound effect on the treatment-seeking population as well as on the treatments being delivered. Researchers must be prepared to describe, investigate, and interpret these trends. For example, the emergence during the 1980s of public interest groups devoted to the prosecution and prevention of drunk driving has placed special demands on treatment services (see Chapters 3 and 4). Legally mandated treatment has raised questions about the appropriateness of using the same conventional approaches that in other contexts rely heavily on individual motivation. Another trend that is affecting the design of treatment services is the increasing health consciousness of the American public, combined with changing norms about the advisability and appropriateness of heavy drinking. As noted in Chapter 4, during the past decade there has been a sharp decline in the public's preference for distilled beverages and a concomitant switch to beers and liquors with lower alcohol contents (Kling, in press). Public awareness of the possible hazards of heavy drinking may increase the acceptability of minimal or brief interventions targeted at the large population of heavy drinkers who are at high risk for alcohol dependence (Babor, Kranzler, and Lauerman, 1987).

Within the alcohol field itself, there have been significant changes in the acceptance of different ideas and concepts. Adult children of alcoholics have received a great deal of attention in the media, which has been fueled in part by advocates of the need for special therapeutic approaches to this population. Similarly, the concept of "codependence" of family members has gained popularity as a clinical entity that is assumed to be partly responsible for maintaining the alcoholic's self-defeating behavior (Cermak, 1986). Little research attention has been devoted to the implications of these new ideas for the improvement of treatment services.

The treatment field has also seen a growing professionalism among alcoholism counselors, as well as an increasing tendency to monitor and coordinate services through managed care systems. These trends will place special demands on the research community, which increasingly is being asked to provide the answers to such complex questions as the relative effectiveness of credentialed versus noncredentialed counselors or the cost savings that can be realized from managed care approaches.

Although other sections of this report address the more traditional types of research opportunities, it is appropriate to begin this discussion of the treatment research agenda with the following recommendations for policy-oriented services research to set the stage for the future:

• Research is needed on the multiple economic forces that shape the demand for, and provision of, treatment services for alcohol-dependent persons and problem drinkers.

• More research is needed, especially at the local level, on the geographic distribution of alcohol treatment. Some of the questions to be answered in this area concern the appropriate and efficient distribution of resources and the social, economic, and geographic factors that affect the development of treatment services.

• Reliable and valid techniques of prevalence assessment that are sensitive to local conditions are needed for health services planning. Researchers should be encouraged to use national sample surveys (e.g., Clark and Midanik, 1982), as well as psychiatric epidemiological methods (e.g., Regier et al., 1984), to develop forecasting models to estimate the need for treatment services.

• The importance of emerging trends in patient characteristics, population demographics, alcohol-use patterns, and service utilization has revealed a need for systematic health services data to describe these trends. Vigorous support should be provided to the national survey of alcoholism, drug abuse, and combined treatment units, which has been conducted for NIAAA and the National Institute on Drug Abuse (NIDA) since 1979. These surveys could be fruitfully expanded with the use of a more intensive data collection procedure and the identification of a representative sample of facilities.

• In addition, other data bases are needed to assess alcohol-related general service and specialty service utilization in ambulatory settings. This research should span a wide range of services such as community mental health centers, family service agencies, prisons, HMOs, primary care clinics, and general hospitals. The development of data bases on ambulatory services will allow more precise estimates of the scope, severity, and cost effects of alcohol use on mental health and general medical problems.

• Both the alcohol and the drug abuse fields have benefited from longitudinal cohort studies of clients sampled from multiple facilities (Armor, Polich, and Stambul, 1978; Hubbard, Marsden, and Allison, 1984). The NIAAA should support major outcome monitoring studies, preferably covering a representative sample of units drawn from the national survey census.

• Researchers should be encouraged to investigate popular trends and concepts in the treatment field--for example, the need for special treatment services for adult children of alcoholics and codependents, and the efficacy of such services once they have been established and marketed.

• Greater attention should be devoted to comparing alternative treatment systems, both in the United States and in other countries. (For example, California's social model program could be compared with other public and private systems in terms of costs and efficacy of both detoxification and rehabilitation treatment.) Detailed historical analyses, contrasting case studies, and large-scale statistical studies are now needed to provide a knowledge base to guide health planning and treatment policy. In a world of great diversity among health systems, all of which seem to be affected by similar economic problems, the promise of comparative treatment systems research both within the United States and internationally is substantial.

• Policy studies should be undertaken to evaluate the impact of recent changes in training, credentialing, and licensing of personnel who treat alcohol problems.

REFERENCES

Armor, D. J., J. M. Polich, and H. B. Stambul. Alcoholism and Treatment. New York: John Wiley and Sons, 1978.

Babor, T. F., H. R. Kranzler, and R. J. Lauerman. Social drinking as a health and psychosocial risk factor: Anstie's limit revisited. Pp. 373-402 in Marc Galanter, ed. Recent Developments in Alcoholism, vol. 5. New York: Plenum Press, 1987.

Borkman, T. A Social-Experiential Model in Programs for Alcoholism Recovery: A Research Report on a New Treatment Design. Washington, DC: NIAAA, 1986.

Cermak, T. L. Diagnosing and Treating Co-Dependence: A Guide for Professionals Who Work with Chemical Dependents, Their Spouses, and Children. Minneapolis, MN: Johnson Institute Books, 1986.

Chafetz, M. From program to people: Toward a national policy for alcoholism services. Alcohol Health and Research World, Summer:14-19, 1975.

Clark, W., and L. Midanik. Alcohol use and alcohol problems among U.S. adults: Results of the 1979 national survey. Pp. 3-52 in National Institute on Alcohol Abuse and Alcoholism. Alcohol Consumption and Related Problems. Alcohol Health Monograph No. 1. USDHHS Publ. No. (ADM)82-1190. Washington, DC: Government Printing Office, 1982.

Hilton, M. E. Drinking patterns and drinking problems in 1984: Results from a general population survey. Alcoholism: Clinical and Experimental Research 11(2):167-175, 1987.

Hubbard, R., M. E. Marsden, and M. Allison. Treatment Outcome Prospective Study: Reliability and Validity of TOPS Data. Research Triangle Park, NC: Research Triangle Institute, April 1984.

Kling, W. Measurement of ethanol consumed in distilled spirits. J. Stud. Alcohol, in press.

Korcor, M. Alcoholism treatment, a growing "product line." American Medical News, October 11, 1985.

Lewis, J. The federal role in alcoholism research, treatment and prevention. Pp. 385-401 in E. L. Gomberg, H. R. White, and J. A. Carpenter, eds. Alcohol, Science and Society Revisited. Ann Arbor: University of Michigan Press, 1982.

Lowman, C. Changes in alcoholism treatment services, 1979-1982. Alcohol Health and Research World 8:2, 1983.

MacIntosh, I. D. Alcohol-related disabilities in general hospital patients: A critical assessment of the evidence. International Journal of Addictions 17(4):609-639, 1982.

Miller, W. R., and R. K. Hester. Matching problem drinkers with optimal treatments. Pp. 175-203 in W. R. Miller and N. Heather, eds. Treating Addictive Behaviors: Processes of Change. New York: Plenum Press, 1986.

National Institute on Alcohol Abuse and Alcoholism. Sixth Annual Report to the U.S. Congress, Fiscal Year. Rockville, MD: NIAAA, 1977.

National Institute on Alcohol Abuse and Alcoholism. Report to the U.S. Congress on Federal Activities on Alcohol Abuse and Alcoholism, Fiscal Year. Rockville, MD: NIAAA, 1980.

National Institute on Alcohol Abuse and Alcoholism. Alcoholism Treatment Impact on Total Health Care Utilization and Costs. Washington, DC: U.S. Department of Health and Human Services, February 1985.

Plotnick, D. E., K. M. Adams, H. R. Hunter, and J. C. Rowe. Alcoholism Treatment Programs Within Prepaid Group Practice HMOs: A Final Report. Rockville, MD: NIAAA, 1982.

Reed, P. G., and D. S. Sanchez. Characteristics of Alcoholism Services in the United States--1984. Rockville, MD: U.S. Department of Health and Human Services, 1986.

Regier, D. A., J. K. Myers, M. Kramer, et. al. The NIMH epidemiologic catchment area program. Arch. Gen. Psych. 41:934-941, 1984.

Robertson, N. The changing world of Alcoholics Anonymous. New York Times Magazine 40-45, February 21, 1988.

Saxe, L., D. Dougherty, K. Esty, and M. Fine. The Effectiveness and Costs of Alcoholism Treatment. Health Technology Case Study 22. Office of Technology Assessment, U.S. Congress. Washington, DC: Government Printing Office, 1983.

U.S. Department of Health and Human Services (OHHS). Fourth Special Report to the U.S. Congress on Alcohol and Health. Washington, DC: National Institute on Alcohol Abuse and Alcoholism, 1981.

U.S. Department of Health and Human Services (OHHS). Fifth Special Report to the U.S. Congress on Alcohol and Health. Washington, DC: National Institute on Alcohol Abuse and Alcoholism, 1983.

Williams, G. D., F. S. Stinson, D. A. Parker, et. al. Demographic trends, alcohol abuse and alcoholism: 1985-1995. Alcohol Health and Research World 2:80-83, 1987.

Yahr, H. T. A national comparison of public and private-sector alcoholism treatment delivery system characteristics. J. Stud. Alcohol 49:233-239, 1988.

8

ISSUES OF ASSESSMENT, METHODOLOGY, AND RESEARCH DESIGN

Despite the practical difficulties of research involving persons with alcohol-related problems, there have been some notable achievements in treatment evaluation in recent years. These accomplishments include conceptual advances, new measurement techniques, the growing sophistication of diagnostic procedures, and improved approaches to research design. In addition to reviewing the opportunities associated with these accomplishments, this chapter also discusses some of the major unresolved evaluation research issues, such as who should be assessed, what variables should be measured, and the validity of current procedures.

RECENT DEVELOPMENTS IN CONCEPTUALIZATION

There are three important conceptual advances relevant to the current status and future conduct of research on the treatment of alcohol-related problems. These advances have guided the development of new assessment procedures that promise to provide a more sophisticated basis for measuring the underlying dynamics of alcohol dependence and its treatment.

The first conceptual development is the description of alcohol dependence as a core syndrome within a broader range of alcohol-related problems. In recent years, research on the alcohol dependence syndrome (Edwards, 1986) has focused on a cluster of biological, psychological, and behavioral elements that are believed to be at the core of pathological alcohol-seeking behavior. With the development of new diagnostic criteria and assessment instruments to measure the presence and severity of alcohol dependence (Rounsaville et al., 1987; Robins et al., 1988), researchers are now in a much better position to evaluate specific treatment interventions that focus on such concomitants of dependence as craving, environmental precipitants, and biological vulnerability factors.

A second development in conceptualization has resulted in a distinction between alcohol dependence and alcohol-related disabilities. Whereas alcohol dependence is seen as a coherent syndrome with signs and symptoms that tend to occur together and mutually reinforce one another, alcohol-related disabilities are now considered to be a rather heterogeneous set of physical, psychological, and social impairments that occur independently of alcohol dependence. In research terms, this distinction means that the assessment of alcoholism should focus both on the underlying dependence and on the problems associated with it. It also means that alcohol-related problems that occur as a result of heavy drinking in the absence of dependence are also the proper targets of treatment prevention efforts. Finally, alcohol dependence is now being conceptualized and measured not as an all-or-none phenomenon but as a continuum that ranges in severity from mild to severe (Edwards, Arif, and Hodgson, 1981).

A third advance in conceptualization concerns new developments in the way treatment evaluation is viewed. Interest in treatment evaluation research has been increasing within the alcohol field over the past 20 years. The dominant approach in both clinical practice and treatment evaluation research has been to ask: Is treatment effective? Traditionally, research has attempted to discover the "main effects" of different treatments relative to the absence of treatment or exposure to some alternative treatment. A more sophisticated model of treatment evaluation, known as the "matching hypothesis," has emerged recently in the fields of drug abuse, alcoholism, and psychotherapy (Luborsky and McLellan, 1981; Moos and Finney, 1985; VandenBos, 1986). This model, which is discussed in detail in Chapter 11, places great demands on the skills, resources, and ingenuity of evaluation researchers.

ADVANCES IN ASSESSMENT TECHNOLOGY

Significant advances have been made in the technology of assessment, which have led to the development of new techniques for screening, diagnosis, and differential assessment. The research opportunities associated with advances in diagnosis and other assessment areas are discussed below. Screening is considered separately in Chapter 10.

Diagnosis

One of the most active areas of development since the last Institute of Medicine report (IOM, 1980) on research opportunities in the alcohol field has been diagnosis, including the tools for diagnostic assessment. The third edition of the American Psychiatric Association's Diagnostic and Statistical Manual of Mental Disorders (DSM-III) (American Psychiatric Association, 1980) was published the same year as the IOM report. DSM-III had a major impact on diagnosis in the mental health field (Spitzer, Williams, and Skodol, 1983) and fostered further development of structured diagnostic interviews. Together, "operational" diagnostic criteria and structured interviews based on those criteria have had a profound effect on the way clinicians conceptualize and determine psychiatric diagnoses. For example, it is now clear that unstructured clinical examinations have major limitations. One problem is reliability among observers. The use of structured interviews has improved the reliability of diagnoses and other clinical assessments in the alcohol field.

On the assumption that some types of information are best gathered by an interviewer, a related issue concerns the degree of clinical expertise the interviewer should possess. Recent research with non-clinically trained (lay) interviewers indicates that if the interview is highly structured, accurate diagnostic information can be gathered by interviewers with little or no clinical experience (Coryell, Cloninger, and Reich, 1978; Helzer et al., 1981).

Some of the commonly employed examinations that are structured enough to be used by nonclinicians include the Diagnostic Interview Schedule (DIS) (Robins et al., 1981) and the Psychiatric Diagnostic Interview (PDI) (Othmer, Powell, and Penick, 1980). These instruments are essentially general diagnostic examinations. Three others that are designed specifically to gather information about substance use are the Composite International Diagnostic Interview, Substance Abuse Module (CIDI-SAM) (Robins et al., 1988), the Addiction Severity Index (ASI) (McLellan et al., 1980), and the Comprehensive Drinker Profile (Marlatt and Miller, 1984).

Related to the development of diagnostic instruments has been a series of ongoing programs of study within NIAAA, the American Psychiatric Association (APA), and the World Health Organization (WHO). These programs have led to recommended revisions in current diagnostic criteria in the Diagnostic and Statistical Manual (DSM-III-R) (APA, 1987), as well as in the International Classification of Diseases (ICD-10) (WHO, 1988). They have also contributed to the development of new diagnostic instruments that are capable of classifying people reliably and quickly, according to the severity of their alcohol dependence (Robins et al., 1988; Wing et al., in press). Moreover, advances in evaluation methodology (Meyer et al., 1985) have stimulated research in this area, and a number of assessment procedures have been developed to measure the severity of alcohol dependence (Stockwell, Murphy, and Hodgson, 1983; Skinner and Horn, 1984). Research suggests that the severity of dependence predicts cravings for alcohol and failure to control drinking following relapse (Polich, Armor, and Braiker, 1981; Babor, Cooney, and Lauerman, 1987). Although further research is called for, it appears that the dependence syndrome construct has considerable promise for early detection, diagnosis, and treatment planning, at least in the European and North American countries in which most of the research has been conducted (Edwards, 1986).

Nevertheless, the concept of the alcohol dependence syndrome has been criticized from a number of points of view, and at present its scientific status as the basis for a worldwide definition of alcohol dependence requires further study. A more systematic program of research using cross-cultural comparative methods could provide useful information. To the extent that consistency is found across disparate samples of alcoholics from different cultures, the case for a core dependence syndrome would be strengthened, thereby facilitating epidemiological research, international communication, and comparisons across treatment evaluation studies.

The following issues and questions offer opportunities for research on diagnosis:

• What is the construct validity of the dependence syndrome concept used as the basis for DSM-III-R and ICD-10? Research should be undertaken on the underlying assumptions of the alcohol dependence syndrome construct, particularly with respect to the relative separation of indicators of dependence from indicators of alcohol-related impairment. Because clinicians are using the same criteria to diagnose all substance abuse disorders, it is crucial to examine the commonalities and distinctions among psychoactive substances. To what extent do differences in severity of dependence represent differences in the abuse liability of different substances?

• Additional cross-cultural research would be useful to identify biobehavioral universals of alcohol dependence. Such research should be encouraged in the context of any program to revise international classification systems (e.g., the ICD-10).

• What is the concordance between current (e.g., DSM-III) and proposed (e.g., DSM-III-R) diagnostic systems, particularly in terms of interrater agreement and test-retest reliability?

• What is the internal and external validity of the new criteria proposed in DSM-III-R and ICD-10? Research should focus on predictive validity (assessing the clinical course of individuals diagnosed according to different diagnostic systems) and diagnostic stability (the persistence of diagnostic symptoms over different periods of the drinking career).

Differential Assessment

Differential assessment is the detailed evaluation of the patient's alcohol-use disorder in terms of etiology, presenting symptoms, substance-use patterns, alcohol-related problems, and other associated features. A variety of purposes can be served by the differential assessment. First, it can help to explain the underlying causes of a disorder. Second, data obtained by careful assessment can serve as both a baseline and a predictor of future behavior. Finally, differential assessment is crucial to individualized treatment planning, which is based on the identification of "matches" between patient characteristics or needs and specific treatment interventions.

There have been some notable advances in basic research that have begun to stimulate new approaches to assessment and patient placement. Laboratory studies of craving, psychological expectancies, and impaired control over drinking have helped to elucidate the natural bases of alcohol dependence (Meyer et al., 1985). With the development of procedures to measure the severity of alcohol dependence, it may soon be possible to assign patients to different types and intensities of treatment, based on their vulnerability to readdiction and the suitability of different therapies for their treatment.

The application of psychological learning theory to the study of relapse (see Chapter 3) has led to the development of specific assessment techniques that are designed to identify the patient's susceptibility to relapse and to minimize the effects of brief lapses (slips) (Annis and Davis, 1987). One of the most promising areas of research related to the development of new assessment procedures is the identification of alcoholic subtypes. For example, there is some evidence to suggest that psychopathology and social instability are associated with poor prognosis, and these types of patients may warrant more individualized treatment (Rounsaville et al., 1987). In addition to structured diagnostic interviews (which allow reliable classification of psychopathology), new approaches to subtyping by personality variables and by other characteristics are being proposed (Cloninger, 1987). Many of these advances have been facilitated by the use of standardized assessment procedures that were developed within other disciplines to measure behavior and symptoms often seen in alcoholics. These techniques include procedures to measure cognitive functioning, affective states, anxiety, depression, social skills, and drug use. Although these procedures appear to be suitable for use with alcoholics, there is also a need to develop measurement techniques that have been designed specifically for alcohol problems and that have been validated by using appropriate patient samples.

A wide range of methods--including interviews, questionnaires, biological tests, performance tests, and clinical examination procedures--has been employed to gather clinical data on substance-use disorders. Clinical instruments vary along several dimensions (e.g., who gathers the information, how detailed it must be), but most interviews rely on the respondent as the main or sole informant. Self-administered instruments are also used; the assumption behind them is that if they are worded carefully enough and the amount of information needed is not lengthy, it is possible to bypass an interviewer altogether. Some commonly used questionnaires include the Michigan Alcoholism Screening Test (MAST) (Hedlund and Vieweg, 1984), the Alcohol Expectancy Questionnaire (Brown et al., 1980), the Alcohol Use Inventory (Wanberg, Horn, and Fisher, 1977), and the Alcohol Dependence Scale (Skinner and Horn, 1984).

In summary, there has been a burgeoning interest in the past decade in the development of questionnaires, interviews, performance tests, personality inventories, and biological tests that have vastly improved the scientist's ability to quantify virtually all of the relevant aspects of alcoholism as a multidimensional clinical disorder. Research instruments such as the MAST, the ASI, and the DIS have gained widespread acceptance among researchers and clinicians (Lettieri, Nelson, and Sayers, 1985). All of these instruments generate reliable, standardized information that could be entered easily into a patient's hospital record to become part of the reporting statistics available to researchers, funding agencies, and health officials. Such data would be extremely useful as a basis for comparing programs and settings in terms of client characteristics and treatment effectiveness, in turn suggesting hypotheses for later clinical trials.

The following research initiatives offer the opportunity to build on recent advances in the technology of differential assessment:

• Appropriate emphasis should be placed on establishing the reliability and validity of various assessment procedures. Clients should be evaluated by using standardized, validated, reliable instruments. Efforts should be made to evaluate the clinical relevance of these instruments for program planning, patient placement, treatment matching, and outcome prediction. Emphasis should be given to measures of treatment readiness, motivation for treatment, alcohol- and drug-use patterns, severity of dependence, alcohol-related disabilities, type and severity of psychopathology, social support networks, and coping skills. In those instances in which instruments have been developed for use with nonalcoholic populations, efforts should be made to validate these measures on alcoholic patient samples.

• The identification of psychiatric comorbidity as a common feature of the clinical picture of alcoholism implies that future research should investigate (a) the relative importance of differentiating alcoholics according to major comorbidities (e.g., antisocial personality, depression, anxiety disorder); and (b) treatment-matching hypotheses that combine new psychiatric assessment procedures with diagnosis-related therapeutic interventions.

• Given the importance of psychiatric interviewing for the development of accurate diagnostic information, the following questions should be pursued. What is the impact of varying degrees of structure in the interview instrument on the quality of clinical data obtained? How do interviews with and without cutoffs compare? How accurate are informants' reports? How much detail can respondents accurately provide about their disorders? Are inaccuracies biased? How do a patient's mental state and level of intoxication or withdrawal affect reporting?

Research on the Reliability and Validity of Assessments

Because patients in treatment for alcohol-related problems have often been found to be defensive, uncooperative, sociopathic, or cognitively impaired, there is reason to be skeptical about the accuracy of the information they provide about themselves for research and clinical purposes. This skepticism has generated a substantial amount of methodological research on the validity of verbal self-report methods; it has also stimulated the search for biological markers and other objective measures of alcohol consumption that are not as susceptible to response distortion (Babor, Stephens, and Marlatt, 1987; O'Farrell and Maisto, 1987). Given the importance of accurate information about the patient's presenting symptoms, drinking history, and treatment outcome, research on the reliability and validity of assessment procedures should receive high priority.

Research on Verbal Report Methods

Verbal report techniques (e.g., interviews, tests, questionnaires) have become the most common method of obtaining clinical data on alcohol abuse and its modification through treatment. Recent research has raised questions about the extent to which this method provides reliable and valid information for research purposes. A review of methodological studies in the alcohol literature (Babor, Stephens, and Marlatt, 1987) shows that, although information obtained from alcoholics tends to be generally reliable and valid, there can be considerable variability in accuracy depending on the sensitivity of the information sought (e.g., arrest records), the specificity of the validation criteria (e.g., archival records, breathalyser readings, informants' reports), the personal characteristics of the respondents (e.g., sober versus intoxicated), the time window of the report (e.g., recent, lifetime), and the demand characteristics of the task situation (e.g., intake interview, research evaluation at follow-up). Verbal data obtained from alcoholic respondents are inherently neither valid nor invalid; they vary with the methodological sophistication of the data gatherer and the personal characteristics of the respondent. These facts suggest that an emphasis on demonstrating whether verbal report data are either valid or invalid is misplaced. A more important issue is how to improve the validity of these procedures.

The variety of verbal report procedures used to assess drinking behavior and alcohol-related problems makes it difficult to evaluate and compare results across studies. Until recently, little attention was focused on the systematic evaluation of measurement procedures, assessment contexts, and response sets. Alcohol research would benefit from a new generation of methodological studies directed at procedures to enhance the validity of verbal report data and at evaluating new procedures that provide objective indicators of recent alcohol consumption.

The generic term for factors that might influence verbal report information in a research context is response effects. Although there has been some general research in this area (Bradburn, 1983), there has been little research focused specifically on substance use or on alcohol-related problems. Such studies are important in the alcohol field because research findings largely depend on the accurate reporting of alcohol problems by study participants.

There are several opportunities for further research in this area. One is the impact of other types of response effects (e.g., accuracy of recall) on the precision of self-reports. There is evidence that the recall of health-related occurrences is inconsistent (Aneshensel et al., 1987) and that, even for such seemingly salient events as hospitalization, there may be underreporting after only one year (Cannell, 1977). Other research questions relate to the costs and sacrifices of various methods of data collection. Pertinent issues include the practical limits on the amount of information that can be obtained with self-report questionnaires and the use of telephone interviews to obtain diagnostic and other clinical data.

The following opportunities may serve as useful guidelines for a research agenda on verbal report methods:

• More studies of assessment contexts and instructional sets are needed. For instance, preliminary results suggest that individual assessments yield more valid results than group assessments (Sobell and Sobell, 1981); that telephone surveying and interviewing may be a reasonably reliable means of obtaining information on drug use (Frank, 1985); that adolescents will give more valid self-reports in private settings (Gfroerer, 1985); and that the use of computerized assessments may yield more valid data than other techniques (Skinner and Allen, 1983).

• Individual difference factors (e.g., social desirability response sets) should be investigated because of their potential influence on validity. Until it can be demonstrated that social desirability scales (e.g., Crowne and Marlowe, 1960) actually measure response bias on alcohol-related assessments, however, their use should not be incorporated automatically into assessment batteries (cf. Bradburn, 1983).

• Some invalid responses may be related to forgetting. In addition, there is a strong relationship between mental status and the validity of self-reports (Miller and Barasch, 1985), suggesting the need for careful assessment of organic impairment in respondents.

• Recently developed time-line follow-back (Sobell et al., 1986) and retrospective diary procedures should be evaluated to assess their ability to improve the reliability and validity of verbal reports by providing recall cues to respondents.

• Because no single measure of alcohol consumption is entirely valid, most researchers recommend the use of convergent lines of evidence to establish drinking status or to measure drinking behavior. Such analytic procedures as the multitrait-multimethod assessment matrix should be used to evaluate the discriminant and convergent validity of verbal report data. Different verbal report strategies for quantifying consumption (e.g., the quantity-frequency question, the diary method/time-line follow-back procedure) should be compared. The use of multiple biological indicators may have promise as a way of corroborating verbal reports, provided sensitivity problems can be overcome (Cushman et al., 1984).

Use of Biological Markers

The presence of alcohol in blood, urine, sweat, or breath is strong evidence that drinking has occurred. Because the duration of abstinence and the amount of drinking following relapse are important criteria for treatment outcome (Babor, Cooney, and Lauerman, 1987), there is great interest in developing laboratory tests (markers) that detect alcohol consumption. An ideal marker would be one that reflected the mean blood alcohol level over several weeks, that did not depend on the presence of organ damage, and that returned to normal relatively quickly with abstinence (O'Farrell and Maisto, 1987).

The major problem with blood, breath, and urine alcohol tests is the relatively short half-life of alcohol after it is ingested. Alcohol is usually not present in any of these fluids hours after ingestion. Thus, a positive alcohol test indicates that drinking occurred that day, but it is not an indication of chronic alcohol use. In this regard, the results of a study by Orrego and colleagues (1979) are important for those interested in alcoholism treatment evaluation. The study was carried out as part of a clinical trial evaluating propylthiouracil treatment of alcoholic hepatitis, in which daily urine specimens were collected and analyzed for ethanol. Of the patients in this study who consistently denied drinking during a six-month period, 25 percent had positive urine specimens. Another 25 percent made claims of abstinence for one week that were refuted by urine tests during the six months.

Because blood, breath, and urine alcohol tests are indicators of recent alcohol use only, one focus of current research is the development of methods to measure alcohol use over longer periods. Phillips (1984) studied a sweat patch that is applied to the skin and cannot be removed without leaving a mark. The patch collects sweat for seven days, which is then analyzed for ethanol. Results showed that 50 percent (11 of 22) of the subjects who returned for follow-up underreported the amount they drank. However, half of the normal volunteers failed to return to have their patches removed; consequently, lack of patient cooperation may present a problem with this method.

Liver enzymes rise with excessive alcohol ingestion and therefore are useful in detecting drinking. Gamma glutamyl transpeptidase (GGT) increases with prolonged heavy drinking to a greater extent than other liver enzymes (Shaw and Lieber, 1980). However, GGT is not a specific marker, because liver injuries other than alcohol abuse also result in increased serum concentrations. Conceivably, isoenzyme profiling techniques may make it possible to distinguish the GGT elevations caused by drinking from those associated with other factors. Recently, Irwin and coworkers (1988) reported that the parallel combination of the percentage of increase in GGT, aspartate aminotransferase (SGOT), and alanine aminotransferase (SGPT) over posttreatment discharge values effectively distinguished recovering alcoholics who remained abstinent for three months from those who resumed drinking.

Another marker involves the mean corpuscular volume (MCV) of red blood cells, which increases with heavy alcohol consumption independent of liver damage (Gheno, Magnabosco, and Mazzei, 1979). Following the cessation of drinking, MCV returns very slowly to normal. Because an alcoholic may have been abstinent for a long period and still have an elevated MCV (Shaw et al., 1979), the usefulness of MCV as a marker for relapse is limited. Laboratory tests for such factors as GGT level and MCV reflect the consequences of alcoholism (i.e., tissue injury) rather than alcohol abuse. The tests of people who are abusing alcohol but have not yet developed organ damage will be normal, a consequence that explains the poor sensitivity of these tests. Other illnesses can also result in test abnormalities. Used by themselves, then, these tests do not have great sensitivity or specificity; however, the combinations used by Cushman and colleagues (1984) and Ryback and coworkers (1982) improve diagnostic accuracy.

High-density lipoprotein cholesterol (HDLC) levels also increase during drinking episodes and return to control levels within one to two weeks after the cessation of drinking (Devenyi et al., 1981). However, HDLC may not be suitable for monitoring drinking in patients with significant liver disease (cirrhosis or alcoholic hepatitis). Haskell, Camargo, and Williams (1984) reported that HDLC also falls significantly when moderate drinkers abstain and rises with the resumption of moderate drinking. Puddy and colleagues (1986) found similar results and, in addition, reported that apoliprotein A-I and A-II declined when moderate drinkers reduced their drinking from five drinks to one per day. Discriminant function analysis showed that a change in the serum apoliprotein A-II was the best of the markers compared by this group (apoliprotein A-I, HDLC, GGT, and MCV) for correctly classifying (with 96 percent accuracy) the category of drinking either five drinks or one.

Platelet monoamine oxidase has been reported to be lower in alcoholics (Wiberg, Gottfries, and Oreland, 1977; Major and Murphy, 1978; Alexopoulos et al., 1981), but this finding was not replicated in a more recent study (Tabakoff et al., 1988). The Tabakoff team also found that platelet adenylate cyclase activity, after stimulation with quanine nucleotide, cesium fluoride, or prostaglandin E, was significantly lower in alcoholics, although the basal platelet adenylate cyclase activity was the same in alcoholics and controls. Because the alcoholics in this study had been abstinent for one to four years, the utility of these markers for treatment outcome evaluation is uncertain.

There is currently considerable interest in two markers: (1) the hemoglobin acetaldahyde adduct (A1) factor and (2) deglycosylated transferrin. In one study (Hoberman and Chiodo, 1982), hemoglobin A1 was significantly elevated in alcoholic patients with and without liver disease compared with normal subjects, but there was some overlap between the two groups and levels returned to normal with abstinence. The duration of abstinence required for hemoglobin A1 to return to normal needs to be defined. Stibler, Borg, and Joustra (1986) have shown that "carbohydrate-deficient" transferrin is a specific marker for chronic drinking with a biologic half-life of approximately 17 days after cessation of alcohol ingestion. Behrens and coworkers (1988) have extended these observations on the specificity of "carbohydrate-deficient" transferrin from Swedish patients to different racial groups in the United States. However, the sensitivity of this marker may be a problem. The Takase research team (1985) found serum desialotransferrin in only 60 percent of Japanese alcoholics.

At this time, with the exception of frequent alcohol tests, biological markers either are not sensitive enough or need further evaluation before they can be used alone to monitor treatment outcome. Markers can be of value as part of an assessment battery that includes self-reports, reports by collateral informants, and official records.

The following opportunities for research on biological markers of treatment outcome should be pursued to improve the validity of treatment evaluation research:

- Researchers should develop and test markers that are sensitive to moderate and heavy alcohol consumption. Markers that return to normal with the cessation of drinking and show prompt elevation at the initiation of drinking would be particularly useful in treatment outcome studies.
- Another type of marker that should be developed and tested is one that is sensitive to cumulative ethanol intake but independent of alcohol-related tissue damage.

Automation of Data Collection

In recent years there has been an increasing trend toward the computerization of diagnostic interviews; that is, rather than using a paper-and-pencil instrument, software programs are written so that interview questions appear on a computer screen. The questions are read to the subject (alternatively, the subject may sit at the terminal and read them), and the response is keyed in, usually with a single number according to a prearranged code. There are numerous advantages to this technology, and it is likely to become increasingly popular.

Additional advantages and savings are realized if computerized interviews can be self-administered by research subjects. These advantages go beyond economy. For example, there is evidence that a computerized, self-administered examination involving interaction with a machine rather than another human may foster a greater degree of respondent candor (Lucas et al., 1977; Duffy and Waterton, 1984). Another possible advantage of the computer in clinical settings--perhaps one of the greatest potential advantages of automation--is in automating the collection of routine data as a research data base for "quasi-experimental" or even true experimental designs. There have been some attempts to form an accumulating data base out of routine examinations, but typically these have depended on the willingness of busy personnel to transfer their clinical observations to computer-readable forms, a labor-intensive rather than a labor-saving effort.

It has been demonstrated that paper-and-pencil structured interviews can be used successfully as a means of routine data collection in clinical settings and can even be acceptable to clinicians in such a context (Helzer et al., 1981). However, computerization does not merely make interviews and questionnaires more accessible and efficient by having structured interviews available for computer administration by lay or clinical interviewers. It also provides an electronic data base without additional labor. If patients can self-administer the interviews, an accumulating electronic data base would be provided at considerable savings of effort.

There are a number of opportunities for research on data collection. Answers to the following questions would be valuable in deciding whether to pursue a policy of increased automation of diagnostic interview data:

• What degree of clinical detail is ascertainable by using a self-administered, computerized format?

• Are subjects more or less likely to remember past symptoms or to report sensitive data when queried by a computer?

• How well do structured interviews perform on a computer administration format?

• Given the opportunity, would clinicians and investigators find self-administered interview data useful?

ASSESSMENT OF TREATMENT PROCESS, QUALITY, AND OUTCOME

Advances in assessment techniques have contributed to a more accurate estimation of the relative contributions of client characteristics, therapeutic interventions, program settings, and environmental variables to the success or failure of treatment.

Treatment Variables

The relevance of treatment research to policy and clinical practice is directly related to the ability of such research to evaluate the costs and effectiveness of different treatment interventions as they relate to specific types of individuals. The complexity of the problem of matching individuals to treatments is related to the complexity of the treatment system in which problem drinkers are typically processed. This system consists of a complex array of treatment settings (e.g., inpatient, outpatient, residential), therapeutic approaches (psychotherapy, AA, peer approaches), and treatment providers (e.g., psychotherapists, recovering alcoholics).

Often, clients are exposed to several different treatment providers and therapeutic approaches in the same setting, after which they move through a series of settings during the course of different stages of treatment and recovery. At the program level of analysis where setting, staff, and therapeutic approaches interact, the mix of experiences may overwhelm the individual contributions of specific treatment variables or components. Specification of treatment is also needed in terms of the duration and quality of exposure. Antabuse patients may have many treatment contacts, but the psychological impact of the contacts may be minimal. Alcoholics Anonymous (AA), on the other hand, may exert a profound effect on attitudes and behavior in a short time as a function of very intensive involvement of the alcoholic in the fellowship's group process.

Recent developments in treatment specification are likely to affect the design of new procedures for the measurement of treatment process and quality (McCrady and Sher, 1985). A number of instruments have been developed and validated for the purpose of studying characteristics of the treatment setting and process (Lettieri, Nelson, and Sayers, 1985). Aspects of treatment specification include the intensity and duration of services received, the type of therapeutic modality the patient is given, the personality and skills of the therapist, the emergence of a "therapeutic alliance" or partnership between patient and therapist, the characteristics of the setting, the competency of the program staff, the degree to which the treatment is delivered as ideally intended (its integrity), and the general atmosphere of the program as experienced by patients. These instruments include rating scales that are designed for trained observers to use to identify unique features of individual and group therapy, client rating forms that are used to assess the qualitative aspects of the services received, and facility inventories that provide a quantitative assessment of the structural properties of a program.

Behavioral and social researchers (McLellan et al., 1983; Pattison, 1985) have argued that traditional outcome assessment methods are too global and imprecise to provide an adequate evaluation of client-treatment matches. This criticism is based on evidence that therapeutic change is multidimensional and that affecting different dimensions requires different types of treatment. There is a growing consensus (Emrick and Hansen, 1983) that, at a minimum, treatment outcome should be evaluated according to the following dimensions: drug and alcohol use, vocational adjustment, psychological problem severity, interpersonal relations, and criminal behavior. Another important trend in the specification of outcome variables has been the growing attention to process measures (Moos and Finney, 1985). Process analysis focuses attention on the causal linkages between treatment components and dimensions of outcome. In general, little research has been devoted to the short-term impact of specific program components such as alcohol education, AA groups, and individual counseling. Short-term gains, such as the information acquired regarding the negative consequences of drinking, changes in attitude toward alcohol, and improvements in psychological adjustment, can be assessed quite readily by means of brief tests and rating scales at the termination of inpatient treatment or immediately following a prescribed period of outpatient treatment.

At present, there is a strong need to apply these newly developed techniques of specifying treatment quality, process, and outcomes to identification of the active ingredients of traditional and experimental treatment interventions. The following areas should be explored in research on treatment process and outcome variables:

- What are the active ingredients of therapeutic interventions, including AA, cognitive-behavioral therapy, and so on?
- Do the various standard components of currently available multimodal rehabilitation programs (e.g., patient education, Twelve Steps groups) produce short-term changes in the patient's attitudes, motivation, and skills that predict long-term remission?
- Markers of compliance with treatment should be developed and tested to facilitate the evaluation of drug therapies. For example, riboflavin markers that can be placed in placebo and active medication can be used to detect compliance with drug therapy. Carbon disulfide breath analysis has a potential for evaluating compliance with disulfiram therapy.

GROWING SOPHISTICATION IN METHODOLOGICAL APPROACHES

In recent years, a variety of research approaches have been developed for use in treatment evaluation. As portrayed in Table 8-1, a basic distinction is often made between two types of research strategies: true experimental designs and quasi-experimental designs (Campbell and Stanley, 1963).

Table 8-1. Methodological Approaches to Alcoholism Treatment Evaluation Research

Populations Sampled From	Research Design	
	Descriptive/Quasi-Experimental	Experimental
One Facility	"Before-After"/ Outcome prediction studies	Preclinical studies Small-scale random assignment studies
Several Facilities	Multisite, multiprogram random sample studies Multisite, multiprogram nonrandom sample studies	Multicenter clinical trials
All Facilities	Aggregate-level descriptive studies	

Experimental Approaches

True experimental designs attempt to rule out all or most of the obvious confounding variables by randomly assigning subjects to experimental and control treatments. Preclinical studies are usually performed on small groups of patients (or animals) to establish a causal linkage between some treatment procedure (e.g., emetine) and a measure that should logically be associated with treatment outcome (e.g., conditioned aversion to alcohol). Small-scale random assignment studies operate at a broader level of analysis, by taking defined treatment modalities or programs and comparing them to no treatment, minimal treatment, or alternative treatments. Multicenter clinical trials represent the culmination of preclinical and small-scale studies.

Quasi-Experimental Approaches

In the alcohol field, true experimental designs, especially multicenter clinical trials, are difficult and expensive to carry out. This may explain why there have been numerous quasi-experimental studies in which researchers have explored treatment questions by weaving a net of circumstantial evidence around the observed associations between client characteristics and differential treatment response. The quasi-experiment is a design in which a variety of strategies other than random assignment are used to minimize the influence of confounding variables. One approach has been to gather treatment and outcome data from a large number of patients who are being treated at different facilities or who have been exposed to different therapeutic modalities (multisite, multiprogram studies). Typically, the patients are not randomly assigned to these conditions, and the research is often designed to answer questions other than those dealing with treatment matching (e.g., Cronkite and Moos, 1980). To control for the influence of major confounding variables, multivariate statistical procedures such as covariance analyses and partial correlation are used.

Although the literature is not lacking in multisite, multiprogram prediction studies (Armor, Polich, and Stambul, 1978; Brown and Lyons, 1981; McLellan et al., 1983), it is important to note the limitations of previous research. First, most prediction studies have been limited to small samples drawn from a small number of unrepresentative treatment settings. Second, even when researchers have sampled patients across multiple settings, only a few studies have considered the characteristics of the setting as well as the quality and types of treatment received; even fewer have conducted extensive evaluations of patient characteristics. Primarily because of logistical problems and the costs of conducting this type of research, there has been an inverse relationship between the number of patients studied and the amount of data collected.

Aggregate-Level Descriptive Studies

In recent years, several attempts have been made to conduct general facility surveys as a means of generating descriptive statistics about the national configuration of alcoholism treatment services (Yahr, 1988). These inventories include the National Drug and Alcoholism Treatment Utilization Survey (NDATUS), the American Hospital Association Annual Survey, and surveys conducted by the National Association of State Alcohol and Drug Abuse Directors and the National Association of Alcoholism Treatment Programs. The most comprehensive aggregate-level descriptive survey is the NDATUS, which has been conducted periodically by NIAAA since 1979. Survey forms for the NDATUS were distributed to all known treatment units in the United States in 1979, 1980, and 1982. A shorter survey, the National Alcoholism and Drug Abuse Program Inventory (NDAPI), was conducted in 1984 to define the universe of facilities that could later be used for more specialized sampling studies.

These surveys have been designed to serve different functions, including resource planning and management on the state and federal levels; the generation of cross-sectional and longitudinal data on treatment utilization, staffing, funding, and length of stay; and the description of characteristics of programs, clients, and ownership of the facilities. In the case of the NDATUS, budgetary considerations have led to a drastic reduction in the amount of data collected; nevertheless, the abbreviated version (the NDAPI) sets the stage for more detailed surveys using random or stratified sampling techniques. The potential for weeding the more intensive, client-focused, multiprogram study designs to large-scale, representative sample surveys could constitute a significant advance in the treatment evaluation knowledge base.

At present, the NDATUS is a brief questionnaire that requires the reporting unit to give its primary orientation (alcoholism, drug abuse, mixed), physical environment or setting (e.g., hospital, freestanding unit), population served (e.g., inner city, suburban), kinds of services provided (e.g., group therapy, education, aftercare), ownership characteristics, staffing patterns, and client census capacity. In addition, current patients are recorded according to race/ethnicity, age, and sex. Descriptive data obtained from the NDATUS applications have been extremely useful in describing characteristics of different treatment systems and identifying changes and trends over time (Yahr, 1988). Although the NDATUS is lacking in most of the client and treatment variables now considered crucial to a proper understanding of treatment efficacy and efficiency, these data could be collected simultaneously from staff, administrators, and clients to provide a more comprehensive description of the services received by different types of clients. The final ingredient of such an approach is the measurement of short-term and long-term treatment gains by using periodic interviews with selected samples of patients at various intervals during and after treatment. Another approach, exemplified in the Epidemiologic Catchment Area Study (Helzer and Pryzbeck, 1988), is to gather data about drinking behavior and treatment use from general published samples and compare these data with those collected from representative treatment settings.

As shown in Table 8-1, the research findings emanating from preclinical, experimental, quasi-experimental, and descriptive research approaches should provide a comprehensive and complementary understanding of the many facets of alcohol problem treatment. Eventually, the active components of the most effective treatment should be identified, leading to a more systematic program of clinical trials that will provide a more definitive test of treatment efficacy, especially in relation to different client types, than has heretofore been possible (Finney and Moos, 1986).

Many opportunities exist for research employing complementary methodologic approaches. The considerations noted above suggest the following programmatic recommendations for funding agencies, research centers, and investigators:

• The new generation of assessment technologies should be employed to evaluate treatment efficacy by means of innovative research methods. Experimental, quasi-experimental, and naturalistic research designs each have their place in treatment evaluation.
• Descriptive studies of the treatment system at the aggregate level of analysis can provide valuable information about changes in the client population, variations in substance-use patterns, trends in program characteristics, and new approaches to treatment. Health services research should be encouraged as the first step toward an integrated program of descriptive and experimental research that will eventually lead to multicenter clinical trials of promising treatment interventions.
• Experimental research designs should be encouraged for alcoholism treatment evaluations whenever appropriate. When experimental designs are employed, there must be adequate specification of the client, program setting, therapist, and treatment variables that affect patient compliance and outcome. When experimental designs are not feasible because of ethical or practical constraints, the new generation of asessment technology should be employed to evaluate treatment efficacy by means of innovative, nonexperimental research methods.
• At times, program evaluation data have been used to support claims that one type of treatment is superior to a lack of treatment or to some comparison treatment. "Success" rates of 80 to 90 percent have been used in media advertisements to solicit patients to proprietary treatment programs. Outcome monitoring studies that do not meet acceptable criteria for making causal inferences have been used to justify requests for insurance reimbursement of unevaluated treatments. At present, there is a significant risk of

misinterpretation in the use of unsound research designs in studies sponsored by individuals or corporations that have a financial interest in the results. Whenever possible, evaluation research should be designed and conducted by investigators who are not likely to benefit from the result either materially or professionally.

REFERENCES

Alexopoulos, G. S., K. Lieberman, I. Frances, and P. Stokes. Platelet MAO during the alcohol withdrawal syndrome. Am. J. Psych. 136:1245-1250, 1981.

American Psychiatric Association. Diagnostic and Statistical Manual of Mental Disorders (DSM-III), 3d ed. Washington, DC: APA, 1980.

American Psychiatric Association. Diagnostic and Statistical Manual of Mental Disorders (DSM-III), 3d ed., rev. Washington, DC: APA, 1987.

Aneshensel, C. S., A. L. Estrada, M. J. H. Hansell et al. Social psychological aspectsof reporting behavior: Lifetime depressive episode reports. J. Health Soc. Behav. 28:232-246, 1987.

Annis, H. M., and C. S. Davis. Assessment of expectancies in alcohol dependent clients. In A. Marlatt and D. Donovan, eds. Assessment of Addictive Behaviors. New York: Guilford Press, 1987.

Armor, D. J., J. M. Polich, and H. B. Stambul. Alcoholism and Treatment. New York: John Wiley and Sons, 1978.

Babor, T. F., N. L. Cooney, and R. J. Lauerman. The drug dependence syndrome concept as a psychological theory of relapse behavior: An empirical evaluation. Br. J. Addiction 82:393-405, 1987.

Babor, T. F., R. S. Stephens, and G. A. Marlatt. Verbal report methods in clinical research on alcoholism: Response bias and its minimalization. J. Stud. Alcohol 48(5):410-424, 1987.

Behrens, U. J., T. M. Worner, L. F. Braly et al. Carbohydrate-deficient transferrin, a marker for chronic alcohol consumption in different ethnic populations. Alcoholism: Clin. Exper. Res. 12:427-432, 1988.

Bradburn, N. M. Response effects. Pp. 289-328 in P. E. Rossi and J. D. Wright, eds. Handbook of Survey Research. New York: Academic Press, 1983.

Brown, J., and J. P. Lyons. A progressive diagnostic schema for alcoholism witevidence of clinical efficacy. Alcoholism: Clinical and Experimental Research 5(1):17-25, 1981.

Brown, S. A., M. S. Goldman, A. Inn et al. Expectations of reinforcement from alcohol: Their domain and relation to drinking patterns. J. Consult. Clin. Psychol. 48:419-426, 1980.

Campbell, D., and J. Stanley. Experimental and Quasi-Experimental Designs for Research. Chicago: Rand McNally, 1963.

Cannell, C. F. A Summary of Studies of Interviewing Methodology. USDHEW Publ. No. (HRA) 77-1343, Series II, No. 69. Washington, DC: U.S. Department of Health, Education, and Welfare, 1977.

Cloninger, C. R. Neurogenetic adaptive mechanisms in alcoholism. Science 236:410-416, 1987.

Coryell, W., C. R. Cloninger, and T. Reich. Clinical assessment: Use of nonphysician interviews. J. Nerv. Ment. Dis. 166:599-606, 1978.

Cronkite, R. C., and R. H. Moos. Determinants of the posttreatment functioning of alcoholic patients: A conceptual framework. J. Consult. Clin. Psychol. 48:305-316, 1980.

Crowne, D. P., and D. Marlowe. A new scale of social desirability independent of psychopathology. J. Consult. Psychol. 24:349-354, 1960.

Cushman, P., G. Jacobson, J. J. Barboriak, and A. J. Anderson. Biochemical markers for alcoholism: Sensitivity problems. Alcohol Clin. Exp. Res. 8:253-257, 1984.

Devenyi, P., G. M. Robinson, B. M. Kapur et al. High density lipoprotein cholesterol in male alcoholics with and without severe liver disease. Am. J. Med. 71:589-594, 1981.

Duffy, J. C., and J. J. Waterton. Under-reporting of alcohol consumption in sample surveys: The effect of computer interviewing in fieldwork. Br. J. Addict. 79:303-308, 1984.

Edwards, G. The alcohol dependence syndrome: A concept as stimulus to enquiry. Br. J. Addict. 81:171-183, 1986.

Edwards, G., A. Arif, and R. Hodgson. Nomenclature and classification of drug and alcohol related problems: A WHO memorandum. Bull. World Health Organization 59(2):225-242, 1981.

Emrick, C. D., and J. Hansen. Assertions regarding effectiveness of treatment for alcoholism: Fact or fantasy? Am. Psychol. 38:1078-1088, 1983.

Finney, J. W., and R. H. Moos. Matching patients with treatments: Conceptual and methodological issues. J. Stud. Alcohol 47:122-134, 1986.

Frank, B. Telephone surveying for drug abuse: Methodological issues and an application. Pp. 71-83 in B. A. Rouse, N. J. Kozel, and L. G. Richards, eds. Self-Report Methods of Estimating Drug Use: Meeting Current Challenges to Validity. NIDA Research Monograph No. 57. Rockville, MD: National Institute for Drug Abuse, 1985.

Gfroerer, J. Influence of privacy on self-reported drug abuse by youths. Pp. 22-30 in B. A. Rouse, N. J. Kozel, and L. G. Richards, eds. Self-Report Methods of Estimating Drug Use: Meeting Current Challenges to Validity. NIDA Research Monograph No. 57. Rockville, MD: National Institute for Drug Abuse, 1985.

Gheno, G., V. Magnabosco, and G. Mazzei. Macrocitosi ed anemia nell'alcoholismo cronico. Min. Med. 3:1301-1306, 1979.

Haskell, W. L., C. Camargo, and P. T. Williams. The effect of cessation and resumption of moderate alcohol intake on serum high density lipoprotein subfractions: A controlled study. New Engl. J. Med. 310:805-810, 1984.

Hedlund, J. L., and B. W. Vieweg. The Michigan Alcoholism Screening Test (MAST): A comprehensive review. J. Operational Psychiat. 15:55-64, 1984.

Helzer, J. E., and T. R. Pryzbeck. The co-occurrence of alcoholism with other psychiatric disorders in the general population and its impact on treatment. J. Stud. Alcohol 49:219-224, 1988.

Helzer, J. E., L. N. Robins, J. L. Croughan et al. Renard Diagnostic Interview: Its reliability and procedural validity with physicians and lay interviewers. Arch. Gen. Psych. 38:393-398, 1981.

Hoberman, H. D., and S. M. Chiodo. Elevation of the hemoglobin A1 fraction in alcoholism. Alcoholism: Clin. Exper. Research 6:260-266, 1982.

Institute of Medicine, Division of Health Promotion and Disease Prevention. Alcoholism, Alcohol Abuse, and Related Problems: Opportunities for Research. Washington, DC: National Academy Press, 1980.

Irwin, M., S. Baird, T. Smith, and M. Schuckit. Use of laboratory tests to monitor heavy drinking by alcoholic men discharged from a treatment program. Am. J. Psych. 145:5, 1988.

Lettieri, D. J., J. E. Nelson, and M. A. Sayers, eds. Alcoholism Treatment Assessment Research Instruments. NIAAA Handbook Series, vol. 2. DHHS Publ. No. (ADM) 85-1380. Washington, DC: NIAAA, 1985.

Luborsky, L., and A. T. McLellan. Optimal matching of patients with types of psychotherapy: What is known and some designs for knowing more. Pp. 51-71 in E. Gottheil, A. T. McLellan, and K. A. Druley, eds. Matching Patient Needs and Treatment Methods in Alcoholism and Drug Abuse. Springfield, IL: Charles C. Thomas, 1981.

Lucas, R. W., P. J. Mullin, C. B. Luna et al. Psychiatrists and a computer as interrogators of patients with alcohol-related illnesses: A comparison. Br. J. Psychiatry 131:160-167, 1977.

Major, L. F., and D. Murphy. Platelet and plasma amine oxidase activity in alcoholic individuals. Br. J. Psychiatry 132:548-554, 1978.

Marlatt, G. A., and W. R. Miller. Comprehensive Drinker Profile. Odessa, FL: Psychological Assessment Resources, 1984.

McCrady, B., and K. Sher. Treatment variables. Pp.48-62 in B. S. McCrady, N. E. Noel, and T. D. Nirenberg, eds. Future Directions in Alcohol Abuse Treatment Research. Research Monograph No. 15. USDHHS Publ. No. (ADM)85-1322. Washington, DC: U.S. Department of Health and Human Services, 1985.

McLellan, A. T., L. Luborsky, F. Erdlen et al. The Addiction Severity Index. Pp. 178-194 in E. Gottheil, A. T. McLellan, and K. D. Druley, eds. Substance Abuse and Psychiatric Illness. New York: Pergamon Press, 1980.

McLellan, A. T., L. Luborsky, G. E. Woody et al. Predicting response to alcohol and drug abuse treatments. Arch. Gen. Psychiatry 40:620-625, 1983.

Meyer, R. E., T. F. Babor, M. Hesselbrock et al. New directions in the assessment of the alcoholic patient. In L. H. Towle, ed. Proceedings: NIAAA-WHO Collaborating Center Designation Meeting and Alcohol Research Seminar. DHHS Publ. No. (ADM)85-1370. Washington, DC: U.S. Department of Health and Human Services, 1985.

Miller, F., and A. Barasch. The under-reporting of alcohol use: The role of organic mental syndromes. Drug Alcohol Depend. 15:347-351, 1985.

Moos, R. H., and J. W. Finney. New directions in program evaluation: Implications for expanding the role of alcoholism researchers. Pp. 173-203 in B. S. McCrady, N. E. Noel, and T. D. Nirenberg, eds. Future Directions in Alcohol Abuse Treatment Research. Research Monograph No. 15. DHHS Publ. No. (ADM)85-1322. Washington, DC: U.S. Department of Health and Human Services, 1985.

O'Farrell, T. J., and S. A. Maisto. The utility of self-report and biological measures of alcohol consumption in alcoholism treatment outcome studies. Adv. Behav. Res. Ther. 9:91-125, 1987.

Orrego, H., L. M. Blendis, J. E. Blake et al. Reliability of assessments of alcohol intake based on personal interviews in a liver clinic. Lancet 2:1354-1356, 1979.

Othmer, E., B. J. Powell, and E. C. Penick. Psychiatric Diagnostic Interview (PDI), 9th rev. Kansas City, KS: University of Kansas Medical Center, 1980.

Pattison, E. M. New directions in alcoholism treatment goals. Pp.7-26 in B. S. McCrady, N. E. Noel, and T. D. Nirenberg, eds. Future Directions in Alcohol Abuse Treatment Research. Research Monograph No. 15. DHHS Publ. No. (ADM)85-1322. Washington, DC: U.S. Department of Health and Human Services, 1985.

Phillips, M. Sweat patch testing detects inaccurate self-reports of alcohol consumption. Alcoholism: Clin. Exper. Research 8:51-53, 1984.

Polich, J. M., D. J. Armor, and H. B. Braiker. The Course of Alcoholism: Four Years After Treatment. New York: John Wiley and Sons, 1981.

Puddy, I. B., J. Masarei, R. Vandongen, and L. J. Beilin. Serum apoliprotein A-II as a marker of change in alcohol intake in male drinkers. Alcohol and Alcoholism 21:375-383, 1986.

Robins, L. N., J. E. Helzer, J. Croughan et al. National Institute of Mental Health Diagnostic Interview Schedule: Its history, characteristics, and validity. Arch. Gen. Psych. 38:381-389, 1981.

Robins, L. N., J. Wing, H. U. Wittchen et al. The Composite International Diagnostic Interview. Arch. Gen. Psych. 45:1069-1077, 1988.

Rounsaville, B. J., Z. S. Dolinsky, T. F. Babor et al. Psychopathology as a predictor of treatment outcome in alcoholics. Arch. Gen. Psych. 44:505-513, 1987.

Ryback, R. S., M. J. Eckhardt, B. Felsher, and R. R. Rawlings. Biochemical and hematological correlates of alcoholism and liver disease. J. Am. Med. Assoc. 248:2261-2265, 1982.

Saunders, S., O. G. Aasland, and M. Grant. AUDIT--The World Health Organization screening instrument for harmful and hazardous alcohol consumption. Br. J. Addiction, in press.

Shaw, S., and C. S. Lieber. Mechanism of increased gamma glutamyl transpeptidase after chronic alcohol consumption: Hepatic microsomal induction rather than dietary imbalance. Substance and Alcohol Actions/Misuse 1:423-428, 1980.

Shaw, S., T. M. Warner, M. F. Borysow et al. Detection of alcoholism relapse: Comparative diagnostic value of MVC, GGTp, and AANB. Alcoholism: Clin. Exper. Research 3:297-301, 1979.

Skinner, H. A., and B. A. Allen. Does the computer make a difference? Computerized versus face-to-face self-report assessments of alcohol, drug and tobacco use. J. Consult. Clin. Psychol. 51:267-275, 1983.

Skinner, H. A., and J. L. Horn. Alcohol Dependence Scale (ADS) User's Guide. Toronto: Addiction Research Foundation, 1984.

Sobell, L. C., and M. B. Sobell Effects of three interview factors on the validity of alcohol abusers' self-reports. Am. J. Drug Alcohol Abuse 8:225-237, 1981.

Sobell, M. B., L. C. Sobell et al. The reliability of timeline method for assessing normal drinker college students' recent drinking history: Utility for alcohol research. Addict. Behav. 11:149-161, 1986.

Spitzer, R. L., J. B. W. Williams, and A. E. Skodol. International Perspectives on DSM-III. Washington, DC: American Psychiatric Press, 1983.

Stibler, H., S. Borg, and M. Joustra. Microanion exchange chromatography of "carbohydrate deficient" transferrin (CDT) in serum in relation to alcohol consumption. Alcoholism: Clin. Exper. Res. 10:535-544, 1986.

Stockwell, T., D. Murphy, and R. Hodgson. The severity of alcohol dependence questionnaire: Its usefulness, reliability and validity. Br. J. Addict. 78:145-155, 1983.

Tabakoff, B., P. L. Hoffman, K. W. Lieberman et al. Differences in platelet enzyme activity between alcoholics and nonalcoholics. New Engl. J. Med. 318:134-139, 1988.

Takase, S., A. Takada, M. Tsutsumi, and Y. Matsuda. Biochemical markers of chronic alcoholism. Alcohol 2:405-410, 1985.

VandenBos, G. R. Psychotherapy research: A special issue. Am. Psychol. 41:111-112, 1986.

Wanberg, K. W., J. L. Horn, and F. M. Fisher. A differential model of alcoholism: The scales of the Alcohol Use Inventory. J. Stud. Alcohol 38:512-543, 1977.

Wiberg, A., C. G. Gottfries, and L. Oreland. Low platelet monamine oxidase activity in human alcoholics. Med. Biol. 55:181-186, 1977.

World Health Organization. Draft revision of Chapter 5, Categories F00-F99, Mental, behavioral, and developmental disorders: Clinical descriptions and diagnostic guidelines. In International Classification of Diseases, 10th ed. Geneva: WHO, 1988.

Yahr, H. T. A national comparison of public and private sector alcoholism treatment delivery system characteristics. J. Stud. Alcohol 49:233-239, 1988.

9

TREATMENT MODALITIES: PROCESS AND OUTCOME

Evaluation research represents a key to the advancement of therapeutic effectiveness in alcohol treatment. Since 1980, more than 250 new studies have been published reporting outcome data on various approaches to the treatment of alcohol problems. This body of research has provided important new knowledge regarding optimal approaches to alcohol treatment, in addition to clarifying areas in which further research is most needed.

A major continuing problem for the field is a gap between available knowledge and current practice. Much of what is presently done in alcohol treatment has not been evaluated; thus, the efficacy of standard components of many current treatment programs has not been established. Other approaches for which there is promising evidence of effectiveness remain largely unused in treatment.

In an effort to close this gap, the sections below survey research focusing on a number of topics of interest: specific treatment approaches, traditional treatment programs, the intensity and duration of treatment, aftercare, and the treatment process itself. In the final section, the committee presents its conclusions and summarizes the opportunities for further progress in treatment research.

OUTCOME RESEARCH ON SPECIFIC TREATMENT APPROACHES

Most of the studies conducted since 1980 have focused on the effectiveness of particular treatment approaches or programs. This research includes many uncontrolled studies but also more than 60 studies that use controlled designs and more methodologically sophisticated approaches. "Controlled" studies comprise those employing randomization or matching procedures to assign individuals to alternative treatment methods or to treatment versus control conditions. Uncontrolled studies typically report outcome data following a single intervention, or employ quasi-experimental designs (Cook and Campbell, 1979) to provide partial control of extraneous variables. Although both types of research can yield informative findings, controlled studies are less subject to confounding and tend to produce more reliable and interpretable results. In this review, therefore, greater emphasis will be placed on the findings of properly controlled evaluations.

Evaluations of interventions for alcohol problems can also be divided according to the point at which intervention occurs. Preventive interventions, generally administered prior to the onset of serious alcohol problems, are discussed in Part I of this report. Within formal treatment, three phases can be distinguished: (1) detoxification, (2) active treatment and rehabilitation, and (3) relapse prevention.

Intervention procedures during the first phase, detoxification, are designed to carry the individual safely through the process of alcohol withdrawal, minimizing the risks associated with the abstinence syndrome for those who are more severely dependent on alcohol. Detoxification typically yields little or no long-term change in alcohol consumption and related problems and is usually viewed as a prelude to active treatment.

Phase 2, active treatment, seeks to bring about change in the individual's use of alcohol and other drugs and to reduce problems associated with that use. Typically, the goal of treatment programs has been total abstention from alcohol and other drugs of abuse. A wide range of treatment strategies is available to achieve this goal, and research on these alternative modalities is discussed in the subsections below. After each discussion are questions that identify opportunities for research in these treatment areas.

During the 1980s, increased attention has been devoted to the importance of relapse prevention as a third phase of treatment. The goal of these efforts is to help the individual avoid a relapse to previous patterns of problematic drinking. When this phase follows inpatient treatment, it is sometimes called aftercare. In essence, relapse prevention is a logical extension of treatment efforts in that it attempts to sustain and stabilize the beneficial changes that have occurred during the initial phases of treatment. Relapse prevention strategies have been incorporated into treatment programs. Principles underlying some of these strategies are described in Chapter 3. In this section of the report, they are discussed among the alternative treatment modalities.

Pharmacotherapies

The use of medications in the treatment of alcohol problems can be divided into three major strategies. Antidipsotropic medications cause adverse results when alcohol is consumed. Their intended effect is to suppress drinking. Effect-altering medications likewise are intended to suppress alcohol consumption but through a different mechanism. Rather than precipitating aversive reactions to alcohol, these medications are designed to diminish the reinforcing or intoxicating properties of ethanol. Psychotropic medications, by contrast, are designed to treat such concomitant disorders as depression, psychosis, or anxiety. Their intended effect is to alleviate psychopathology that may accompany alcohol abuse, thereby diminishing the likelihood of relapse to drinking and improving the person's overall functioning.

Antidipsotropics

Within the United States, the principal antidipsotropic agent is disulfiram (Antabuse). Taken on a regular basis, disulfiram induces an adverse reaction of variable severity if the person consumes alcohol. New studies have provided mixed evidence regarding the usefulness of disulfiram in promoting improvement. Like earlier research, recent studies (e.g., Duckert and Johnsen, 1987; Thurston, Alfano, and Nerviano, 1987) have reported a relationship between voluntary compliance with disulfiram and favorable treatment outcome. In such investigations, however, medication effects were confounded with individual difference variables affecting motivation and compliance.

Several new controlled trials have failed to show benefits from disulfiram. Powell and colleagues (1985) found no differences in outcome over 12 months of follow-up among groups that were assigned at random to receive medication (disulfiram plus the option of chlordiazepoxide), medication plus supportive counseling, or a control group receiving only monitoring of medical problems. In studies of alcoholics who were being treated in Veterans Administration methadone clinics, Ling and coworkers (1983) observed no differences in abstinence, treatment compliance, or breath test results between groups that were randomly assigned to receive disulfiram and those assigned to receive a placebo.

Schuckit (1985) also reported no difference in the 12-month outcome between alcoholics who were prescribed and agreed to take disulfiram and those who refused to take it.

Recent research further suggests that most or all of the therapeutic impact of disulfiram prescription (at least without compliance assurance) may not be attributable to specific medication effects. Fuller and Williford (1980), in a urinalysis of a randomized clinical trial, reported that two groups of alcoholics who were given disulfiram showed significantly higher abstinence rates at 12 months, compared with those who were given no disulfiram. Only one of the two medicated groups received a therapeutic dose, however, whereas the other was given only 1 milligram (mg), an inert dose. Thus, both groups who believed they were receiving disulfiram showed higher abstinence rates.

In the largest and most carefully designed clinical trial of disulfiram to date, Fuller and coworkers (1986) replicated their earlier study in a nine-site collaborative research program. Outpatient alcoholics were again randomly assigned to receive 250 mg (therapeutic) doses, 1 mg (inert) doses of disulfiram, or a vitamin supplement and no disulfiram. Over 12 months of follow-up, the three groups did not differ on measures of total abstinence, employment, or social stability. Compliance with medication (even the inert dose or the vitamin supplement) was highly associated with abstinence. Within the subgroup of individuals who were highly compliant with research procedures and provided complete data, those given the therapeutic dose reported significantly fewer drinking days than their counterparts in the two control groups.

Other studies have employed the surgical implantation of disulfiram in an attempt to avoid problems with compliance. Wilson, Davidson, and Blanchard (1980) found a substantially higher rate of abstinence in two groups undergoing surgical operations--one for the implantation of disulfiram, the other for an inert implant-- relative to a random control group that was given no operation. No difference in outcome was observed between the disulfiram and inert implant groups. Johnsen and colleagues (1987) similarly found no differences in a double-blind randomization study comparing disulfiram and inert implantation. The failure of disulfiram implants to show a specific medication effect, however, may be due to the low probability of a disulfiram-ethanol reaction, even when the person drinks (Wilson et al., 1984; Johnsen et al., 1987). Future research may discover more effective methods administering long-acting doses of disulfiram. A danger attached to long-acting parenteral administration, however, is the difficulty of reversing an acute disulfiram-ethanol reaction if the individual consumes alcohol.

Thus, at present, oral administration is the standard procedure for administering antidipsotropics in the United States, and compliance is a crucial issue in the effectiveness of oral disulfiram. Recent studies have found few or no differences between disulfiram accepters and refusers on the basis of personality and demographic variables (O'Neil et al., 1982; Schuckit, 1985), which suggests that contextual or attitudinal factors may be important determinants of compliance (Brubaker, Prue, and Rychtarik, 1987). Motivational strategies to promote medication compliance appear to increase the impact of disulfiram treatment. Azrin and coworkers (1982) tested a simple disulfiram assurance procedure whereby the alcoholic took the medication daily in the presence of a significant other who provided praise and support for compliance. At the six-month follow-up point, those in the disulfiram assurance group showed substantially better outcomes than randomly chosen controls for whom disulfiram was prescribed but who were given no compliance intervention. The difference was greatest for married persons, perhaps because of the spouse's availability to serve as the reinforcing partner.

In another study, Kofoed (1987) found that a chemical monitoring system to verify disulfiram intake increased medication compliance in a controlled trial but did not affect compliance with other aspects of treatment. Keane and colleagues (1984) reported favorable results with a home-based disulfiram compliance program that involved monitoring and contracting with the spouse. Determination of the effects of mandated monitoring of disulfiram compliance on long-term outcomes, either by chemical testing or by direct observation (e.g., Sereny et al., 1986), has not yet been evaluated in a properly controlled trial.

Calcium carbimide, an alternative antidipsotropic medication, has been tested in other countries but has not yet been approved for therapeutic use in the United States. A pharmacologic comparison of carbimide and disulfiram indicated similar adverse reactions when alcohol is consumed, with the carbimide-ethanol reaction being somewhat more severe (Peachey et al., 1983). However, the pharmacodynamics of carbimide differ significantly from those of disulfiram. The more rapid onset and increased intensity of aversive effect with carbimide may offer advantages for certain therapeutic applications. Peachey and Annis (1985) proposed its use as part of a relapse prevention procedure whereby an individual could take it acutely in anticipation of a high-risk situation. Furthermore, carbimide appears to be less toxic and to yield fewer side effects than disulfiram (Peachey and Annis, 1984). Well-controlled clinical trials of carbimide have not yet been reported. If future trials reflect positive outcomes, however, carbimide should be made available in the United States as an alternative pharmacotherapeutic agent for the treatment of alcohol problems.

The potential benefits of antidipsotropics must be weighed against their side effects and the potential hazards associated with their longer term use, particularly in light of studies reflecting no differences between medication and control groups. Recent reports suggest that antidipsotropic medication may increase sexual dysfunction (Snyder, Karacan, and Salis, 1981; Jensen, 1984) and a craving for alcohol (Nirenberg et al., 1983; Stockwell, Sutherland, and Edwards, 1984), in addition to other commonly reported side effects. However, at least one double-blind study found no differences in side effects between disulfiram and placebo groups (Christensen, Ronsted, and Vaag, 1984).

The following questions represent opportunities for research on antidipsotropic medications:

• What motivational procedures most effectively increase compliance with antidipsotropic medications?
• What are optimal combinations of antidipsotropic medication with other treatment strategies?
• What are the characteristics of individuals who accept and respond favorably to the various classes of antidipsotropic medications?
• What are the effects of mandatory monitoring of compliance with antidipsotropics? Does this procedure increase abstinence during and after the period of mandatory monitoring?
• What are the effects of various antidipsotropic medications on subjective desire and craving for alcohol?
• What methods of administration, if any, could be used safely to sustain effective and long-acting doses of antidipsotropic medications?

Effect-Altering Medications

Effect-altering medications reduce the reinforcing properties of ethanol without producing illness. Rockman and coworkers (1979) reported that zimelidine, a serotonin uptake inhibitor, diminished alcohol intake by animals in a free-choice drinking paradigm. Similar results have been reported in rodent studies of other serotonin uptake inhibitors including norzimelidine, citalopram, alaproclate, fluoxetine, indalpine, viqualine, and fluvoxamine. In studies with nondepressed, nondependent, heavy-drinking humans, zimelidine and citalopram have been found to reduce alcohol intake (Naranjo et al., 1984, 1987).

The principal effect of zimelidine was found to be an increase in the number of abstinent days for heavy drinkers. Moreover, zimelidine was effective within the first two weeks of treatment, before its antidepressant effects normally occur (Naranjo et al., 1984). Amit and colleagues (1985) found that drinkers given a single dose of zimelidine reported a reduced euphoriant effect from alcohol as well as a decreased desire to drink. These effects of zimelidine may be due to an effect on the reinforcing properties of ethanol or to a generalized suppressant effect on both food and alcohol consumption (Gill and Amit, 1987).

Because zimelidine produced flulike symptoms and neuropathy in a significant number of subjects who were being treated for depression, it has been withdrawn from human use. Other serotonin uptake inhibitors such as fluoxetine and fluvoxamine would appear to be reasonable candidates for therapeutic trial in alcoholic patients (Linnoila, et al., 1987) but thus far have been tested only in heavy drinkers. Fluoxetine does not act synergistically with alcohol on physiologic, psychometric, or psychomotor activity; it also does not increase blood alcohol levels (Lemberger et al., 1985). Recent work by E. M. Sellers of the Addiction Research Foundation of Ontario (personal communication, 1988) suggests that fluoxetine affects the initiation of drinking behavior as opposed to moderating drinking episodes. Fluvoxamine is approximately three times as selective in serotonin uptake inhibition (relative to norepinephrine reuptake) as zimelidine. At the time of this report, one serotonin uptake inhibitor (fluoxetine) has been approved for the treatment of depressive disorders in the United States.

Effect-altering medications could be used in the treatment of alcohol-dependent persons much as opiate antagonists have been used in treating opiate addiction. It may be useful to combine such pharmacotherapy with psychological interventions designed to enhance motivation and medication compliance.

The following questions represent opportunities for research on effect-altering medications:

   • What is the impact of various effect-altering medications on subjective desires and cravings for alcohol and on the perceived reinforcing effects of alcohol consumption?
   • What motivational procedures most effectively increase compliance with effect-altering medications?
   • What are the side effects and long-term risks involved in the use of various effect-altering medications?
   • Do effect-altering medications promote long-term sobriety?
   • What is an optimal duration for treatment with effect-altering medications to maximize therapeutic effects while minimizing side effects and medication-related risks?

• What are the characteristics of individuals who accept and respond favorably to various classes of effect-altering medications?

• What are optimal combinations of effect-altering medications and other treatment strategies?

Psychotropics

Psychotropic medications have three potential uses in the treatment of alcohol problems. First, certain medications are of demonstrated utility during alcohol detoxification (Liskow and Goodwin, 1987). The usefulness of such medications during acute withdrawal is now generally accepted, although detoxification can often be accomplished without medication in nonhospital settings (Whitfield et al., 1978; Whitfield, 1980; Sparadeo et al., 1982).

Second, as indicated in the discussion of effect-altering drugs, it has been suggested that some psychotropic medications may decrease the desire for and use of alcohol (McMillan, 1981). In addition to the antidepressants and serotonin uptake inhibitors discussed earlier, lithium has been investigated in this regard. Fawcett and colleagues (1987) found no differences on drinking measures between alcoholics given lithium and alcoholics given a placebo. Compliance with either medication was highly associated with abstinence. Among compliant individuals, those sustaining high blood levels of lithium did show a higher rate of abstinence than those with low lithium levels or placebo doses. No differences were observed between depressed and nondepressed alcoholics. Other investigations, including a major Veterans Administration collaborative study, have found no therapeutic impact of lithium on the drinking outcomes of either depressed or nondepressed alcoholics (Peck et al., 1981; Pond et al., 1981; Powell et al., 1986; Dorus, 1988). A variety of other psychotropic medications have been tested for their effects on drinking behavior and the desire to drink (Liskow and Goodwin, 1987).

A third potential use of psychotropic medications is in the treatment of "dual diagnosis" individuals, who manifest both alcohol abuse and another significant form of psychopathology. Current evidence indicates that untreated concomitant psychopathology generally predicts a poor prognosis for alcoholics (Rounsaville et al., 1987) and is associated with a high rate of treatment dropout (Kofoed et al., 1986). It is logical (although not yet conclusively demonstrated) that alcoholics with major depression that persists into sobriety would be significantly more likely to remain sober if their depression could be treated effectively by antidepressant medication or other means. Similarly, it is quite plausible that individuals with concomitant alcohol abuse and schizophrenia would benefit from antipsychotic medication and that alcoholics with bipolar affective disorder would have an improved prognosis if given lithium.

It is important to note here that apparent psychopathology that coincides with active alcohol and drug abuse frequently remits during the early weeks of sobriety (Nakamura et al., 1983). Sufficient time should be allowed for full withdrawal from abused drugs, and the diagnosis should be firmly established before psychotropic medication is considered. Nonpharmacological alternatives should also be considered in treating concomitant psychopathology (e.g., depression or anxiety). Extreme caution is warranted in the prescription of psychiatric medications with a high potential for abuse and dependence. However, many medications of known therapeutic value for other conditions (e.g., lithium, antipsychotic and antidepressant agents) pose few risks of abuse or dependence. Given proper consideration and precautions, there is no persuasive reason to deny such medications to alcoholics who manifest concomitant psychopathology for which these drug treatments are known to be effective therapeutic agents.

Finally, it is worth noting that no medication currently constitutes a primary treatment for alcohol problems. Pharmacotherapy is only an adjunctive treatment that is best used in combination with other strategies. Medications are not regarded as a "cure" for alcohol problems, but when properly used, they may be valuable aids in the recovery process.

The following questions represents opportunities for research on psychotropic medications:

• For persons with dual diagnoses (e.g., major depression, bipolar disorder, schizophrenia), does appropriate psychotropic medication reduce the risk of relapse and improve other aspects of outcome?

• What is the relative effectiveness in reducing relapse potential of psychotropic medication versus alternative drug-free strategies of treatment (e.g., cognitive-behavioral therapy) for individuals with concomitant psychopathology?

• Are certain psychotropic medications of value in reducing drinking or the desire to drink among alcoholics without concomitant psychopathology?

• What therapeutic doses, verified by appropriate means (e.g., serum monitoring), are essential to produce improvement in treatment outcome?

• When are the optimal time (in the continuum of detoxification, active treatment, and relapse prevention) and duration for administering psychotropic medications as an aid to recovery?

Aversion Therapies

Aversion therapy for alcohol abuse is based on the principle of counterconditioning. Attraction to, and positive associations with, alcohol are replaced by conditioned aversive reactions. Unlike the antidipsotropic medications, aversion therapy is designed to produce an enduring adverse reaction to alcohol in the absence of medication. In aversion therapy, alcohol is associated with unpleasant experiences or images. The typical and intended effects are a loss of desire for alcohol and avoidance of drinking.

Various methods have been used to produce conditioned aversive responses to alcohol. Electrical and apneic aversion have fallen into justifiable disuse, and no new studies have appeared since 1980 (Miller and Hester, 1986a; Wilson, 1987). Chemical aversion pairs alcohol with nausea and vomiting induced by emetic drugs. Aversion therapy is a mainstay of alcohol treatment in the Soviet Union and continues to be used in some U.S. treatment centers.

In the 1980s, however, chemical aversion therapy has come under sharp attack (National Center for Health Care Technology, 1981; Wilson, 1987). Although uncontrolled studies have reported relatively high rates of abstinence (Miller and Hester, 1980; Neuberger et al., 1980, 1981, 1982), support from controlled studies has been weak, and the absolute impact of chemical aversion treatment beyond or in the absence of adjunctive therapeutic approaches is unclear. Cannon, Baker, and Wehl (1981) found no long-term differences between a group treated with chemical aversion and a control group receiving only standard hospital treatment, although both fared better than a group that received electrical aversion. Richard (1983) found no effects of an aversion procedure based on nausea induced by motion sickness. Thurber (1985) expressed cautious optimism based on a meta-analysis of controlled studies of chemical aversive counterconditioning. The Council on Scientific Affairs of the American Medical Association (1987) likewise found "positive results" from aversion therapies but called for further controlled trials. Wilson (1987), in contrast, concluded that the use of chemical aversion therapy for alcoholism is unwarranted, given its stressful and potentially hazardous nature and the absence of clear evidence for its efficacy.

One strength of the chemical aversion approach is its foundation in basic research and learning theory. Acquired and persistent taste aversion is a well-established phenomenon in mammals, including humans. Elkins (1984) demonstrated a strong relationship between the intensity of induced nausea and the persistence of taste aversion. Elkins and Hobbs (1982) likewise demonstrated a potent genetic influence on the susceptibility to taste aversion learning, perhaps mirroring human individual differences in response to this treatment modality. This inherited susceptibility factor appears to be quite specific to taste aversion and is not generalized to other learning paradigms such as electric shock aversion (Hobbs and Elkins, 1983; Elkins, 1986). Recent human research has demonstrated that chemical aversion therapy does produce a conditioned aversive response to alcohol and that the strength of conditioning is predictive of treatment outcome (Cannon and Baker, 1981; Cannon, Baker, and Wehl, 1981; Baker et al., 1984; Cannon et al., 1986). The robustness of these experimental findings and of the taste aversion conditioning phenomenon itself warrants further investigation of taste aversion therapy for alcohol problems.

Covert sensitization is an alternative aversive counterconditioning procedure employing only imagery. It requires no use of drugs or shock, is less physically stressful, and can be administered in outpatient treatment. Recent studies have demonstrated that conditioned aversion to alcohol can be produced by covert sensitization and that (as with chemical aversion) the strength of conditioning is predictive of treatment outcome (Elkins, 1980; Miller and Dougher, 1984). Olson and colleagues (1981) demonstrated greater suppression of drinking among alcoholics assigned at random to receive behavior therapy (including covert sensitization), relative to two groups receiving transactional analysis or milieu treatment alone. Covert sensitization administered in groups was found in two studies to be ineffective (Sanchez-Craig and Walker, 1982; Telch, Hannon, and Telch, 1984).

Finally, it should be noted that certain therapeutic procedures for alcohol problems (including some aversion therapies) require the administration of small amounts of alcohol to those undergoing treatment. Certain relapse prevention and cue exposure procedures may require exposure to the sight, smell, or taste of alcohol (see Chapter 12). Research on these procedures may thus require the presentation of alcohol to alcohol-dependent persons. Recent reports have specified clear ethical guidelines for the administration or exposure to alcohol of persons with alcohol problems, for research purposes (NIAAA, 1988). Available evidence indicates that when such guidelines are carefully followed, the administration of alcohol during research or treatment poses no significant risks to the individual's welfare.

The following questions represent opportunities for research on aversion therapies:

• Does the addition of chemical aversion therapy to an alcohol treatment program significantly improve long-term outcomes?
• Does covert sensitization suppress urges to drink and have beneficial effects on long-term outcomes?

• Do chemical aversion and covert sensitization differ in their relative impact on drinking behavior and on urges or the craving to drink?

• What individual factors predict the establishment of conditioned aversion and of favorable responses to aversion therapy?

Psychotherapy and Counseling

Controlled treatment outcome studies prior to 1980 failed to yield persuasive evidence for the effectiveness of psychodynamic psychotherapy with alcoholics (Miller and Hester, 1980). Recent controlled studies have not substantially altered this trend, although more promising results have been obtained in drug abuse populations (see Chapter 12). Olson and colleagues (1981) found that insight-oriented psychotherapy yielded no increase in effectiveness when added to a milieu treatment program and was less effective than behavioral approaches. Brandsma, Maultsby, and Welsh (1980) found somewhat fewer drinking days among mandated individuals assigned at random to either cognitive-behavioral or insight-oriented therapy, relative to untreated controls after one year. Braunstein et al. (1983) observed no differences in outcome between those assigned at random to aftercare that included individual counseling and group psychotherapy and two control groups that were given only medical monitoring. Annis and Chan (1983) similarly found no effect of confrontational group therapy in a random assignment design with incarcerated alcohol-related offenders. Individuals low in self-esteem, however, showed detrimental effects from confrontational psychotherapy, whereas those higher in self-esteem evidenced some benefit. In another randomized trial, Swenson and Clay (1980) observed no differences at an eight-month follow-up interval between drunk-driving offenders assigned to confrontational group therapy and those given only a home-study course.

There has been increased interest in and research on cognitive-behavioral therapy with alcoholics, although the results of outcome studies to date have been mixed. Oei and Jackson (1982) found significantly greater improvement among two groups of alcoholics that were randomly assigned to receive cognitive restructuring, relative to controls who received the same residential treatment without cognitive therapy. Modeling and reinforcement of positive self-statements appear to be important to the effectiveness of cognitive therapy with alcoholics (Oei and Jackson, 1984). Positive results have been reported from a prevention program based on cognitive-behavioral procedures (Botvin et al., 1984a). Other randomized clinical trials have reported no significant effect of cognitive therapies with drunk-driving offenders (Rosenberg and Brian, 1986) or halfway house residents (Sanchez-Craig and Walker, 1982; Walker, Sanchez-Craig, and Bornet, 1982).

Psychotherapy is also used in the treatment of concomitant psychopathology. For example, two types of psychotherapy (interpersonal and cognitive-behavioral) have been evaluated rigorously for their effectiveness in the treatment of outpatients with major depression; generally positive results have been reported (Elkin et al., 1989). For alcoholics with concomitant depression, then, psychotherapy may be effective not only in treating depression, but also in diminishing the likelihood of relapse to drinking. Such therapeutic effects with alcoholics, however, have not yet been demonstrated in properly controlled studies.

A common problem in research on psychotherapy and counseling is the definition and integrity of interventions. What constitutes the "psychotherapy" or "counseling" given? Evaluations should, as much as possible, specify and standardize the treatment being studied. Efforts should also be made to ensure the integrity and consistency of delivery of the specified psychotherapeutic procedures.

The following questions represent opportunities for research on psychotherapy and counseling:

• Are certain therapies (e.g., cognitive-behavioral therapy) differentially effective in preventing relapse to drinking for persons manifesting concomitant psychopathology (e.g., depression) for which the therapy is an effective treatment?

• In treating psychopathology concomitant to alcohol abuse, do psychotherapy and psychotropic medication differ in their impact on drinking?

• What are the components and processes of counseling as typically administered by alcohol counselors?

• What approaches to or components of alcohol counseling significantly improve treatment outcome?

• Are there additive effects of psychotherapy or counseling in combination with other therapeutic strategies (e.g., pharmacotherapy)?

• Within the continuum of detoxification, active treatment, and relapse prevention, when is the optimal time to initiate psychotherapeutic intervention?

• What individual difference variables (e.g., degree of residual cognitive impairment) are predictive of response to psychotherapy?

Didactic Approaches

Treatment programs frequently include educational lectures on alcohol and related problems. Interventions with drunk-driving offenders sometimes rely solely on educational strategies. Siegal (1985a,b) reported lower recidivism in two educational intervention groups than in a nonrandom control group whose members apparently were given jail sentences. Yet controlled research to date has failed to yield any persuasive evidence of the impact of such educational strategies on drinking behavior among problem drinkers or alcoholics (Uecker and Solberg, 1973; Swenson and Clay, 1980; Miller and Hester, 1986a). One concern here is whether cognitive impairment from excessive drinking may deter alcoholics from comprehending and retaining information presented in traditional educational approaches. Two studies reported very poor retention of treatment-relevant information by alcoholics (Sanchez-Craig and Walker, 1982; Becker and Jaffe, 1984).

The following questions represent opportunities for research on didactic approaches:

• What contributions to treatment outcome are made by educational lectures within the context of a multimodal treatment program?

• Does the level of cognitive impairment predict the response of alcoholics to educational interventions?

• What short-term changes, if any (e.g., information gain, attitude shifts, motivation increases) are predictive of long-term behavior change following educational interventions?

• What elements of newly developed educational technologies could be tested that might increase the effectiveness of traditional classes?

Mutual Help Groups

Although it has been in existence since 1935 and has been an important shaping force in alcohol treatment in the United States, Alcoholics Anonymous (AA) has been subjected to surprisingly little scientific study. In the 1980s, contributions to the literature on AA have continued to consist primarily of commentaries and summaries of available correlational data (Glaser and Ogborne, 1982; Kurtz, 1982; Emrick, 1987). Some progress has been made toward identifying the characteristics of individuals who are most likely to maintain affiliation with AA (Boscarino, 1980; Ogborne and Glaser, 1981), although favorable outcomes in AA are by no means limited to particular types of persons (Emrick, 1987). Correlational studies continue to support a relationship between abstinence and AA attendance (Alford, 1980; Polich, Armor and Braiker, 1980; Hoffman, Harrison, and Belille, 1983). Both correlational and controlled studies have suggested a relationship between AA attendance and greater severity of symptomatology if subsequent drinking does occur (Brandsma, Maultsby, and Welsh, 1980; Ogborne and Bornet, 1982; Walker, Sanchez-Craig and Bornet, 1982; Stimmel et al., 1983).

The findings of correlational investigations are difficult to interpret because differences (e.g., between AA attenders and nonattenders) may be attributable to a variety of factors that are confounded in such studies. Treatment-compliant individuals, for example, generally show better prognosis than those who are less compliant (Fuller et al., 1986; Fawcett et al., 1987). An observed relationship between treatment exposure and outcome, then, may be due not to specific characteristics of the treatment but to nonspecific individual difference factors that drive compliance.

Prior to 1980 only one controlled study had been conducted of outcomes of AA (Ditman et al., 1967). Only two controlled outcome studies of AA have appeared in the 1980s. Brandsma, Maultsby, and Welsh (1980) found no long-term differences between problem drinkers who were court-mandated to participate in AA and those who were assigned at random to a no-treatment condition. A second controlled evaluation (Stimmel et al., 1983) compared outcomes of alcohol-abusing methadone maintenance patients assigned at random to an AA-based therapy group, a controlled drinking training group, or a control group (no additional treatment beyond the methadone program). Among treatment completers (fewer than 20 percent), the controlled drinking and control groups showed decreased drinking on a measure of peak use, whereas the AA abstinence-focused group reported an increase on the same measure. (The relevance of this study for the principal target population of AA, namely alcoholics without other substance abuse problems, remains in doubt.)

Given its great importance in U.S. treatment programs, it is unfortunate that AA has not been the subject of more empirical research. The inherent anonymity of the treatment group presents special but not insurmountable challenges in studying its effectiveness. Advances in outcome assessment and in program evaluation methodology have increased the feasibility of conducting meaningful research on AA processes and effectiveness (Glaser and Ogborne, 1982). Alcoholics Anonymous is available in nearly every U.S. city, offering a free and highly accessible support system for recovering alcoholics. Because it is free, on a cost-effectiveness basis AA is likely to compare favorably with alternative intervention approaches. Furthermore, the enduring success of this organization in attracting alcoholics to recovery is itself worthy of study. There is, therefore, a pressing need for high-quality research on the impact and mechanisms of AA.

In addition to AA, other U.S. mutual help movements currently include AlAnon, Women for Sobriety, and Adult Children of Alcoholics. The impact of affiliation on members of these groups and their families is unknown. Systematic outcome research on mutual help groups for alcoholics and their families represents a promising avenue for future study.

The following questions represent opportunities for research on mutual help groups:

- What are the long-term impact and cost-effectiveness of participation in mutual help groups, relative to alternative approaches? There is a particular need for outcome research employing a range of contemporary treatment assessment approaches.
- What role does mutual help group participation play in the context of multimodal treatment programs?
- What are the characteristics of individuals who maintain a stable affiliation with mutual help groups and experience favorable outcomes?
- What is the impact of mandated mutual help group attendance among offenders, relative to alternative interventions or legal sanctions alone?
- What are the key mechanisms of effective change for those who maintain successful affiliation with mutual help groups?
- What differentiates long-term affiliates from those who do not attend or who drop out after brief attendance?
- What common stages or processes of change may underlie (a) remission without formal treatment, (b) remission following formal treatment, and (c) remission associated with participation in mutual help groups?

Behavioral Self-Control Training

Behavioral self-control training (BSCT) as applied to the treatment of alcoholism consists of a set of self-management procedures that are intended to help problem drinkers reduce or stop alcohol consumption (Sanchez-Craig, 1984). Since 1980 there have been more studies on the effectiveness of BSCT than on any other single treatment modality for alcohol abuse.

A number of controlled studies compared alternative BSCT procedures or contrasted BSCT with other approaches. Brown (1980) found significantly greater reductions in drinking among driving-while-intoxicated (DWI) offenders who were given BSCT than among those receiving conventional alcohol education. Connors, Maisto, and Ersner-Hershfield (1986), who also worked with DWI offenders, reported that BSCT resulted in significantly reduced consumption, whereas two random control groups showed no change. Four controlled studies offering BSCT to outpatient problem drinkers and randomly assigning them to abstinence versus moderation goals found no long-term differences in outcome based on the assigned goal (Sanchez-Craig, 1980; Stimmel et al., 1983; Sanchez-Craig et al., 1984; Orford and Keddie, 1986; Graber and Miller, 1988)

Other research efforts have produced somewhat different results. Foy, Nunn, and Rychtarik (1984), working with inpatient alcoholics, assigned them at random to receive or not receive moderation-oriented BSCT training in addition to the abstinence-based award program. Those given the additional moderation training fared worse at short-term follow-up but showed no different long-term outcome from those receiving only abstinence-oriented treatment (Rychtarik et al., 1987). Other studies found comparable impacts from therapist-administered and self-administered BSCT (Miller and Taylor, 1980; Miller, Taylor, and West, 1980; Miller, Gribskov, and Mortell, 1981; Carpenter, Lyons, and Miller, 1985; Berg and Skutle, 1986; Skutle and Berg, 1987).

The outcomes of BSCT, even in controlled trials, have thus ranged from significant benefit (e.g., Brown, 1980) to a detrimental effect (Foy, Nunn, and Rychtarik, 1984). Comparisons with alternative treatment modalities have sometimes but not always yielded differences favoring BSCT. A plausible reason for this diversity of findings is the heterogeneity of populations included in these studies. Other causes of diversity include variations in content and in implementation effectiveness of the BSCT method. Treated populations have included inpatients on an alcohol unit (Foy, Nunn, and Rychtarik, 1984), heroin addicts on methadone maintenance (Stimmel et al., 1983), drunk-driving offenders (Brown, 1980), and self-referred problem drinkers from the community (Miller, Taylor, and West, 1980; Miller, Gribskov, and Mortell, 1981). Further study should be directed toward an examination of the characteristics of individuals and populations for whom BSCT procedures are optimally effective.

The following opportunities exist for research on behavioral self-control training:

- Studies are needed to address the following question: How effective is abstinence-oriented BSCT, relative to other approaches to abstinence?

Conjoint Therapies

Recent research supports a strong association between favorable family adjustment and sustained abstinence or problem-free drinking after treatment (Moos, Finney and Gamble, 1982; Billings and Moos, 1983; Moos and Moos, 1984). This association suggests that interventions to improve the relationship functioning of couples and families may enhance treatment outcome.

New data are available regarding conjoint couples therapy as an adjunct to alcohol treatment. One study found that, over six months of follow-up, alcoholics given behavioral marital therapy showed more rapid reductions in drinking and somewhat better maintenance of sobriety than two control groups (McCrady et al., 1987). Similarly, Stout and colleagues (1988) reported that alcoholics who undertook behavioral marital therapy showed superior outcomes at longer follow-up points, relative to those treated with only an alcohol problem focus. However, a four-year follow-up study supported earlier findings that joint hospitalization of alcoholics and their spouses did not improve outcome relative to hospitalization of the alcoholics alone (McCrady et al., 1982).

Conjoint therapy has also been found to decrease the probability of treatment dropout (Noel et al., 1987; Weidman, 1987). O'Farrell, Cutter, and Floyd (1985) compared group behavioral marital therapy with an "interactional" couples group focusing on mutual support, discussion of feelings, and insights. Couples in behavioral marital therapy showed greater improvement in marital functioning than those in the interactional group, relative to controls who received no marital therapy. On a measure of alcohol-free days, all groups showed improvement, but individuals in behavioral marital therapy improved significantly more than those treated by interactional couples group therapy.

Interventions with spouses of alcoholics have also been tested. In one controlled study (Dittrich and Trapold, 1984), wives of alcoholics who were given eight weeks of treatment showed significantly greater reductions in anxiety and enabling behavior and significantly enhanced self-concepts relative to a random waiting list control group.

Although recent studies provide support for the effectiveness of behavioral marital therapy, current alcohol treatment programs include a much wider range of interventions for couples and families. These include confrontational family sessions, AlAnon and AlaTeen meetings, groups for young and adult children of alcoholics, and a variety of other conjoint and group approaches to marital and family counseling. The effectiveness of these approaches, however, is unknown. Reports of studies that compare alternative approaches have only recently begun to appear (e.g., Zweben, Pearlman and Li, 1988).

Current research has focused largely on couples in which both spouses were cooperative and willing to participate in treatment. Yet a common problem in treatment is the uncooperative partner. Unilateral interventions have been described for working with one spouse (Thomas and Santa, 1982; Thomas et al., in press). The effectiveness of such unilateral marital/family therapy interventions, with either the alcoholic or the alcoholic's spouse, is unclear at present.

Furthermore, only couples therapies have been systematically evaluated (most evaluations have focused on behavioral marital therapy), and the effectiveness of treating alcoholics within the context of the whole family is unknown. New research is needed to explore the effects of conjoint therapies, not only on the drinking of the alcoholics but also on the adjustment of spouses, children, and other family members.

The following questions represent opportunities for research on conjoint therapies:

   •   What couples and family therapy approaches contribute significantly to favorable outcomes for treated alcoholics and their families?
   •   What is the relative effectiveness of treating the individual alcoholic, the couple, or the entire family?
   •   In what ways and by what processes do conjoint therapies contribute to long-term favorable outcomes?
   •   What dimensions of adjustment should be assessed as prognostic and outcome measures in family members?
   •   For what subpopulations is conjoint therapy effective, ineffective, or contraindicated?
   •   In the continuum of detoxification, active treatment, and relapse prevention, at what point is it most effective to introduce conjoint therapy?
   •   When the spouse (without alcohol problems) is unwilling to enter treatment, what unilateral interventions are effective in improving relationship functioning for the couple or family and in decreasing the likelihood of relapse?

Broad-Spectrum Treatment Strategies

The term "broad spectrum" applies to treatment strategies that address not only alcohol consumption but other problem areas that may be functionally related to alcohol abuse. Broad-spectrum treatments have been generally (although not necessarily) derived from a social learning theory approach to alcohol problems. Evidence increasingly indicates that appropriately planned broad-spectrum treatment is associated with lower rates of relapse to alcohol abuse (Miller and Hester, 1986a). Broad-spectrum treatment strategies should not be seen as treating an "underlying cause" of alcohol problems. Rather, these strategies appear to be useful in relapse prevention after the stabilization of alcohol problems. This is consistent with other findings which suggest that posttreatment problems and experiences are major determinants of long-term outcomes (Cronkite and Moos, 1980; Finney, Moos, and Mewborn, 1980).

Social skills training appears to be an effective adjunct in promoting sobriety among alcoholics who are deficient in social skills. Oei and Jackson (1980) found significantly greater improvement on drinking and other measures among those assigned at random to receive social skills training, relative to those assigned to traditional supportive therapy. These findings were replicated in a later study that showed significant beneficial effects of both social skills training and cognitive restructuring, with an apparent additive effect of the two interventions (Oei and Jackson, 1982). Ferrell and Galassi (1981) reported substantially higher one-and two-year abstinence rates among alcoholics given assertiveness training in addition to standard treatment procedures.

A Norwegian study similarly found that inpatients given social skills training, relative to controls who received only standard hospital treatment, had twice as many days of sobriety and employment in the subsequent year, sustained abstinence for longer periods, and experienced fewer than one-fourth as many days of institutionalization (Eriksen, Bjornstad, and Gotestam, 1986). Jones, Kanfer, and Lanyon (1982) reported that both a social skills training program and a social coping discussion group significantly improved drinking outcomes for inpatient alcoholics, relative to controls who received only hospital treatment. Chick and his colleagues (1988) found that alcoholics who received "extended treatment" that included group social skills training showed significantly greater reductions in alcohol-related problems at the one-year follow-up point, relative to two control groups who received brief "advice" interventions. Skills training has also been found to be effective in substance abuse prevention (Botvin et al., 1984a,b; Gilchrest et al., 1987).

Stress management training likewise may be helpful to alcoholics in staying sober, particularly when anxiety is a significant concomitant problem (Miller and Hester, 1986a). Although three studies found no overall effect of relaxation training on drinking measures (Miller and Taylor, 1980; Miller, Taylor, and West, 1980; Sisson, 1981), Rosenberg (1979) found that biofeedback-assisted relaxation training did contribute to reductions in drinking, but only for individuals who were high in anxiety. Controlled studies with nonalcoholic drinkers have found modest short-term suppression of alcohol consumption through aerobic exercise but not through meditation (Murphy, Pagano, and Marlatt, 1986), although uncontrolled studies suggest a correlation between the long-term practice of meditation and a reduction in substance abuse (Aron and Aron, 1980, 1983). A general stress management training program has also produced promising results (Rohsenow, Smith, and Johnson, 1985).

The community-reinforcement approach (CRA) is a comprehensive broad-spectrum treatment strategy that addresses many life-style areas related to alcohol abuse, including unemployment, marital problems, isolation, use of leisure time, and social support. The CRA combines a variety of behavioral strategies in an attempt to make the person's nondrinking life-style more rewarding than drinking. It includes job-search training, behavioral marital therapy, monitored disulfiram, and counseling focused on alcohol-free social and recreational activities. Prior evaluations of the CRA (Hunt and Azrin, 1973; Azrin, 1976) indicated a large effect on treatment outcome. More recently, Azrin and coworkers (1982) randomly assigned alcoholics to a CRA group versus traditional outpatient treatment. At the six-month follow-up point, the CRA group showed nearly total abstinence and employment, whereas most controls had relapsed and showed high rates of drinking and unemployment. In another controlled experiment, Mallams and colleagues (1982) found that one specific component of the CRA, the encouragement to attend an alcohol-free social club, likewise led to greater sobriety.

The following questions represent opportunities for research on broad-spectrum treatment strategies:

• What broad-spectrum treatment strategies (social skills training, stress and mood management training, etc.) effectively decrease the likelihood of relapse following treatment?

• Is a high level of pretreatment distress, life problems, or skills deficits a differential predictor of favorable outcome for broad-spectrum interventions?

• At what point in the treatment and relapse prevention process is it optimal to undertake broad-spectrum treatment strategies?

Relapse Prevention

In the early 1980s Marlatt introduced a conceptual model and new treatment procedures that were broadly described as "relapse prevention." Marlatt suggested that relapse was best understood not as a sudden discrete event but rather as a developmental process. He described a sequence of cognitive and behavioral events that lead to relapse and a set of strategies that might be used to decrease its likelihood (Cummings, Marlatt, and Gordon, 1980; Marlatt and Gordon, 1985). Other cognitive-behavioral models for relapse prevention have been introduced more recently, including Annis's self-efficacy approach (1986b) and Litman's "survival" model (1986). As discussed in the writings of Gorski (e.g., Gorski and Miller, 1982), relapse prevention strategies have been popularized and integrated into the 12 step approach used by AA.

The approach's intended effect is that the addition of relapse prevention procedures to a treatment program will reduce the probability and rapidity of relapse. At present, only three controlled studies of cognitive-behavioral relapse prevention procedures with problem drinkers have been reported. Rosenberg and Brian (1986) reported no differences on drinking outcome measures between an "unstructured therapy" control group and two treatment groups for DWI offenders, one of which was based on Marlatt's relapse prevention model. Missing data from the control group, however, compromised the interpretability of this study. In a large, controlled evaluation, Annis and coworkers (1988) found a modest impact of cognitive relapse prevention procedures on treatment outcome. However, Ito, Donovan, and Hall (1988) found no differences in outcome between groups given a cognitive-behavioral relapse prevention program based on Marlatt's model and an interpersonal process aftercare program based on a more psychodynamic approach.

Reactivity to alcohol stimuli has been found to be predictive of relapse. A plausible but still experimental relapse prevention strategy is cue exposure, in which the goal is to diminish alcoholics' responsivity to cues that may precipitate the desire to drink or relapse to drinking (Rankin, 1986). Empirical support for the cue exposure approach is currently limited to case reports (Blakey and Baker, 1980) and evidence that cue exposure decreases the subjective desire to drink and reduces the perceived difficulty of resisting relapse (Rankin, Hodgson, and Stockwell, 1983).

The following questions represent opportunities for research on relapse prevention:

• What relapse prevention procedures--when added to alcohol treatment programs significantly reduce the frequency, severity, or duration of posttreatment relapses?
• Are cue exposure strategies effective in reducing the desire for and relapse to drinking after treatment?
• At what point in the treatment process are relapse prevention strategies best taught? Is it more effective to offer relapse prevention training during intensive treatment or after formal treatment as a follow-up strategy?
• What individual characteristics most strongly predict relapse and which traits predict a favorable response to relapse, prevention procedures?
• What change processes do individuals use successfully to avoid or cope with relapses?
• Do relapse prevention strategies constitute an effective treatment in themselves? What is the optimal combination of relapse prevention strategies with other procedures?

RESEARCH ON TRADITIONAL TREATMENT PROGRAMS

In practice, alcoholism treatment programs in the United States typically offer a combination of modalities that includes detoxification and health care, AA groups, lectures and films, group therapy, individual counseling, recreational and occupational therapy, medication, and aftercare group meetings. Claims of high success rates are sometimes made for such programs. For example, in testimony before the Senate Committee on Governmental Affairs, McElrath (1988) stated that the Hazelden approach (the Minnesota model) "is the most successful form of treatment for chemical dependency in recorded history."

Scientific evidence regarding traditional multicomponent programs thus far has been limited to uncontrolled studies, several of which have been reported since 1980. Gilmore, Jones, and Tamble (1986) reported the results of 6-and 12-month follow-up questionnaires completed by patients of Hazelden and two other treatment facilities. Excluded from the study were short-stay patients, those who were deceased or absent without leave, and those who refused to complete the questionnaire. In the remaining Hazelden sample, 70 percent of the 6-month follow-up questionnaires were completed, among which 73 percent (51 percent of the total sample) reported abstinence from alcohol. At 12 months (74 percent completed), 58 percent (43 percent of the total sample) reported continuing abstinence. Validity checks were made by interviewing significant others in an unspecified number of cases.

A similar uncontrolled study by CompCare (1988) reported a telephone follow-up survey of 1,002 patients discharged from 50 care units. Short-stay patients not receiving normal discharge were excluded from the study. At 12 to 15 months after discharge, with a 72 percent follow-up completion rate, 43 percent (31 percent of the total sample) reported continuous abstinence from alcohol and drugs, with an additional 18 percent (13 percent of the sample) having had one to four relapses. These two groups were combined to constitute a 61 percent "recovering" rate (44 percent of the total sample). No verification of the accuracy of the self-reports of the respondents was included in the report of the study. Compliance with treatment and aftercare recommendations was reported to be a strong predictor of favorable outcome.

A third recent study was an uncontrolled evaluation of patients treated at Edgehill Newport, a private for-profit hospital (Wallace, et al.). From a target treated sample of 380, an interviewer was able to screen 257 (68 percent) eligible respondents for the study. Of these, 65 cases (25 percent) were excluded because they were unmarried, were living apart from their spouses, or failed to complete treatment; 11 others refused to participate. Of the remaining 181, 169 were interviewed by telephone during a follow-up survey six months later. This figure represents 93 percent of the attempted interviews, although only 44 percent of the original target sample. A collateral informant was interviewed in 98 percent of the found cases, and the less optimistic report of outcome was accepted as accurate. The reported rate of abstinence varied, depending on the criteria used, from 57 percent (continuous abstinence from alcohol and other drugs for six months) to 72 percent (current abstinence from alcohol only). Rate of abstinence was found to be correlated with the frequency of attendance at meetings of Alcoholics Anonymous or Narcotics Anonymous.

Two recent studies employed more conservative methodological standards. Alford (1980) reported two-year follow-up data for 56 patients who completed 5 to 11 weeks of inpatient treatment and received staff-approved discharges. Verification of self-reports was obtained from significant others, and evaluation focused on employment and social stability as well as drinking variables. At two years, 66 percent were reported to be either "essentially abstinent" (51 percent) or light to moderate drinkers (15 percent). When more stringent criteria were employed that required abstinence with few slips, employment, and good social adjustment, 41 percent were rated as successful at two years.

In the second study, Pettinati and coworkers (1982) accounted for 100 percent of 255 patients who were followed annually for four years after inpatient treatment at the Carrier Foundation. As in the Alford study, collateral verification was obtained, and evaluation included a broad range of outcome dimensions. Abstinence (allowing for a few slips) was reported in 40, 45, 51, and 55 percent of cases at one-, two-, three-, and four-year follow-ups, respectively. When cases that showed "drinking with good adjustment" were included, these figures rose to 48, 51, 56, and 60 percent. However, about half of the cases in the study showed fluctuation in outcome status over follow-up points, and only 22 percent evidenced continuous abstinence (29 percent were mostly abstinent with slips) over the four-year period. These studies exemplify how reported success rates are significantly influenced by the stringency of outcome criteria.

Reports of uncontrolled studies pose difficulties in interpretation. Because random assignment and control groups are absent (they are often regarded as unacceptable in traditional treatment settings), the absolute effectiveness of treatment cannot be inferred. Positive outcomes may be attributable, at least in part, to favorable pretreatment characteristics or posttreatment experiences of the clinical population (Finney, Moos, and Mewborn, 1980). Consequently, despite some very useful information that can be gleaned from uncontrolled program evaluations (e.g., predictors of outcome within a program), such studies cannot support causal inferences or yield reliable estimates of the absolute or relative magnitude of treatment effects. Furthermore, it is difficult to determine which elements of a multicomponent program may account for the positive outcomes that are observed.

Methodological shortcomings can also inflate the reported rates of favorable outcomes. For example, patients who cannot be located for follow-up generally have a poorer prognosis than those who participate in follow-up studies; thus, the exclusion of the cases that are lost to follow-up is likely to yield overestimates of success within the total population. The exclusion of short-stay and noncompliant cases, dropouts, and irregular discharges likewise biases a study sample toward inflated remission rates in that compliance with treatment recommendations is known to be a favorable prognostic indicator regardless of treatment modality. Some studies have also eliminated unmarried or less stable cases, again with the likely effect of inflating success rates (e.g., Wallace et al., in press). The reliability and validity of self-reports (e.g., questionnaires or telephone interviews) without objective verification are also questionable.

As a quasi-experimental alternative to a randomized design, Grenier (1985) contrasted AA-based residential treatment for adolescents with a waiting list group. For the treated group, a 65.5 percent abstinence rate was estimated, based on two multiple choice questions administered to parents by telephone. The report did not specify the duration of reported abstinence, the length of follow-up, the percentage of cases that were not interviewed, or whether lost cases were included among nonabstinent cases. The waiting list group consisted of parents who had contacted the treatment center expressing a "sincere interest in admitting an alcohol-or drug-abusing adolescent for treatment" (p. 383), but who for unstated reasons had not done so for 3 to 18 months after initial contact. The telephone follow-up completion rate for this group was reported to be 36 percent, although outcome data were reported for only 26 percent. Among the waiting list parents, 47 percent reported improvement, including 20 percent who reported total abstinence. Several abstinent cases were excluded because they had received alternative treatment, leaving a 14 percent abstinence rate among located, untreated cases.

Contrasting the study's 65.5 and 14 percent abstinence rates, Grenier (1985, p.389) concluded that residential treatment for adolescents "was a significant causal factor in the reduction of chemical use." Causal interpretations of such findings, however, cannot be made with confidence. Individuals who remain on a waiting list for 18 months do so for a wide variety of reasons, which introduces substantial selection differences between treated and "control" groups. In addition, the accuracy of unverified self-reports is impossible to ascertain--perhaps even more so when data are gathered by mailed questionnaires or by telephone rather than in personal interviews. A high rate of uncompleted interviews also introduces interpretation difficulties because unlocated cases are not likely to be representative of those interviewed.

Uncontrolled and quasi-experimental designs may yield useful information about treatment impact, particularly when controllable methodological problems are properly addressed. Important new knowledge may be obtained regarding predictors of outcome. In addition, special populations that are seen in private treatment programs may not be found in public programs in which controlled research is more commonly conducted. Yet uncontrolled studies cannot substitute for properly controlled, randomized designs in determining the absolute and relative effectiveness of treatment programs and modalities. Increased attention should be devoted to the possibility of conducting controlled trials in a broader range of treatment facilities. Even in cases in which conditions constrain randomization to untreated or alternative treatment groups, it may be feasible to conduct well-controlled evaluations by comparing the addition or deletion of specific treatment components designed to enhance motivation or prevent relapse (Miller, 1980, 1985). Such studies yield information of immediate clinical utility by indicating the value of adding specific components to ongoing treatment programs.

The following types of studies, which offer opportunities for research on traditional treatment programs, are particularly needed at this time:

- evaluations conducted in ongoing treatment settings, involving collaborations of research teams with traditional treatment personnel and programs;
- specification of the treatment methods and procedures that constitute typical and traditional alcohol treatment programs;
- evaluations of the effectiveness of generic, traditional treatment procedures as offered by typical U.S. programs;
- controlled additive designs evaluating the effectiveness of traditional treatment programs with and without additional innovative treatment strategies; and
- unpackaging designs to identify the "active ingredients" of traditional treatment programs.

RESEARCH ON THE INTENSITY AND DURATION OF TREATMENT

It is a commonsense assumption that if one kind of treatment is longer, more intensive, offered in a hospital, or more expensive than another, that treatment should also be more effective than the other. Reimbursement policies of health care insurers have often followed this maxim, paying preferentially for more intensive and expensive forms of alcohol treatment.

Uncontrolled studies have long reported a positive correlation between length of stay in treatment and favorable outcome, and studies since 1980 have continued this trend (e.g., Finney, Moos, and Chan, 1981; McLellan et al., 1982), although there are exceptions (e.g., Booth, 1981). As discussed earlier, however, such correlational findings confound treatments with important individual determinants of outcome (e.g., compliance) and thus are difficult to interpret.

Fortunately, more than two dozen controlled studies have addressed this issue. In the typical study, individuals eligible for either form of care (excluding those who urgently need intensive treatment) have been assigned at random to more versus less intensive treatments or settings or to longer versus shorter treatment. With great consistency, these controlled studies have found no differences in outcome based on the duration or intensity of treatment or the setting (e.g., inpatient versus outpatient) in which it is offered (for reviews, see U.S. Congress, Office of Technology Assessment, 1983; Annis, 1986a; Miller and Hester, 1986b). Recent studies continue to find no overall advantage of residential treatment over nonresidential alternatives (McLachlan and Stein, 1982; Longabaugh et al., 1983; Eriksen, 1986; Chapman and Huygens, 1988). Similarly, recent controlled studies have found that increasing the length of alcohol treatment does not result in improved outcomes relative to briefer interventions (Miller and Baca, 1983; Walker et al., 1983; Powell et al., 1985; Eriksen, 1986; Zweben, Pearlman, and Li, in press).

Treatment settings may differ importantly, however, in cost and cost-effectiveness. Treatment is often substantially more expensive in residential and longer treatment programs. Several studies have reported that individuals treated in residential settings show increased future use of hospital-based treatment with no offsetting advantage in long-term outcome, relative to those treated in nonresidential settings (Miller and Hester, 1986b). If these increased costs are not offset by superior outcomes, less expensive forms of treatment are preferable on a cost-effectiveness basis.

Even if there is no <u>overall</u> advantage in outcome from longer, more intensive, or hospital-based treatment programs, <u>there remains the question of whether certain subpopulations of alcoholics may benefit differentially from such approaches.</u> Currently available data are limited but suggest that intensive residential treatment may be warranted for socially unstable individuals (e.g., unemployed or homeless persons; drinkers with more severe psychopathology) and for individuals with more severe alcohol dependence. Socially stable and less severely dependent persons, by contrast, appear to do as well or better in less intensive treatment (Miller and Hester, 1986b). The interactions of severity and treatment approaches are complex, however (see McLellan et al., 1983), and require further investigation.

The following questions represent opportunities for research on the intensity and duration of treatment:

• For what types of individuals is residential treatment differentially effective or more cost-effective than nonresidential alternatives?
• For particular treatment approaches, what minimum length or intensity is sufficient to yield most of the benefits attendant to the treatment? What length and setting are optimal for maximum cost-effectiveness?
• What is the relative cost-effectiveness of different treatment settings (e.g., residential, day hospital, social model, outpatient) when consistent content is offered?

RESEARCH ON AFTERCARE

Relapse prevention as more broadly conceived includes any intervention that is designed to diminish, forestall, or attenuate relapses following treatment. Program components that are referred to as "aftercare" have traditionally been designed to promote this same goal of maintaining gains following treatment. Aftercare is not itself a form of treatment but rather a phase of treatment--continued contact with, and services to, clients or patients following the termination of a formal phase of treatment. The term is typically used only in conjunction with residential treatment, in which discharge is a discrete event. Research on aftercare, then, is essentially research on the optimal timing of various treatment procedures. Most of the treatment strategies previously discussed in this section could, in this sense, be offered as "aftercare."

Progress has been made toward defining interventions that decrease relapse during the aftercare period. Correlational and quasi-experimental studies generally point to a strong relationship between aftercare attendance and sustained remission (Costello, 1980; Ornstein and Cherepon, 1985; Ito and Donovan, 1986) although there are exceptions (Gilbert, 1988). Experimental studies of aftercare procedures have begun to appear. In a randomized trial (Ahles et al., 1983), individuals who were given a behavioral contracting intervention and a calendar designating scheduled aftercare sessions were significantly more likely to attend, to be abstinent at 3-, 6-, and 12-month follow-ups, and to sustain continuous abstinence. In that study, this simple intervention doubled the treatment success rate during the first year (after residential treatment) from 39 to 78 percent. One placebo-controlled study reported that acupuncture significantly suppressed drinking episodes, readmissions, and urges to drink following treatment (Bullock et al., 1987). However, the effectiveness of specific alternative aftercare approaches may vary with the pretreatment characteristics of participants (e.g., McLachlan, 1972, 1974), which suggests a need for individualized matching of aftercare strategies.

Other studies have failed to support the impact of aftercare procedures. Fitzgerald and Mulford (1985), in a randomized trial, found no effect of biweekly telephone contacts over a year of follow-up after inpatient treatment. Another controlled study found no differences in outcome between inpatients assigned at random to medical monitoring only versus aftercare that consisted of biweekly group therapy, individual counseling, family therapy, and social service support (Braunstein et al., 1983). Ito, Donovan, and Hall (1988) found no differences in outcomes from two alternative aftercare programs based on cognitive-behavioral versus interpersonal process models.

Although controlled and correlational studies now indicate that participation in aftercare increases the effectiveness of residential treatment, it is unclear to what extent hospital treatment contributes to long-term prognosis above and beyond the effects of aftercare itself (Miller and Hester, 1986b).

The following questions offer opportunities for research on aftercare:

- What variables predict and what interventions increase aftercare participation?
- Do alternative aftercare procedures differ in their impact or cost-effectiveness?
- Is there an optimal sequencing for specific treatment interventions? Are certain modalities best offered after a period of prior detoxification and treatment?
- What characteristics of individuals predict differential response to alternative aftercare approaches?
- What are the relative contributions of residential treatment versus outpatient aftercare procedures to long-term outcome? Does a preceding period of inpatient treatment improve prognosis, given an effective "aftercare" program? If so, for what types of individuals are there differential benefits?

TREATMENT PROCESS RESEARCH

Whereas outcome research provides data regarding the overall impact of therapeutic interventions, process research yields information about the active ingredients of treatment efficacy. Process and outcome research are not wholly separable approaches and in fact are best conducted conjointly. The central concern of the former, however, is to investigate the underlying processes involved in treatment. Three emerging areas of treatment process research are considered here: (1) mechanisms of treatment efficacy, (2) therapist variables, and (3) motivation.

Mechanisms of Treatment Efficacy

Most therapeutic interventions include at least three kinds of components: (1) active ingredients that have specific and direct effects on outcome, (2) placebo or nonspecific elements that also contribute to outcome but are not unique to the particular treatment, and (3) inert components that have no impact on outcome. Treatment interventions may also inadvertently contain components that are detrimental to recovery. Such research strategies as dismantling or additive designs can be used to identify which elements of treatment are crucial to positive outcomes.

Research on brief-treatment strategies indicates that, for some individuals, sufficient conditions for change can be contained within relatively minimal interventions. Common elements within currently documented brief-treatment strategies appear to be (1) motivational feedback to increase the perception of risk, (2) clear advice or guidelines for change, and (3) an empathic approach that fosters self-efficacy and perceived choice (Miller, 1985; Orford, 1986; Miller, Sovereign and Krege, in press).

Within particular treatment modalities, specific mechanisms of efficacy can be tested for consistency with the theoretical model underlying the treatment. A client-centered treatment perspective, for example, would posit a strong relationship between treatment outcome and the level of "critical conditions" (e.g., empathy) offered by the therapist during therapy. Empirical support exists for this position (Miller, Taylor and West, 1980; Valle, 1981; Miller and Sovereign, 1988). Oei and Jackson (1984) found that therapist self-disclosure and reinforcement of positive client self-statements are crucial components of cognitive therapy with alcoholics. The effectiveness of social skills training would presumably rely on the improvement of the individual's interpersonal skills (e.g., Greenwald et al., 1980). In treatment programs that subscribe to a traditional disease model, it would be predicted that certain processes (e.g., reduction of denial, acceptance of oneself as alcoholic, recognition of alcoholism as a disease, working the early steps of AA's "Twelve Steps" program) would be crucial prerequisites for recovery.

The Pavlovian learning theory basis of aversion therapies would require the establishment of a conditioned aversion response to alcohol as a precondition for successful outcome. Studies of both chemical aversion (Baker et al., 1984; Cannon et al., 1986) and covert sensitization (Elkins, 1980; Miller and Dougher, 1984) show a strong relationship between treatment outcome and the strength of the conditioning that is established during treatment. When administered in a manner that is unlikely to produce conditioned aversion, covert sensitization appears to be ineffective (Telch, Hannon and Telch, 1984). This type of process research supports the integrity of a specific treatment approach and clarifies the critical elements that should be included when the treatment is replicated.

A limited but nonetheless potentially fruitful strategy for clarifying treatment process is to ask treated individuals which elements of the program they have found most useful or have continued to use during the follow-up period. Self-reports do not necessarily identify the true determinants of outcome, but such inquiries can provide useful leads for further exploration.

The following questions represent opportunities for research on the mechanisms of treatment efficacy:

- For a particular treatment approach (e.g., cognitive therapy, marital/family therapy, AA), what are predicted to be the necessary and sufficient conditions for recovery to occur? Do these process dimensions, when operationally defined and measured, prove to be strong predictors of treatment outcome?
- What do those who have been treated perceive to be the crucial elements of treatment that is, the elements that most account for their outcomes?

Therapist Variables

Although therapist skills and characteristics have long been regarded as important factors in treatment outcome, these variables have remained largely unexamined within the alcohol treatment field (Cartwright, 1981). A few studies prior to 1980 pointed to important relationships between therapist attributes and treatment motivation, dropout, or outcome (Miller, 1985).

Some studies have focused on client/patient perceptions of therapist empathy, a variable with a plausible but still unclear relationship to treatment outcome. Two studies (Lawson, 1982; Kirk, Best, and Irwin, 1986) reported that alcoholics' perceptions of counselor empathy were unaffected by whether the counselor was a recovering alcoholic, although other perceived therapist dimensions may be influenced by this factor (Lawson, 1982). Recent reports continue to reflect no significant difference in treatment outcomes between treatment by counselors who are themselves recovering substance abusers and treatment by those who are not (Aiken et al., 1984).

Other research has included direct measures of the interpersonal functioning of therapists. One therapist characteristic that appears to be related to favorable motivation and treatment outcomes is therapist empathy. "Empathy" in this context refers not to the ability to identify with others based on similar personal experiences but rather empathic understanding as operationally defined by Carl Rogers and his students (Truax and Carkhuff, 1967). A therapist attitude of empathic understanding has been a common element in brief interventions that have been reported to have substantial impact on alcohol problems (Chafetz, 1961; Chafetz et al., 1962; Edwards et al., 1977; Kristenson et al., 1983). In a study assigning alcoholics at random to different counselors, Valle (1981) found a significant relationship between therapist empathy skill and treatment outcomes at 6, 12, 18, and 24 months. Miller, Taylor, and West (1980) found that therapist empathy during behavioral treatment accounted for two-thirds of the variance in 6-month treatment outcome (r = .82) and that a strong relationship persisted in outcomes measured at 12 and 24 months (Miller and Baca, 1983). Analyzing tapes of therapeutic interventions, Miller and Sovereign (1988) found that confrontive and directive therapist behaviors (experimentally controlled) were associated with increased client/patient resistance and higher rates of drinking at the 12-month follow-up point, whereas therapist supportive and listening behaviors were associated with lower resistance and more positive outcomes.

Other therapist behaviors may be important determinants of outcome. As noted in the previous discussion on mechanisms of treatment efficacy, Oei and Jackson (1984), in an experimental study, found greater improvement among individuals whose therapists practiced self-disclosure and reinforced clients' positive self-statements. Cartwright (1980) reported a relationship between therapist self-esteem and positive attitudes toward alcoholics. McLachlan (1972, 1974) reported differential effects of therapist "conceptual level" (directiveness versus nondirectiveness), depending on a corresponding personality type among alcoholic patients. A variable found to be important in research on the treatment of other problems (e.g., depression) is the extent to which the therapist consistently adheres to specific treatment procedures. Still another dimension for exploration is the impact of the therapist's personal history of alcoholism.

The following questions represent opportunities for research on therapist characteristics:

• What role do therapist characteristics (e.g., empathy, self-disclosure, optimism, confrontiveness) play in influencing client/patient dropout, motivation for change, and treatment outcome?
• Do certain types of people respond better to therapists with particular characteristics or styles (e.g., empathic versus confrontational)?

- Is therapist effectiveness influenced by the consistency with which the therapist adheres to specific treatment strategies?
- How great are differences in therapist effectiveness within specific treatment strategies?
- What factors influence client/patient perceptions of therapist empathy, likability, and effectiveness? Are such perceptions predictive of long-term outcome?
- Do recovering persons differ from others in their effectiveness as therapists? If so, in what ways do they use their recovering status in the process of treatment?
- What forms of training or credentialing for treatment providers will improve the effectiveness of their services?

Motivation

Motivation has long been recognized as a key factor in recovery. Early writings conceptualized motivation in alcoholics as a trait or personal characteristic of the individual. Consistent with this perspective, many studies continue to focus on dispositional or demographic predictors of treatment noncompliance (e.g., Bander et al., 1983; Beck et al., 1983; Ornstein and Cherepon, 1985). Yet the dispositional markers of compliance identified in such studies have shown few consistencies, suggesting that individual pretreatment characteristics interact with attributes of the particular treatment setting (Fink et al., 1984).

Research has generally failed to support a trait view of alcoholics as poorly motivated, prone to particular defense mechanisms (e.g., denial), inherently resistive, or possessing a characteristic personality. Rather, motivation or resistance appears to be determined by a range of factors in the treatment situation, many of which are influenced by the therapist (Miller, 1985). Studies do, however, continue to find positive relationships between treatment compliance and outcome (Finney, Moos, and Chan, 1981; Westermeyer and Neider, 1984; Fuller et al., 1986; Fawcett et al., 1987). Consequently, the emphasis in research has shifted from alcoholic traits to a search for intervention procedures that increase compliance and the motivation for change.

Interventions that provide personal feedback about risk appear to have a particular impact on motivation and may be sufficient to induce change in many problem drinkers (Kristenson et al., 1983; Miller, 1985). Two recent controlled evaluations of a "Drinker's Checkup" intervention indicate that problem drinkers significantly reduce their alcohol consumption after receiving feedback about personal harm and risks (Miller and Sovereign, 1988; Miller, Sovereign, and Krege, in press). Such interventions appear to interact with therapist style as well. Risk feedback that is given in a supportive, empathic style appears to induce more change than risk feedback presented in a confrontational and directive style (Miller, 1983; Miller and Sovereign, 1988).

Compliance

Relatively simple interventions have been demonstrated in controlled studies to have powerful effects on treatment entry, persistence, and compliance (Miller, 1985). Moreover, recent studies have added new tools to the armamentarium of motivation-boosting techniques. Pretreatment exposure to videotape role modeling (Craigie and Ross, 1980), participation in a prescreening group (Olkin and Lemle, 1984), and participation in an orientation group (Panepinto et al., 1980) have been found to increase the frequency of return for treatment. Zweben and Li (1981) found that a "role induction" preparation for treatment increased continuation in therapy. For white-collar workers, a role induction conducted by an ex-patient proved less effective than inductions administered by a therapist or by staff using videotape.

In another study, Ossip-Klein and colleagues (1984) provided a wall calendar marked with the dates of aftercare meetings and negotiated a behavioral contract for aftercare attendance. This simple intervention doubled the rate of aftercare compliance, relative to a random control group. Procedures adapted from Azrin's community reinforcement approach were found in three studies to increase treatment entry (Sisson and Azrin, 1986), attendance at AA and AlAnon meetings (Sisson and Mallams, 1981), and medication compliance with subsequent abstinence (Azrin et al., 1982). In another controlled study, a simple contingency contracting procedure substantially increased aftercare participation (Ahles et al., 1983). Correlational studies point to the potential importance of other variables in precipitating or preventing dropout: staff attitudes toward alcoholics (Velleman, 1984), the length of delay between appointments (Leigh, Ogborne and Cleland, 1984), spouse involvement in treatment (Zweben, Pearlman, and Li, 1983), and the availability of treatment groups that include peers of one's own gender or age (Duckert, 1987; Kofoed et al., 1987). Other studies have contributed to our knowledge of motivation by finding a surprising lack of beneficial impact from what would be expected to be an effective intervention. Rees (1985), for example, demonstrated that health beliefs predicted treatment compliance and outcome; in a subsequent experimental study, however, the same investigator found that an intervention which increased the relevant health beliefs had no impact on compliance (Rees, 1986).

Mandated Treatment

An increasingly common practice is the mandating of treatment interventions by requiring individuals to choose between accepting treatment or suffering adverse consequences (e.g., imprisonment, loss of employment). Despite their widespread current use, intervention strategies such as "constructive confrontation" (Trice and Beyer, 1984) and group confrontational intervention (Johnson, 1980) have not as yet been subjected to adequately controlled evaluations of their impact on outcome.

Uncontrolled studies reflect roughly comparable outcomes among mandated and voluntary participants in treatment (Freedberg and Johnston, 1980). Yet direct comparisons of mandated interventions with control groups have yielded inconsistent results. Salzberg and Klingberg (1983), replicating the findings of two previous studies, found that DWI offenders who were given deferred sentencing and then referred for alcohol treatment, showed significantly higher rates of recidivism relative to a comparison group that was given only legal sanctions. Swenson and colleagues (1981) found no differences between two treatment programs for DWI offenders and a home-study control group given a single 30-minute session and educational reading matter. With few exceptions (e.g., Brown, 1980), educational and treatment intervention have not been shown in properly controlled trials to improve long-term outcome and to suppress recidivism to a greater extent than such ordinary legal sanctions as monitored probation (cf. Brandsma et al., 1980; Ditman et al., 1967).

With increasing frequency, employee assistance programs (EAPs) refer employees to treatment when an alcohol or other drug problem is detected, often with the condition that continued employment depends on participation and improvement. Uncontrolled studies of EAPs (e.g., Spickard and Tucker, 1984) continue to report high rates of favorable outcomes in such programs. Several recent studies have focused in particular on the outcomes of impaired physicians who seek treatment in order to retain or regain their license to practice. Among those completing such programs, reported "success" rates near 80 percent are not uncommon (Shore, 1982, 1987; Gualtieri, Cosentino, and Becker, 1983; Morse et al., 1984). Such rates are sometimes inflated by the exclusion of lost, deceased, or uncooperative cases (e.g., Morse et al., 1984).

The contribution of particular intervention components is difficult to assess in this context. Improvement may be motivated simply by the crisis of being identified as having a problem or by the desire to maintain employment, license, or liberty. Morse and coworkers (1984) found that physicians who were closely monitored and in jeopardy of loss of license showed a higher improvement rate than a comparison group of nonphysicians in treatment for alcohol and drug dependence without such scrutiny and contingencies. As with court probation cases, formal treatment may make little or no contribution to outcome above the effects attributable to the threatened loss of liberty or livelihood. Another important factor to consider is the extent to which threatened penalties for noncompliance in "mandated" programs are actually enforced. Perceived stringency of enforcement may be an important determinant of the impact of mandatory treatment. Thus, the level of enforcement of participation should be documented, and perceived enforcement should be assessed.

The following questions represent opportunities for research on motivation, compliance, and mandated treatment:

- What interventions, therapist characteristics, or situational factors increase the probability that a problem drinker will enter, continue, and comply with treatment?
- What measures of motivation best predict a favorable response to treatment? What proportion of variance in outcome is accounted for by dispositional versus situational aspects of motivation and by compliance with specific components of treatment?
- What approaches will instill a motivation for change in individuals who display hazardous alcohol consumption patterns but do not regard themselves as problem drinkers or in need of treatment?
- What are the short-and long-term effects on outcome of coercive motivational strategies (e.g., court-mandated treatment, employee assistance programs, confrontational interventions), relative to less coercive or intrusive alternatives?

CONCLUSIONS

The foregoing discussion constitutes a comprehensive review, within the context of knowledge from earlier research, of what has been learned in treatment outcome studies since 1980. In this section, specific conclusions based on the preceding review will be drawn in order to summarize the opportunities for further progress in treatment research.

Does Treatment Work?

As an introduction to such conclusions, it is important to address what is an inevitable and broader question: Does treatment work? Although attention to this issue was not part of the committee's specific charge, this fundamental question necessarily underlies any consideration of research opportunities. Indeed, the answer to this question may be what many readers of this report most wish to obtain through an examination of well-designed research.

Clearly, clinicians believe sincerely in the efficacy of their interventions; otherwise they would probably not be involved in the treatment enterprise. The history of medicine, as well as recent psychological and medical research, however, abundantly shows that clinician confidence in a treatment is not a reliable indicator of its specific effectiveness. Judgments of whether treatment works must rely on more valid criteria than the certitude of treatment agents or the testimonials of clients or patients.

Given the hundreds of clinical studies now available, what meaningful answer can be given to this question? The answer depends, of course, on what is meant by the question. The first problem to be considered in seeking an answer is the great heterogeneity of treatments for alcohol problems. A very broad array of different treatment approaches has been evaluated in clinical research, and a still wider range has been implemented in practice. If the question, Does treatment work? is understood to mean, Do all of these treatments work?, the answer is plainly, no. Some methods (several of which remain in widespread use) have consistently failed to show a significant impact on alcohol problems. Other currently or previously used treatment methods remain unproved. More than half of controlled clinical trials of alcohol treatment approaches have yielded negative results; that is, no significant differences in outcome among groups. Clearly, no blanket blessing can be given to all or unspecified treatments as "effective."

If, on the other hand, the question is taken to mean, Are any of these treatments effective?, one can more confidently answer, Yes. Several different treatment modalities have been found in a number of clinical trials to produce significantly better outcomes than occur in the absence of the treatment or with alternative treatment. Thus, we are in the happy position of having at our disposal a variety of promising treatment strategies with a positive record of success in well-designed studies.

A third interpretation of the question might be: Is there a single treatment of choice that is superior to all other approaches? Here, the answer is an unambiguous no. No treatment method is universally effective. Few have been found to yield favorable outcomes in even a majority of cases over the long run. Some approaches have poor records of success, whereas others have demonstrated encouragingly consistent benefits, but no particular treatment can lay justifiable claim to superiority over all others. Instead of a single outstandingly effective strategy, there are a number of promising alternatives, each of which appears to be effective with different types of individuals. Behavioral self-control training, for example, appears to be most effective with individuals showing less severe alcohol-related problems and dependence, whereas AA tends to be more effective with individuals who have histories of more severe alcohol problems and dependence.

This picture is consistent with human therapeutics in other fields. In medicine, for example, no single medication is effective against all infections. Nevertheless, the judicious use of the entire range of available medications, effectively deployed on an individual case basis, produces an excellent record against infection. There is no one therapeutic method for dealing with cancer, but the combined use of surgery, chemotherapy, and radiation in differing degrees in individual cases has produced notable reductions in suffering and mortality. Likewise, there are now not one but multiple potentially effective ways to treat diabetes mellitus, depression, anxiety disorders, heart disease, and hypertension. All of these examples are no longer regarded as uniform or unitary problems; rather, each is properly regarded as a family of related disorders that are diverse in etiology as well as optimal treatment. Alcohol problems are fruitfully understood in this same light as heterogeneous disorders, admitting of variety in etiology and proper treatment.

Thus, depending on the meaning of the question, Does treatment work?, the answer can be gloomy or optimistic. The grounds for optimism are not to be found in the efficacy of all treatments or in the established superiority of any particular approach. Instead, this committee, in reviewing its charge, is optimistic about the encouraging array of promising treatment procedures that have been identified through research and about the opportunities for continued research to improve the effectiveness of treatment. The following conclusions should be read within this general context.

Specific Conclusions

Significant progress has been made in alcohol treatment research since 1980. Based on currently available empirical research, the nine following conclusions appear to be supported:

1. The provision of appropriate, specific treatment modalities can substantially improve outcome. A variety of specific alcohol treatment methods have been associated with increased improvement, relative to no treatment or alternative treatments, in controlled studies. Future research should continue to evaluate the effectiveness of alternative current and new treatment modalities.

2. There is no single superior treatment approach for all persons with alcohol problems. Although a number of different treatment methods show promise with particular groups, no single approach stands out as significantly more effective overall. Reason for optimism about alcohol treatment lies in the range of promising alternatives that are available, each of which may be optimal for different types of individuals. Rather than seeking to establish the superiority of a single approach by testing specific interventions in heterogeneous populations, treatment outcome studies should delineate the characteristics of the subpopulation for whom particular modalities are maximally effective.

3. Therapist characteristics have been underestimated as determinants of outcome. Treatment is not offered by neutral agents. Therapist skills and attributes appear to be important factors that influence treatment outcome. Interactions of therapist factors with treatment and client/patient variables, as well as the main effects of therapist characteristics, may account for a substantial amount of variance in client/patient motivation, dropout, compliance, and outcome. Future research should examine the impact of therapist attributes and behaviors on treatment outcome.

4. Alcoholics Anonymous, one of the most widely used approaches to recovery in the United States, remains one of the least rigorously evaluated. Given its widespread availability and potential cost- effectiveness, there is a need for well-designed studies to elucidate the impact and mechanisms of change within AA. There is a particular need for outcome research that employs a range of contemporary treatment assessment strategies.

5. Treatment of other life problems related to drinking can improve alcohol treatment outcome. Posttreatment problems and experiences have been shown to be important determinants of outcome. Social skills training, marital and family therapy, antidepressant medication, stress management training, and the community reinforcement approach all show promise for promoting and prolonging sobriety. Such broad-spectrum strategies appear to affect sobriety by helping to resolve other significant problems that, left untreated, could precipitate relapse. Future research should continue to explore the impacts of posttreatment adjustment and the treatment of other life problems on outcome.

6. Outcome may be predictable from treatment process factors. Individual difference variables that are nonspecific (e.g., resistance) or specific to particular approaches (e.g., the establishment of a conditioned aversion response) may predict treatment outcome. Future studies should seek to clarify treatment process factors that are key determinants

of outcome within specific treatment modalities and to build stronger theoretical models of treatment efficacy.

7. The overall effectiveness of treatment with unselected patients appears to be no different in residential versus nonresidential programs or in longer versus shorter inpatient programs. Although health care reimbursement systems have emphasized more expensive forms of treatment, studies to date fail to show an offsetting increase in overall effectiveness relative to less expensive alternative forms of intervention. Residential care may be differentially effective for individuals who are socially unstable (e.g., homeless, unemployed) as well as those who have more severe levels of alcohol dependence and psychopathology. Socially stable individuals without severe alcohol dependence or psychopathology appear to be treatable by less intensive approaches without compromising effectiveness and at substantially less cost. The validation of differential criteria for admission to various treatment settings and for flexible movement between them during the course of an individual's treatment is an important task for future research.

8. Both experimental and quasi-experimental designs contribute important new knowledge regarding treatment outcome. Randomized, controlled trials yield data from which conclusions of specific effectiveness can be drawn more confidently than from uncontrolled demonstrations; moreover, such studies have tended to yield more consistent results. Experimental studies may be more expensive (although a number of published controlled trials have been conducted at relatively low cost), but given the incremental new knowledge they yield, well-designed controlled clinical trials remain a cost-effective investment of research funds. Contemporary quasi-experimental designs offer sound alternatives in instances in which controlled trials are not feasible. Properly designed nonexperimental studies likewise can yield useful incremental information regarding treatment outcome.

9. The implementation of any treatment procedure warrants careful consideration of the relative risks and benefits that are likely to be derived. A treatment is justifiable when the probable benefits demonstrably outweigh the risks and costs involved in the proposed treatment procedures. Probable benefits may be judged, in general or for specific subpopulations, from the weight of current evidence in treatment outcome research. Treatments with documented special risks merit particular consideration of the risk-benefit balance. Future research should address the relative benefits, risks, and costs attached to specific alternative treatment modalities.

REFERENCES

Ahles, T. A., D. G. Schlundt, D. M. Prue et al. Impact of aftercare arrangements on the maintenance of treatment success in abusive drinkers. Addict. Behav. 8:53-58, 1983.

Aiken, L. S., L. A. LoSciuto, M. A. Ausetts et al. Paraprofessional versus professional drug counselors: The progress of clients in treatment. Int. J. Addict. 19:383-401, 1984.

Alford, G. Alcoholics Anonymous: An empirical study. Addict. Behav. 5:359-370, 1980.

Amit, Z., Z. Brown, A. Sutherland et al. Reduction in alcohol intake in humans as a function of treatment with zimelidine: Implications for treatment. In C. A. Naranjo and E. A. Sellers, eds. Research Advances in New Psychopharmacological Treatments for Alcoholism. Amsterdam: Elsevier, 1985.

Annis, H. M. Is inpatient rehabilitation of the alcoholic cost effective? Con position. Advances in Alcohol and Substance Abuse 5:175-190, 1986a.

Annis, H. M. A relapse prevention model for treatment of alcoholics. Pp. 407-433 in W. R. Miller and N. Heather, eds. Treating Addictive Behaviors: Processes of Change. New York: Plenum, 1986b.

Annis, H. M., and D. Chan. The differential treatment model: Empirical evidence from a personality typology of adult offenders. Criminal Justice and Behav. 110:159-173, 1983.

Annis, H. M., C. S. Davis, M. Graham et al. A controlled trial of relapse prevention procedures based on self-efficacy theory. Unpublished manuscript. Toronto: Addiction Research Foundation, 1988.

Aron, A., and E. N. Aron. The transcendental meditation program's effect on addictive behavior. Addict. Behav. 5:3-12, 1980.

Aron, E. N., and A. Aron. The patterns of reduction of drug and alcohol use among transcendental meditation participants. Bull. Soc. Psychol. Addict. Behav. 2:8-33, 1983.

Azrin, N. H. Improvements in the community-reinforcement approach to alcoholism. Behav. Res. Ther. 14:339-348, 1976.

Azrin, N. H., R. W. Sisson, R. Meyers et al. Alcoholism treatment by disulfiram and community reinforcement therapy. J. Behav. Ther. Exp. Psychiatry 13:105-112, 1982.

Baker, T. B., D. S. Cannon, S. T. Tiffany et al. Cardiac response as an index of the effect of aversion therapy. Behav. Res. Ther. 22:403-411, 1984.

Bander, K. W., N. A. Stilwell, E. Fein et al. Relationship of patient characteristics to program attendance by women alcoholics. J. Stud. Alcohol 44:318-327, 1983.

Beck, N. C., W. Shekin, C. Fraps et al. Prediction of discharges against medical advice from an alcohol and drug misuse treatment program. J. Stud. Alcohol 44:171-180, 1983.

Becker, J. T., and J. H. Jaffe. Impaired memory for treatment-relevant information in inpatient men alcoholics. J. Stud. Alcohol 45:339-343, 1984.

Berg, G., and A. Skutle. Early intervention with problem drinkers. Pp. 205-220 in W. R. Miller and N. Heather, eds. Treating Addictive Behaviors: Processes of Change. New York: Plenum, 1986.

Billings, A. G., and R. H. Moos. Psychosocial processes of recovery among alcoholics and their families: Implications for clinicians and program evaluators. Addict. Behav. 8:205-218, 1983.

Blakey, R., and R. Baker. An exposure approach to alcohol abuse. Behav. Res. Ther. 18:319-326, 1980.

Booth, R. Alcohol halfway houses: Treatment length and treatment outcome. Int. J. Addict. 16:927-934, 1981.

Boscarino, J. Factors related to "stable" and "unstable" affiliation with Alcoholics Anonymous. Int. J. Addict. 15:839-848, 1980.

Botvin, G. J., E. Baker, N. L. Renick et al. A cognitive-behavioral approach to substance abuse prevention. Addict. Behav. 9:137-148, 1984a.

Botvin, G. J., E. Baker, E. M. Botvin et al. Prevention of alcohol misuse through the development of personal and social competence: A pilot study. J. Stud. Alcohol 45:550-552, 1984b.

Brandsma, J. M., M. C. Maultsby, and R. J. Welsh. The Outpatient Treatment of Alcoholism: A Review and Comparative Study. Baltimore, MD: University Park Press, 1980.

Braunstein, W. B., B. J. Powell, J. F. McGowan et al. Employment factors in outpatient recovery of alcoholics: A multivariate study. Addict. Behav. 8:345-351, 1983.

Brown, R. A. Conventional education and controlled drinking education courses with convicted drunken drivers. Behav. Ther. 11:632-642, 1980.

Brubaker, R. G., D. M. Prue, and R. G. Rychtarik. Determinants of disulfiram acceptance among alcohol patients: A test of the theory of reasoned action. Addict. Behav. 12:43-52, 1987.

Bullock, M. L., A. J. Umen, P. D. Culliton et al. Acupuncture treatment of alcoholic recidivism: A pilot study. Alcoholism Clin. Exp. Res. 11:292-295, 1987.

Cannon, D. S., and T. B. Baker. Emetic and electric shock alcohol aversion therapy: Assessment of conditioning. J. Consult. Clin. Psychol. 49:20-33, 1981.

Cannon, D. S., T. B. Baker, and C. K. Wehl. Emetic and electric shock alcohol aversion therapy: Six-and twelve-month follow-up. J. Consult. Clin. Psychol. 49:360-368, 1981.

Cannon, D. S., T. B. Baker, A. Gino et al. Alcohol-aversion therapy: Relation between strength of aversion and abstinence. J. Consult. Clin. Psychol. 54:825-830, 1986.

Carpenter, R. A., C. A. Lyons, and W. R. Miller. Peer-managed self-control program for prevention of alcohol abuse in American Indian high school students: A pilot evaluation study. Int. J. Addict. 20:299-310, 1985.

Cartwright, A. K. J. The attitudes of helping agents towards the alcoholic client: The influence of experience, support, training, and self-esteem. Br. J. Addict. 75:413-431, 1980.

Cartwright, A. K. J. Are different therapeutic perspectives important in the treatment of alcoholism? Br. J. Addict. 76:347-361, 1981.

Chafetz, M. E. A procedure for establishing therapeutic contact with the alcoholic. Q. J. Stud. Alcohol 22:325-328, 1961.

Chafetz, M. E., H. T. Blane, H. S. Abram et al. Establishing treatment relations with alcoholics. J. Nerv. Ment. Dis. 134:395-409, 1962.

Chapman, P. L. H., and I. Huygens. An evaluation of three treatment programmes for alcoholism: An experimental study with six and 18-month follow-ups. Br. J. Addict. 83:67-81, 1988.

Chick, J., B. Ritson, J. Connaughton et al. Advice versus extended treatment for alcoholism: A controlled study. Br. J. Addict. 83:159-170, 1988.

Christensen, J. K., P. Ronsted, and U. H. Vaag. Side effects after disulfiram: Comparison of disulfiram and placebo in a double-blind multicentre study. Acta Psychiatr. Scand. 69:265-273, 1984.

CompCare. Care Unit Evaluation of Treatment Outcome. Newport Beach, CA: Comprehensive Care Corporation, 1988.

Connors, G. J., S. A. Maisto, and S. M. Ersner-Hershfield. Behavioral treatment of drunk-drinking recidivists: Short-term and long-term effects. Behav. Psychotherapy 14:34-35, 1986.

Cook, T. D., and D. T. Campbell. Quasi-experimentation: Design and Analysis Issues for Field Settings. Boston: Houghton-Mifflin, 1979.

Costello, R. M. Alcoholism aftercare and outcome: Cross-lagged panel and path analyses. Br. J. Addict. 75:49-53, 1980.

Council on Scientific Affairs, American Medical Association. Aversion therapy. J. Am. Med. Assoc. 258:2562-2566, 1987.

Craigie, F. C., Jr., and S. M. Ross. The use of a videotape pre-therapy training program to encourage treatment-seeking among alcohol detoxification patients. Behav. Ther. 11:141-147, 1980.

Cronkite, R. C., and R. H. Moos. Determinants of the posttreatment functioning of alcoholic patients: A conceptual framework. J. Consult. Clin. Psychol. 48:305-316, 1980.

Cummings, C., G. A. Marlatt and J. R. Gordon. Relapse: Prevention and prediction. In W. R. Miller, ed. The Addictive Behaviors: Treatment of Alcoholism, Drug Abuse, Smoking, and Obesity. Oxford: Pergamon Press, 1980.

Ditman, K. S., G. G. Crawford, E. W. Forgy et al. A controlled experiment on the use of court probation for drunk arrests. Am. J. Psychiatry 124:160-163, 1967.

Dittrich, J. E., and M. A. Trapold. A treatment program for wives of alcoholics: An evaluation. Bull. Soc. Psychol. Addict. Behav. 3:91-102, 1984.

Dorus, W. Lithium carbonate treatment of depressed and non-depressed alcoholics in a double-blind, placebo-controlled study. Presented at the annual meeting of the Research Society on Alcoholism, June 3, 1988.

Duckert, F. Recruitment into treatment and effects of treatment for female problem drinkers. Addict. Behav. 12:137-150, 1987.

Duckert, F., and J. Johnsen. Behavioral use of disulfiram in the treatment of problem drinking. Int. J. Addict. 22:445-454, 1987.

Edwards, G., J. Orford, S. Egert et al. Alcoholism: A controlled trial of "treatment" and "advice." J. Stud. Alcohol 38:1004-1031, 1977.

Elkin, I., M. T. Shea, J. T. Watkins et al. National Instiute of Mental Health Treatment of Depression Collaborative Research Program: General Effectiveness of Treatments. Arch. Gen. Psychiatry 46:971-982, 1989.

Elkins, R. L. Covert sensitization treatment of alcoholism: Contributions of successful conditioning to subsequent abstinence maintenance. Addict. Behav. 5:67-89, 1980.

Elkins, R. L. Taste-aversion retention: An animal experiment with implications for consummatory-aversion alcoholism treatments. Behav. Res. Ther. 22:179-186, 1984.

Elkins, R. L. Separation of taste-aversion-prone and taste-aversion-resistant rats through selective breeding: Implications for individual differences in conditionability and aversion-therapy alcoholism treatment. Behav. Neuroscience 100:121-124, 1986.

Elkins, R. L., and S. H. Hobbs. Taste aversion proneness: A modulator of conditioned consummatory aversion in rats. Bull. Psychonomic Soc. 20:257-260, 1982.

Emrick, C. D. Alcoholics Anonymous: Affiliation processes and effectiveness as treatment. Alcoholism Clin. Exp. Res. 11:416-423, 1987.

Eriksen, L. The effect of waiting for inpatient treatment after detoxification: An experimental comparison between inpatient treatment and advice only. Addict. Behav. 10:235-248, 1986.

Eriksen, L., S. Bjornstad, and K. G. Gotestam. Social skills training in groups for alcoholics: One-year treatment outcome for groups and individuals. Addict. Behav. 11:309-330, 1986.

Fawcett, J., D. C. Clark, C. A. Aagesen et al. A double-blind, placebo-controlled trial of lithium carbonate therapy for alcoholism. Arch. Gen. Psychiatry 44:248-256, 1987.

Ferrell, W. L., and J. P. Galassi. Assertion training and human relations training in the treatment of chronic alcoholics. Int. J. Addict. 16:959-968, 1981.

Fink, E. B., S. Rudden, R. Longabaugh et al. Adherence in a behavioral alcohol treatment program. Int. J. Addict. 19:709-719, 1984.

Finney, J. W., R. H. Moos, and D. A. Chan. Length of stay and program component effects in the treatment of alcoholism: A comparison of two techniques for process analyses. J. Consult. Clin. Psychol. 49:120-131, 1981.

Finney, J. W., R. H. Moos, and C. R. Mewborn. Posttreatment experiences and treatment outcome of alcoholic patients six months and two years after hospitalization. J. Consult. Clin. Psychol. 48:17-29, 1980.

Fitzgerald, J. L., and H. A. Mulford. An experimental test of telephone aftercare contacts with alcoholics. J. Stud. Alcohol 46:418-424, 1985.

Foy, D. W., B. L. Nunn, and R. G. Rychtarik. Broad-spectrum behavioral treatment for chronic alcoholics: Effects of training in controlled drinking skills. J. Consult. Clin. Psychol. 52:218-230, 1984.

Freedberg, E. J., and W. E. Johnston. Outcome with alcoholics seeking treatment voluntarily or after confrontation by their employer. J. Occup. Med. 22:83-86, 1980.

Fuller, R. K., and W. O. Williford. Life-table analysis of abstinence in a study evaluating the efficacy of disulfiram. Alcoholism Clin. Exp. Res. 4:298-301, 1980.

Fuller, R. K., L. Branchey, D. R. Brightwell et al. Disulfiram treatment of alcoholism: A Veterans Administration cooperative study. J. Am. Med. Assoc. 256:1449-1455, 1986.

Gilbert, F. S. The effect of type of aftercare follow-up on treatment outcome among alcoholics. J. Stud. Alcohol 49:149-159, 1988.

Gilchrest, L. D., S. P. Schinke, J. E. Trimble et al. Skills enhancement to prevent substance abuse among American Indian adolescents. Int. J. Addict. 22:869-879, 1987.

Gill, K., and Z. Amit. Effects on serotonin uptake blockade on food water and ethanol consumption in rats. Alcoholism Clin. Exp. Res. 11(5):444-449, 1987.

Gilmore, K., D. Jones, and L. Tamble. Treatment Benchmarks. Center City, MN: Hazelden, 1986.

Glaser, F. B., and A. C. Ogborne. Does A.A. really work? Br. J. Addict. 77:123-129, 1982.

Gorski, T. T., and M. Miller. Counseling for Relapse Prevention. Independence, MO: Herald House-Independence Press, 1982.

Graber, R. A., and W. R. Miller. Abstinence and controlled drinking goals in behavioral self-control training of problem drinkers: A randomized clinical trial. Psychol. Addict. Behav. 2:20-33, 1988.

Greenwald, M. A., J. D. Kloss, M. E. Kovaleski et al. Drink refusal and social skills training with hospitalized alcoholics. Addict. Behav. 5:227-228, 1980.

Grenier, C. Treatment effectiveness in an adolescent chemical dependence treatment program: A quasi-experimental design. Int. J. Addict. 20:381-391, 1985.

Gualtieri, A. C., J. P. Cosentino, and J. S. Becker. The California experience with a diversion program for impaired physicians. J. Am. Med. Assoc. 249:226-229, 1983.

Hobbs, S. H., and R. L. Elkins. Operant performance of rats selectively bred for strong or weak acquisition of conditioned taste aversions. Bull. Psychonomic Soc. 21:303-306, 1983.

Hoffman, N. B., P. A. Harrison, and C. A. Belille. Alcoholics Anonymous after treatment: Attendance and abstinence. Int. J. Addict. 18:311-318, 1983.

Hunt, N. H., and N. H. Azrin. A community-reinforcement approach to alcoholism. Behav. Res. Ther. 11:91-104, 1973.

Ito, J. R., and D. M. Donovan. Aftercare in alcoholism treatment: A review. Pp.435-456 in W. R. Miller and N. Heather, eds. Treating Addictive Behaviors: Processes of Change. New York: Plenum, 1986.

Ito, J. R., D. M. Donovan, and J. J. Hall. Relapse prevention and alcohol aftercare: Effects on drinking outcome, change process, and aftercare attendance. Br. J. Addict. 83:171-181, 1988.

Jensen, S. B. Sexual function and dysfunction in younger married alcoholics. Acta Psychiatr. Scand. 69:543-549, 1984.

Johnsen, J., A. Stowell, J. Bache-Wiig et al. A double-blind placebo controlled study of male alcoholics given a subcutaneous disulfiram implantation. Br. J. Addict. 82:607-613, 1987.

Johnson, V. I'll Quit Tomorrow. New York: Harper and Row, 1980.

Jones, S. L., R. Kanfer, and R. I. Lanyon. Skill training with alcoholics: A clinical extension. Addict. Behav. 7:285-290, 1982.

Keane, T. M., D. W. Foy, B. Nunn et al. Spouse contracting to increase Antabuse compliance in alcoholic veterans. J. Clin. Psychol. 40:340-344, 1984.

Kirk, W. G., J. B. Best, and P. Irwin. The perception of empathy in alcoholism counselors. J. Stud. Alcohol 47:834-838, 1986.

Kofoed, L. L. Chemical monitoring of disulfiram compliance: A study of alcoholic outpatients. Alcoholism Clin. Exp. Res. 11:481-485, 1987.

Kofoed, L. L., J. Kania, T. Walsh, and R. Atkinson. Outpatient treatment of patients with substance abuse and coexisting psychiatric disorders. Am. J. Psych. 143:867-872, 1986.

Kofoed, L. L., R. L. Tolson, R. M. Atkinson et al. Treatment compliance of older alcoholics: An elder-specific approach is superior to "mainstreaming." J. Stud. Alcohol 48:47-51, 1987.

Kristenson, H., H. Ohlin, M. B. Hulten-Nosslin et al. Identification and intervention of heavy drinking in middle-aged men: Results and follow-up of 24-60 months of long-term study with randomized controls. Alcoholism Clin. Exp. Res. 7:203-209, 1983.

Kurtz, E. Why A.A. works: The intellectual significance of Alcoholics Anonymous. J. Stud. Alcohol 43:38-80, 1982.

Lawson, G. Relation of counselor traits to evaluation of the counseling relationship by alcoholics. J. Stud. Alcohol 43:834-838, 1982.

Leigh, G., A. C. Ogborne, and P. Cleland. Factors associated with patient dropout from an outpatient alcoholism treatment service. J. Stud. Alcohol 45:359-362, 1984.

Lemberger, L., H. Rowe, R. F. Bergstrom et al. The effect of fluoxetine on psychomotor performance, physiologic response, and kinetics of ethanol. Clin. Pharmacol. Ther. 37:658-64, 1985.

Ling, W., D. G. Weiss, V. C. Charuvastra et al. Use of disulfiram for alcoholics in methadone maintenance programs: A Veterans Administration cooperative study. Arch. Gen. Psychiatry 40:851-861, 1983.

Linnoila, M., M. Eckardt, M. Durcan et al. Interactions of serotonin with ethanol: Clinical and animal studies. Psychopharm. Bull. 23:452-457, 1987.

Liskow, B. I., and D. W. Goodwin. Pharmacological treatment of alcohol intoxication, withdrawal and dependence: A critical review. J. Stud. Alcohol 48:356-370, 1987.

Litman, G. Alcoholism survival: The prevention of relapse. Pp. 391-405 in W. R. Miller and N. Heather, eds. Treating Addictive Behaviors: Processes of Change. New York: Plenum, 1986.

Longabaugh, R., B. McCrady, E. Fink et al. Cost-effectiveness of alcoholism treatment in partial vs. inpatient settings: Six-month outcomes. J. Stud. Alcohol 44:1049-1071, 1983.

Mallams, J. H., M. D. Godley, G. M. Hall et al. A social-systems approach to resocializing alcoholics in the community. J. Stud. Alcohol 43:1115-1123, 1982.

Marlatt, G. A., and Gordon, J. Relapse prevention: Maintenance strategies in the treatment of addictive behaviors. New York: Guilford Press, 1985.

McCrady, B. S., J. Moreau, T. J. Paolino, Jr., et al. Joint hospitalization and couples therapy for alcoholism: A four-year follow-up. J. Stud. Alcohol 43:1244-1250, 1982.

McCrady, B. S., N. E. Noel, D. B. Abrams et al. Comparative effectiveness of three types of spouse involvement in outpatient behavioral alcoholism treatment. J. Stud. Alcohol 47:459-467, 1986.

McElrath, D. The Hazelden treatment model. Testimony before the U.S. Senate Committee on Governmental Affairs, Washington DC, June 16, 1988.

McLachlan, J. F. C. Benefit from group therapy as a function of patient-therapist match on conceptual level. Psychother. 9:317-323, 1972.

McLachlan, J. F. C. Therapy strategies, personality orientation, and recovery from alcoholism. Can. Psychiatr. Assoc. J. 19:25-30, 1974.

McLachlan, J. F. C., and R. L. Stein. Evaluation of a day clinic for alcoholics. J. Stud. Alcohol 43:261-272, 1982.

McLellan, A. T., L. Luborsky, C. O'Brien et al. Is treatment for substance abuse effective? J. Am. Med. Assoc. 247:1423-1428, 1982.

McLellan, A. T., G. E. Woody, L. Luborsky et al. Increased effectiveness of substance abuse treatment: A prospective study of patient-treatment "matching." J. Nerv. Ment. Dis. 171:597-605, 1983.

McMillan, T. M. Lithium and the treatment of alcoholism: A critical review. Br. J. Addict. 76:245-258, 1981.

Miller, W. R. Maintenance of therapeutic change: A usable evaluation design. Prof. Psychol. 41:773-775, 1980.

Miller, W. R. Motivational interviewing with problem drinkers. Behavioral Psychotherapy 11:147-172, 1983.

Miller, W. R. Motivation for treatment: A review with special emphasis on alcoholism. Psychol. Bull. 98:84-107, 1985.

Miller, W. R., and L. M. Baca. Two-year follow-up of bibliotherapy and therapist-directed controlled drinking training for problem drinkers. Behav. Ther. 14:441-448, 1983.

Miller, W. R., and M. J. Dougher. Covert sensitization: Alternative treatment approaches for alcoholics. Paper presented at the Second Congress of the International Society for Biomedical Research on Alcoholism, Santa Fe, 1984.

Miller, W. R., and R. K. Hester. Treating the problem drinker: Modern approaches. In W. R. Miller, ed. The Addictive Behaviors: Treatment of Alcoholism, Drug Abuse, Smoking, and Obesity. Oxford: Pergamon Press, 1980.

Miller, W. R., and R. K. Hester. The effectiveness of alcoholism treatment: What research reveals. Pp. 121-174 in W. R. Miller and N. Heather, eds. Treating Addictive Behaviors: Processes of Change. New York: Plenum, 1986a.

Miller, W. R., and R. K. Hester Inpatient alcoholism treatment: Who benefits? American Psychologist 41(7):794-805, 1986b.

Miller, W. R., and R. G. Sovereign. A comparison of two styles of therapeutic confrontation. Unpublished manuscript, University of New Mexico, 1988.

Miller, W. R., and C. A. Taylor. Relative effectiveness of bibliotherapy, individual and group self-control training in the treatment of problem drinkers. Addict. Behav. 5:13-24, 1980.

Miller, W. R., C. J. Gribskov, and R. L. Mortell. Effectiveness of a self-control manual for problem drinkers with and without therapist contact. Int. J. Addict. 16:1247-1254, 1981.

Miller, W. R., K. A. Hedrick, and C. A. Taylor. Addictive behaviors and life problems before and after behavioral treatment of problem drinkers. Addict. Behav. 8:403-412, 1983.

Miller, W. R., A. L. Leckman, and M. Tinkcom. Long-term follow-up of controlled drinking therapies, unpublished, 1988.

Miller, W. R., R. G. Sovereign, and B. Krege. Motivational interviewing with problem drinkers. II. The drinker's check-up as a preventive intervention. Behav. Psychother, in press.

Miller, W. R., C. A. Taylor, and J. C. West. Focused versus broad-spectrum therapy for problem drinkers. J. Consult. Clin. Psychol. 48:590-601, 1980.

Moos, R. H., and B. S. Moos. The process of recovery from alcoholism. III. Comparing functioning in families of alcoholics and matched control families. J. Stud. Alcohol 45:111-118, 1984.

Moos, R. H., J. W. Finney, and W. Gamble. The process of recovery from alcoholism. II. Comparing spouses of alcoholic patients and matched community controls. J. Stud. Alcohol 43:888-909, 1982.

Morse, R. M., M. A. Martin, W. M. Swenson et al. Prognosis of physicians treated for alcoholism and drug dependence. J. Am. Med. Assoc. 251:743-746, 1984.

Murphy, T. J., R. R. Pagano, and G. A. Marlatt. Lifestyle modification with heavy alcohol drinkers: Effects of aerobic exercise and meditation. Addict. Behav. 11:175-186, 1986.

Nakamura, M., J. E. Overall, L. E. Hollister et al. Factors affecting outcome of depressive symptoms in alcoholics. Alcoholism Clin. Exp. Res. 7:188-193, 1983.

Naranjo, C. A., E. A. Sellers, C. A. Roach et al. Zimelidine-induced variations in alcohol intake by non-depressed heavy drinkers. Clin. Pharm. Ther. 35:374-381, 1984.

Naranjo, C. A., E. A. Sellers, J. T. Sullivan et al. The serotonin uptake inhibitor citalopram attenuates ethanol intake. Clin. Pharmaco. Ther. 41:266-274, 1987.

National Center for Health Care Technology. Assessment of Chemical Aversion Therapy for Alcoholism. Washington DC: National Center for Health Care Technology, 1981.

National Institute on Alcohol Abuse and Alcoholism. Draft recommended council guidelines on ethyl alcohol administration in human experimentation. Washington, DC: NIAAA, November 1988.

Neuberger, O. W., J. D. Matarazzo, R. E. Schmitz et al. One-year follow-up of total abstinence in chronic alcoholic patients following emetic counterconditioning. Alcoholism Clin. Exp. Res. 4:306-312, 1980.

Neuberger, O. W., N. Hasha, J. D. Matarazzo et al. Behavioral-chemical treatment of alcoholism: An outcome replication. J. Stud. Alcohol 42:806-810, 1981.

Neuberger, O. W., S. I. Miller, R. E. Schmitz et al. Replicable abstinence rates in an alcoholism treatment program. J. Am. Med. Assoc. 248:960-963, 1982.

Nirenberg, T. D., L. C. Sobell, S. Ersner-Hershfield et al. Can disulfiram use precipitate urges to drink alcohol? Addict. Behav. 8:311-313, 1983.

Noel, N. E., B. S. McCrady, R. L. Stout et al. Predictors of attrition from an outpatient alcoholism treatment program for couples. J. Stud. Alcohol 48:229-235, 1987.

Oei, T. P. S., and P. R. Jackson. Long-term effects of group and individual social skills training with alcoholics. Addict. Behav. 5:129-136, 1980.

Oei, T. P. S., and P. R. Jackson. Social skills and cognitive behavioral approaches to the treatment of problem drinking. J. Stud. Alcohol 43:532-547, 1982.

Oei, T. P. S., and P. R. Jackson. Some effective therapeutic factors in group cognitive-behavioral therapy with problem drinkers. J. Stud. Alcohol 45:119-123, 1984.

O'Farrell, T. J., H. S. G. Cutter, and F. J. Floyd. Evaluating behavioral marital therapy for male alcoholics: Effects on marital adjustment and communication before and after treatment. Behav. Ther. 16:147-167, 1985.

Ogborne, A. C., and A. Bornet. Abstinence and abusive drinking among affiliates of Alcoholics Anonymous: Are these the only alternatives? Addict. Behav. 7:199-202, 1982.

Ogborne, A. C., and F. B. Glaser. Characteristics of affiliates of Alcoholics Anonymous: A review of the literature. J. Stud. Alcohol 42:661-675, 1981.

Olkin, R., and R. Lemle. Increasing attendance in an outpatient alcoholism clinic: A comparison of two intake procedures. J. Stud. Alcohol 45:465-468, 1984.

Olson, R. P., R. Ganley, V. T. Devine et al. Long-term effects of behavioral versus insight-oriented therapy with inpatient alcoholics. J. Consult. Clin. Psychol. 49:866-877, 1981.

O'Neil, P. M., J. C. Roitzsch, J. P. Glacinto et al. Disulfiram acceptors and refusers: Do they differ? Addict. Behav. 7:207-210, 1982.

Orford, J. Critical conditions for change in the addictive behaviors. Pp. 91-108 in W. R. Miller and N. Heather, eds. Treating Addictive Behaviors: Processes of Change. New York: Plenum, 1986.

Orford, J., and A. Keddie. Abstinence or controlled drinking in clinical practice: A test of the dependence and persuasion hypotheses. Br. J. Addict. 81:495-504, 1986.

Ornstein, P., and J. A. Cherepon. Demographic variables as predictors of alcoholism treatment outcome. J. Stud. Alcohol 46:425-432, 1985.

Ossip-Klein, D. J., W. VanLandingham, D. M. Prue et al. Increasing attendance at alcohol aftercare using calendar prompts and home based contracting. Addict. Behav. 9:85-90, 1984.

Panepinto, W., M. Galanter, M. Bender et al. Alcoholics' transition from ward to clinic: Group orientation improves retention. J. Stud. Alcohol 41:940-944, 1980.

Peachey, J. E., and H. M. Annis. Pharmacologic treatment of chronic alcoholism. Psych. Clin. N. Am. 7:745-756, 1984.

Peachey, J. E., and H. M. Annis. New strategies for using the alcohol-sensitizing drugs. Pp. 199-216 in C. A. Naranjo and E. M. Sellers, eds. Research Advances in New Psychopharmacological Treatments for Alcoholism. Amsterdam: Excerpta Medica, 1985.

Peachey, J. E., D. H. Zilm, G. M. Robinson et al. A placebo-controlled double-blind comparative clinical study of the disulfiram-and calcium carbimide-acetaldehyde mediated ethanol reactions in social drinkers. Alcoholism Clin. Exp. Res. 7:180-187, 1983.

Peck, C. C., S. M. Pond, C. E. Becker et al. An evaluation of the effects of lithium in the treatment of chronic alcoholism. II. Alcoholism Clin. Exp. Res. 5:252-255, 1981.

Pettinati, H. M., A. A. Sugerman, N. DiDonato et al. The natural history of alcoholism over four years after treatment. J. Stud. Alcohol 43:201-215, 1982.

Polich, J. M., D. J. Armor, and H. B. Braiker. Patterns of alcoholism over four years. J. Stud. Alcohol 41:397-416, 1980.

Pond, S. M., C. E. Becker, R. Vandervoort et al. An evaluation of the effects of lithium in the treatment of chronic alcoholism: I. Clinical results. Alcoholism Clin. Exp. Res. 5:247-251, 1981.

Powell, B. J., E. C. Penick, M. R. Read et al. Comparison of three outpatient treatment interventions: A twelve-month follow-up of men alcoholics. J. Stud. Alcohol 46:309-312, 1985.

Powell, B. J., E. C. Penick, S. Rahaim et al. The dropout in alcoholism research: A brief report. Int. J. Addict. 22:283-287, 1986.

Rankin, H. Dependence and compulsion: Experimental models of change. Pp. 361-374 in W. R. Miller and N. Heather, eds. Treating Addictive Behaviors: Processes of Change. New York: Plenum, 1986.

Rankin, H., R. Hodgson, and T. Stockwell. Cue exposure and response prevention with alcoholics: A controlled trial. Behav. Res. Ther. 21:435-446, 1983.

Rees, D. W. Health beliefs and compliance with alcoholism treatment. J. Stud. Alcohol 46:517-524, 1985.

Rees, D. W. Changing patients' health beliefs to improve compliance with alcoholism treatment: A controlled trial. J. Stud. Alcohol 47:436-439, 1986.

Richard, G. P. Behavioral treatment of excessive drinking. Unpublished dissertation, University of New South Wales, 1983.

Rockman, G. E., Z. Amit, G. Carr et al. Attenuation of ethanol intake by 5-hydroxytryptamine uptake blockade in laboratory rats. I. Involvement of brain 5-hydroxytryptamine in the mediation of the positive reinforcing properties of ethanol. Arch. Int. Pharmacodyn. Ther. 241:245-259, 1979.

Rohsenow, D. J., R. E. Smith, and S. Johnson. Stress management training as a prevention program for heavy social drinkers: Cognitive, affect, drinking, and individual differences. Addict. Behav. 10:45-54, 1985.

Rosenberg, H., and T. Brian. Cognitive-behavioral group therapy for multiple-DUI offenders. Alcoholism Treat. Q. 3:47-65, 1986.

Rosenberg, S. D. Relaxation training and a differential assessment of alcoholism. Unpublished doctoral dissertation (University Microfilms No. 8004362), California School of Professional Psychology, San Diego, 1979.

Rounsaville, B. J., Z. S. Dolinsky, T. Babor et al. Psychopathology as a predictor of treatment outcome in alcoholics. Arch. Gen. Psychiatry 44:505-513, 1987.

Rychtarik, R. G., D. W. Foy, T. Scott et al. Five-year follow-up of broad-spectrum behavioral treatment for alcoholism: Effects of training controlled drinking skills. J. Consult. Clin. Psychol. 55:106-108, 1987.

Salzberg, P. M., and C. L. Klingberg. The effectiveness of deferred prosecution for driving while intoxicated. J. Stud. Alcohol 44:299-306, 1983.

Sanchez-Craig, M. Random assignment to abstinence or controlled drinking in a cognitive-behavioral program: Short-term effects on drinking behavior. Addict. Behav. 5:35-39, 1980.

Sanchez-Craig, M. Therapist's Manual for Secondary Prevention of Alcohol Problems: Procedures for Teaching Moderate Drinking and Abstinence. Toronto: Addiction Research Foundation, 1984.

Sanchez-Craig, M., and K. Walker. Teaching coping skills to chronic alcoholics in a coeducational halfway house. I. Assessment of programme effects. Br. J. Addict. 77:35-50, 1982.

Sanchez-Craig, M., H. M. Annis, A. R. Bornet et al. Random assignment to abstinence and controlled drinking: Evaluation of a cognitive-behavioral treatment program for problem drinkers. J. Consult. Clin. Psychol. 52:390-403, 1984.

Schuckit, M. A. A one-year follow-up of men alcoholics given disulfiram. J. Stud. Alcohol 46:191-195, 1985.

Sereny, G., V. Sharma, J. Holt et al. Mandatory supervised antabuse therapy in an outpatient alcoholism program: A pilot study. Alcoholism Clin. Exp. Res. 10:290-292, 1986.

Shore, J. H. The impaired physician: Four years after probation. J. Am. Med. Assoc. 248:3127-3130, 1982.

Shore, J. H. The Oregon experience with impaired physicians on probation: An eight-year follow-up. J. Am. Med. Assoc. 257:2931-2934, 1987.

Siegal, H. A. The intervention approach to drunk driver rehabilitation. I. Evolution, operations, and impact. Int. J. Addict. 20:661-673, 1985a.

Siegal, H. A. The intervention approach to drunk driver rehabilitation. II. Evaluation. Int. J. Addict. 20:675-689, 1985b.

Sisson, R. W. The effect of three relaxation procedures on tension reduction and subsequent drinking of inpatient alcoholics. Unpublished doctoral dissertation (University Microfilms No. 8122668), Southern Illinois University at Carbondale, 1981.

Sisson, R. W., and N. H. Azrin. Family-member involvement to initiate and promote treatment of problem drinkers. J. Behav. Ther. Exp. Psychiatry 17:15-21, 1986.

Sisson, R. W., and J. H. Mallams. The use of systematic encouragement and community access procedures to increase attendance at Alcoholics Anonymous and Al-Anon meetings. Am. J. Drug Alcohol Abuse 8:371-376, 1981.

Skutle, A., and G. Berg. Training in controlled drinking for early-stage problem drinkers. Br. J. Addict. 82:493-501, 1987.

Snyder, S., I. Karacan, and P. J. Salis. Disulfiram and nocturnal penile tumescence in the chronic alcoholic. Biol. Psychiatry 16:399-406, 1981.

Sparadeo, F. R., W. R. Zwick, S. D. Ruggiero et al. Evaluation of a social-setting detoxification program. J. Stud. Alcohol 43:1124-1136, 1982.

Spickard, W. A., and P. J. Tucker. An approach to alcoholism in a university medical center complex. J. Am. Med. Assoc. 252:1894-1897, 1984.

Stimmel, B., M. Cohen, V. Sturiano et al. Is treatment of alcoholism effective in persons on methadone maintenance? Am. J. Psychiatry 140:862-866, 1983.

Stockwell, T., G. Sutherland, and G. Edwards. The impact of a new alcohol sensitized agent (nitrefazole) on craving in severely dependent alcoholics. Br. J. Addict. 79:403-409, 1984.

Stout, R. L., B. S. McCrady, R. Longabaugh et al. Marital therapy helps enhance the long-term effectiveness of alcohol treatment. (Abstract) Alcoholism: Clin. and Exper. Res. 11:213,1987.

Swenson, P. R., and T. R. Clay. Effects of short-term rehabilitation on alcohol consumption and drinking-related behaviors: An eight-month follow-up study of drunken drivers. Int. J. Addict. 15:821-838, 1980.

Swenson, P. R., D. L. Struckman-Johnson, V. Ellingstad et al. Results of a longitudinal evaluation of court-mandated DWI treatment programs in Phoenix, Arizona. J. Stud. Alcohol 42:642-653, 1981.

Telch, M. J., R. Hannon, and C. F. Telch. A comparison of cessation strategies for outpatient alcoholism. Addict. Behav. 9:103-109, 1984.

Thomas, E. J., and C. A. Santa. Unilateral family therapy for alcohol abuse: A working conception. Am. J. Fam. Ther. 10:49-60, 1982.

Thomas, E. J., C. A. Santa, D. Bronson et al. Unilateral family therapy with spouses of alcoholics. J. Soc. Serv. Res., in press.

Thurber, S. Effect size estimates in chemical aversion treatments of alcoholism. J. Clin Psychol. 41:285-287, 1985.

Thurston, A. H., A. M. Alfano, and V. J. Nerviano. The efficacy of A.A. attendance for aftercare of inpatient alcoholics: Some follow-up data. Int. J. Addict. 22:1083-1090, 1987.

Trice, H. M., and J. M. Beyer. Work-related outcomes of the constructive-confrontation strategy in a job-based alcoholism program. J. Stud. Alcohol 45:251-259, 1984.

Traux, C. B., and R. R. Carkhuff. Toward Effective Counseling and Psychotherapy. Chicago: Aldine, 1967.

Uecker, A. E., and K. B. Solberg. Alcoholics' knowledge about alcohol problems: Its relationship to significant attitudes. Q. J. Stud. Alcohol 34:509-513, 1973.

U.S. Congress, Office of Technology Assessment (OTA). The Effectiveness and Costs of Alcoholism Treatment. Washington, D.C.: OTA, 1983.

Valle, S. K. Interpersonal functioning of alcoholism counselors and treatment outcome. J. Stud. Alcohol 42:783-790, 1981.

Velleman, R. The engagement of new residents: A missing dimension in the evaluation of halfway houses for problem drinkers. J. Stud. Alcohol 45:251-259, 1984.

Walker, K., M. Sanchez-Craig, and A. Bornet. Teaching coping skills to chronic alcoholics in a coeducational halfway house. II. Assessment of outcome and identification of outcome predictors. Br. J. Addict. 77:185-196, 1982.

Walker, R. D., D. M. Donovan, D. R. Kivlahan et al. Length of stay, neuropsychological performance, and aftercare: Influences on alcohol treatment outcome. J. Consult. Clin. Psychol. 51:900-911, 1983.

Wallace, J., D. McNeill, D. Gilfillan et al. Six-month treatment outcomes in socially stable alcoholics: Abstinence rates. J. Substance Abuse Treatment, in press.

Weidman, A. Family therapy and reductions in treatment dropout in a residential therapeutic community for chemically dependent adolescents. J. Substance Abuse Treat. 4:21-28, 1987.

Westermeyer, J., and J. Neider. Predicting treatment outcome after ten years among American Indian alcoholics. Alcoholism Clin. Exp. Res. 8:179-184, 1984.

Whitfield, C. L. Non-drug treatment of alcohol withdrawal. Curr. Psychiatr. Ther. 19:101-119, 1980.

Whitfield, C. L., G. Thompson, A. Lamb et al. Detoxification of 1,024 alcoholic patients without psychoactive drugs. J. Am. Med. Assoc. 239:1409-1410, 1978.

Wilson, A., W. J. Davidson, and R. Blanchard. Disulfiram implantation: A trial using placebo implants and two types of controls. J. Stud. Alcohol 41:429-436, 1980.

Wilson, A., R. Blanchard, W. J. Davidson et al. Disulfiram implantation: A dose response trial. J. Clin. Psychiatry 45:242-247, 1984.

Wilson, G. T. Chemical aversion conditioning as a treatment for alcoholism: A re-analysis. Behav. Res. Ther. 25:503-516, 1987.

Zweben, A., and S. Li. The efficacy of role induction in preventing early dropout from outpatient treatment of drug dependency. Am. J. Drug Alcohol Abuse 8:171-183, 1981.

Zweben, A., S. Pearlman, and S. Li. Reducing attrition from conjoint therapy with alcoholic couples. Drug Alcohol Depend. 11:321-331, 1983.

Zweben, A., S. Pearlman, and S. Li. A comparison of brief advice and conjoint therapy in the treatment of alcohol abuse: The results of the marital systems study. Br. J. Addict., 83(8):899-916, 1988.

EARLY IDENTIFICATION AND TREATMENT

Since 1980, increased attention has been given to the identification and treatment of individuals early in their development of alcohol problems. Indeed, people who are unlikely to meet the diagnostic criteria for alcohol dependence actually experience the largest proportion of society's alcohol problems (Moore and Gerstein, 1981). Like many other health problems, alcohol problems may be treated more easily and successfully if they are detected early. The growth of employee assistance programs, student assistance programs, and health maintenance organizations has increased access to populations within which early identification and intervention are feasible. This identification effort represents an overlap of "treatment" with "secondary prevention" of alcohol problems.

To implement a public health approach to the secondary prevention of alcohol-related problems, programs are now under way in several countries to link a new generation of screening technologies to low-cost early intervention strategies (Babor, Ritson, and Hodgson, 1986). Part of the impetus for these programs comes from a broader public health concern with the relationship between life-style-related behavioral risk factors and disease prevalence (IOM, 1982). Because life-style risk factors such as heavy or intensive drinking are often amenable to behavioral interventions, a number of innovative clinical trials, demonstration projects, and early intervention programs have been initiated. An underlying assumption of such efforts is that regular drinking and frequent alcohol intoxication increase substantially the risk of social, medical, and psychological problems (Babor, Kranzler, and Lauerman, 1987). Promising research opportunities in this domain are noted as questions to be investigated.

CONTROLLED TRIALS AND PROGRAM EVALUATIONS

During the 1970s there were a number of research reports evaluating the effectiveness of behavioral treatments for problem drinkers who were recruited from the community rather than from traditional treatment settings (Miller, 1983). In general, the early studies of less dependent problem drinkers were encouraging, with success rates at the one-year follow-up point averaging between 60 and 70 percent (Miller and Hester, 1980). The broad-spectrum treatment methods used in some of these early studies, however, were time-consuming, sometimes requiring as much as 45 hours per client. Studies reported in the 1980s have tended to employ less time-consuming approaches that can be grouped under the heading of behavioral self-control training (see Chapter 9). Such an approach typically includes specific behavioral goal setting, self-monitoring, modulation of the rate of consumption, functional analysis of drinking behavior, self-reinforcement training, and the learning of alternative behavioral competencies to substitute for previous functions of drinking (Miller and Munoz, 1982).

One unexpected finding that emerged from the research of Miller and his colleagues was that a self-help manual may be as effective as self-control training provided by a therapist (Miller and Taylor, 1980; Miller, Taylor, and West, 1980; Miller, Gribskov, and Mortell, 1981). Subsequently, several research teams have systematically investigated the effectiveness of minimal treatment interventions using self-help manuals, simple advice, and brief time-limited counseling (Babor, Ritson, and Hodgson, 1986). The effectiveness of manual-based self-help approaches has been supported in several recent controlled trials (Buck and Miller, 1981; Heather, 1986; Heather et al., 1986). These findings suggest that low-cost interventions based on a manual or brief counseling may be appropriate and effective as a first attempt to intervene with the large number of people who drink heavily but show little or no dependence on alcohol.

The results of several other studies support this conclusion. Kristenson and his colleagues in Malmo, Sweden, studied a group of 529 middle-aged men who had been identified as at-risk drinkers during a general community-wide health screening project (Kristenson, Trell, and Hood, 1982; Kristenson et al., 1983). Men with an elevated liver enzyme (gamma-glutamyl transpeptidase, or GGT) were randomly allocated either to a brief counseling group or to a control group. Although the GGT scores of both groups decreased significantly over the six-year follow-up period, the group given the brief intervention showed greater reductions in absenteeism, sick days, and days hospitalized.

A related Scottish study was conducted at the Royal Edinburgh Infirmary to assess the impact of brief counseling and a self-help manual on socially stable problem drinkers who had been identified in a general hospital (Chick, Lloyd, and Crombie, 1985). Screening was conducted by a trained nurse using a 10-minute interview covering drinking habits, medical history, and social background. Although both the counseled and the control group reported significantly less alcohol consumption at the one-year follow-up point, the group that was given a single brief intervention showed fewer alcohol-related problems, greater reductions in GGT values, and better performance on a global outcome measure. Elvy and colleagues (1988) similarly reported a significant impact of a brief referral intervention with alcohol-impaired patients treated on orthopedic and surgical wards.

Perhaps the most ambitious program of early intervention with heavy drinkers was initiated in France as part of a national policy to deal with alcohol problems in specialized outpatient clinics rather than in primary care settings and hospitals. Beginning in 1970, the French Health Ministry established a system of outpatient clinics as part of a national program to prevent alcohol problems. These clinics respond to the needs of habitual excessive drinkers who do not have serious psychological problems (LeGo, 1977). More than 140 Centers of Nutritional Hygiene have now been established, reaching every major city in France. Although a randomized clinical trial has not been conducted, two critical reviews (Babor et al., 1983; Chick, 1984) concur that this program merits careful attention because of its low cost (relative to inpatient treatment), widespread accessibility, and apparent effectiveness in reaching large numbers of problem drinkers.

BRIEF INTERVENTIONS AND TREATMENT RESEARCH

Current data indicate that brief interventions are superior to no treatment or to waiting list status. The assumption is made that some proportion of those on a waiting list would respond favorably to a brief intervention and not require treatment, leaving a subpopulation that was more in need of therapeutic assistance. The apparent effectiveness of certain brief interventions also suggests a more feasible alternative to no-treatment controls in experimental designs. Justification for the use of an alcoholism treatment method could be based on its ability to exceed the effectiveness of a well-implemented brief intervention. The use of research-supported brief intervention comparison groups can avert some of the ethical concerns regarding refusal of treatment to control groups.

Alternatively, a brief intervention can be used to remove from a clinical population those individuals who respond to simpler strategies. Such a design provides a reasonable analogue to a procedure sometimes used in drug research, whereby "placebo responders" are first removed from a population before the specific effect of a drug is tested. Although a true placebo therapy is difficult if not impossible to achieve, those individuals who respond to brief intervention can be successfully treated and then removed from the sample, leaving a subpopulation that is not responsive to minimal intervention. Such a subpopulation may be particularly useful in evaluating the true specific impact of particular treatment interventions.

A variety of brief intervention strategies have emerged in recent efforts to encourage behavior change in at-risk drinkers (Hodgson and Miller, 1982; Miller and Munoz, 1982; Skinner and Holt, 1983; Miller, 1985; Babor, Ritson, and Hodgson, 1986; Berg and Skutle, 1986; Heather, 1986; Heather, Whitton, and Robertson, 1986). As evaluation research and program planning become more sophisticated, it is important to develop a more systematic understanding of the common processes that underlie effective brief interventions. It appears at present that the more promising approaches use a combination of intervention strategies that address various aspects of problems and resistance (Miller, 1985; Miller and Sanchez, in press).

The following questions represent opportunities for research on brief interventions:

- What brief intervention procedures effectively reduce the probability and severity of future alcohol abuse? How much reduction in drinking and related problems can be accomplished through brief interventions?
- How do brief intervention procedures compare, in absolute impact, with more intensive treatment alternatives?
- What kinds of drinkers respond best to brief intervention programs? Do persons who fail to respond to brief intervention show more receptiveness to further treatment? Do they achieve more favorable outcomes when treated subsequently with more intensive approaches?
- Are there identifiable pretreatment characteristics (e.g., family history, sociopathology, depression) that are prognostic of poor response to brief interventions and that justify more intensive initial treatment?
- What are the key ingredients of an effective brief intervention strategy? Are there unique contributions of screening, assessment, feedback, and advice elements of brief intervention programs?

RESEARCH ON INTERVENTIONS WITH PREGNANT WOMEN

Interest in brief and early intervention has also increased because of concerns regarding the effects of alcohol on the fetus when pregnant women drink (see the discussion of this problem in Chapter 2). Research on the prevention of fetal alcohol effects has developed during the last 15 years following the reports of Jones and Smith (1973) and Jones and colleagues (1973). These authors reported on eight children born to alcoholic mothers, all of whom displayed a similar pattern of craniofacial, limb, and cardiovascular defects that were associated with growth deficiency and developmental delay. They called this constellation of abnormalities the fetal alcohol syndrome (FAS). In 1980, minimal criteria were established for the diagnosis of FAS (Rosett and Weiner, 1985).

Prevention of FAS and of less serious but possibly significant fetal effects of maternal drinking has focused heavily on reductions in alcohol intake by pregnant women. Prevention has taken the form of educational activities, social support, and efforts to identify problem drinkers among pregnant women.

As with the findings from studies of early intervention with problem drinkers, there are some grounds for optimism regarding the prevention of adverse fetal alcohol effects. Two programs have reported successful impacts--one at Boston City Hospital (Rosett et al., 1983) and the other in Sweden (Larsson, 1983). Each program systematically evaluated all pregnant women who attended the prenatal clinic, checking for excessive alcohol intake by means of interviews and questionnaires. The women in the study by Rosett and colleagues (1983) were told that they had a better chance of having a healthy baby if they abstained from alcohol use during pregnancy. Supportive therapy with a psychiatrist or counselor was provided one to four times a month in conjunction with prenatal visits. Treatment stressed a positive approach to reducing heavy drinking while avoiding the induction of guilt. About two-thirds of the women who participated in at least three sessions appeared to have stopped heavy drinking before the third trimester. The five cases of FAS diagnosed in this population were all associated with women who continued to drink heavily.

Larsson (1983) implemented a similar program with 464 women at four maternal health centers in Stockholm. Alcohol abuse was identified in 4 percent of these women, according to criteria established by Rosett and coworkers (1983). Rosett's counseling intervention was offered to all women (not only those identified as problem drinkers) who attended the centers. Reduction in alcohol use was observed for all women classified as excessive drinkers, and for 78 percent of those diagnosed as showing alcohol abuse. More infants from mothers classified as excessive drinkers or abusers (33 percent) were placed in the intensive care nursery than were infants born to mothers who were social drinkers (12 percent). The two babies born to mothers who continued to drink heavily exhibited significant growth retardation, and one was diagnosed as having FAS.

The following questions represent opportunities for research on intervention to prevent fetal alcohol effects:

   • What interventions are effective in suppressing drinking behavior among pregnant women?
   • Do drinking-focused interventions with pregnant women yield significant reductions in risk for their infants?
   • Is it warranted and effective to include family members or significant others in interventions designed to reduce alcohol-related fetal risk?

RESEARCH ON NONABSTINENCE OUTCOMES AND GOALS

The development of the prevention and early intervention efforts discussed in this chapter implies that the reduction of alcohol consumption to low-risk levels is a worthwhile goal within certain contexts and populations. Achieving this goal necessitates a more careful examination of nonabstinence outcomes and goals in addressing alcohol problems.

The occurrence of moderate and problem-free drinking outcomes following treatment is a complex, emotionally charged, and highly controversial issue within the alcohol treatment community (Miller, 1983). Total abstinence from alcohol and other drugs of abuse has been the consensus goal of most treatment personnel. Nevertheless, it has become normative in the 1980s for outcome studies to report alcohol consumption and its sequelae among individuals who continue to drink after treatment. A majority of studies likewise now employs such data to classify various proportions of nonabstinent outcomes as "improved," "controlled," "moderate," or "asymptomatic."

An important research development in the 1980s has been the emergence of new data regarding the long-term stability of nonabstinent outcomes. Many of the studies relevant to this issue are epidemiological or natural history studies rather than treatment outcome studies. Helzer and colleagues (1985), for example, evaluated 5- to 7-year outcomes among alcoholics who received unspecified treatment at medical and psychiatric facilities. They reported that 15 percent were totally abstinent for at least the 3 years prior to the interview, 1.6 percent sustained moderate drinking for that period, 4.2 percent were mostly abstinent with occasional moderate alcohol consumption, 12 percent were drinking heavily but without evidence of problems, and 66 percent continued heavy drinking with alcohol-related problems. A 15- to 32-year prospective study (Nordstrom and Berglund, 1987) reported that, among 55 alcoholics evidencing good social adjustment (by Swedish public health records), 11 (20 percent) were abstainers, 21 (38 percent) were drinking without problems, and 23 (40 percent) showed continuing evidence of alcohol abuse. Alford (1980) studied 56 (of 68) alcoholics who completed inpatient treatment based on Alcoholics Anonymous and were discharged with staff approval. At the 2-year follow-up point, 15 percent were reported to have sustained moderate drinking for the previous year, and 51 percent were reported to have been "essentially abstinent" (no more than two slips) during the same period. Two older reports of moderation outcomes were subjected to independent retrospective follow-ups at 10 years (Pendery, Maltzman, and West, 1982) and 29 to 34 years (Edwards, 1985). Both provided evidence that questioned the stability of controlled drinking outcomes in the cases studied.

New data likewise have appeared regarding long-term outcomes following treatments with a goal of moderation. Research teams have reported long-range outcome data for behavioral self-control training programs after two years (Miller and Baca, 1983; Sanchez-Craig et al., 1984), five to six years (Foy, Nunn, and Rychtarik, 1984), and five to eight years (Miller, Leckman, and Tinkcom, 1988). These studies reported that between 10 and 37 percent of individuals who were treated in a program with a goal of moderation sustained moderate drinking at long-term follow-up intervals. All of the controlled studies thus far in which problem drinkers have been allocated at random to abstinence versus moderation goal conditions have reported no differences in outcome based on the assigned goal (Sanchez-Craig, 1980; Stimmel et al., 1983; Sanchez-Craig et al., 1984; Orford and Keddie, 1986b; Graber and Miller, 1988).

The verification of self-reports of moderation is a concern that has been addressed thus far through the use of collateral reports, serum chemistries, and neuropsychological assessment (e.g., Babor, Kranzler and Lauerman, 1989). More aggressive verification procedures (e.g., daily breath or urine testing) have not been used in studies to document either moderation or abstinence goals.

In some outcome studies, treated individuals who showed stable abstinence and those who evidenced stable, problem-free drinking outcomes have constituted groups of roughly equal size (Booth, Dale, and Ansari, 1984; Helzer et al., 1985; Rychtarik et al., 1987); in other studies, however, either abstainers (Taylor et al., 1985; Chapman and Huygens, 1988; Miller, Leckman, and Tinkcom, 1988) or moderate drinkers (Bernadou et al., 1981, cited by Babor et al., 1983; Gottheil et al., 1982; Nordstrom and Berglund, 1987) have been more numerous. In any event, the assessment of a full spectrum of alcohol use outcomes following treatment (from abstinence through moderation to excessive drinking) is now clearly accepted in practice as an important element of alcoholism treatment evaluation (Gottheil et al., 1982).

With the recognition that some individuals do sustain moderate and problem-free drinking after treatment, another important question has been the focus of a number of studies: What differentiates these people either from those who sustain abstinence or from those who remain unremitted? This question has been addressed within programs that emphasize a goal of abstinence (Finney and Moos, 1981; Polich, Armor, and Braiker, 1981; Edwards et al., 1983) and in treatment programs with a goal of moderation (Maisto, Sobell, and Sobell, 1980; Miller and Baca, 1983; Miller, Leckman, and Tinkcom, 1988). Although findings have not been wholly consistent (Elal-Lawrence, Slade, and Dewey, 1987a,b), U.S. studies generally indicate stable moderation to be most likely for those with less severe alcohol problems and dependence, whereas those with more severe problems are most likely to succeed in abstinence. Several European studies, however, have reported no relationship between the severity of dependence and different outcome patterns (Orford and Keddie, 1986a,b; Nordstrom and Berglund, 1987). Peele (1987) has speculated that this discrepancy may be attributable to cross-cultural differences in beliefs about alcoholism. Two studies (Booth, Dale, and Ansari, 1984; Miller, Leckman, and Tinkcom, 1988) reported individual goal preference to be predictive of outcome (abstinence versus moderation). Other investigators have pointed to a relationship between outcome type and the individual's beliefs about alcoholism (Pfrang and Schenk, 1985; Orford and Keddie, 1986b), although Watson and coworkers (1984) found no such relationship. Ogborne (1987) reported that alcohol abusers who self-select a moderation goal resemble the profile of optimal responders to this treatment approach. The general picture is one of a continuum of severity of alcohol problems, with moderation being most feasible toward the lower end, abstinence most vital toward the upper end, and a large gray area in between. Contraindications for specific treatment goals remain an important area for future research (cf. Miller and Caddy, 1977).

The following questions represent opportunities for research on abstinence outcomes and goals:

• What are the characteristics of individuals who sustain moderate and problem-free drinking over extended spans of time after treatment? How do they differ from those who successfully sustain abstinence or who fail to show improvement?
• Are there significant differences between stable abstainers and stable moderate drinkers on other important outcome dimensions (e.g., neuropsychological functioning, physical health, family and social adjustment)?
• With less dependent problem drinkers, what are the positive or negative effects of openly negotiating the treatment goal, as compared with permitting only a goal of total abstention?
• What treatment or prevention procedures are effective in establishing stable, moderate, and problem-free drinking outcomes among less dependent problem drinkers?

SCREENING, RECRUITMENT, AND IMPLEMENTATION

Although the concepts of brief intervention and secondary prevention are attracting widespread interest, the development of effective, inexpensive, early interventions is still in the beginning stages. Programs to date have been experimental or demonstration projects. Some have not been evaluated with sufficient rigor to provide more than a suggestion of their efficacy. The only major long-term clinical trial to date (Kristenson et al., 1983) produced highly encouraging results on the ability of early intervention to reduce alcohol-related morbidity and mortality. Other program evaluations have indicated that modest but reliable effects on drinking behavior and related problems can follow from brief interventions, especially among less severe problem drinkers. Before these findings can be applied to the design of large-scale secondary prevention programs, however, further research is needed to clarify the behavioral processes that underlie the effectiveness of such programs and the barriers that may limit widespread initiation of early intervention. Specific research needs include further exploration of screening, recruitment, and implementation processes.

Screening

Screening is designed to differentiate among apparently well people, separating those who probably have the condition of interest from those who probably do not. It is equally applicable either to conditions that are categorical entities (i.e., conditions that are present versus not present) or to conditions that exist on a continuous scale of severity. The latter requires an operational threshold for a "case," that is, the point on the continuum at which treatment becomes preferable to no treatment.

Implicit in the concept of screening is the assumption that the health and well-being of the individual will benefit significantly from early detection of the condition. Screening is thus conceptually different from "detection" or "case finding," although these terms are sometimes used interchangeably. The aim of case finding is to identify active cases that have already developed a diagnosable disorder.

A variety of assessment procedures have been developed in recent years to facilitate the early identification of persons with harmful or potentially harmful alcohol consumption. Job performance criteria are used in industry, blood alcohol concentrations are employed in the courts, biochemical tests and brief questionnaires are used in health settings, and population surveys are conducted in the community. Although most of these procedures have been developed to identify active cases of alcohol dependence or "alcoholism," many are useful for early identification as well. These procedures include self-report instruments like the Michigan Alcohol Screening Test (MAST) and the CAGE questions, objective blood tests like those for GGT and mean corpuscular volume (MCV), and clinical examinations (Babor and Kadden, 1985). Because verbal report methods such as the MAST and CAGE can be falsified easily by defensive individuals, there has been strong interest in the development of biological markers that reflect recent heavy drinking or the early onset of physical consequences. Measures of GGT and MCV have been used for both screening and confirmatory diagnosis, but their values are affected by substances other than alcohol, as well as by physical conditions that are not related to drinking; furthermore, they are not invariably elevated in heavy drinkers. Serum transferrin and new immunological tests that have been developed to measure acetaldehyde bound to hemoglobin show promise as more specific markers of heavy drinking, but further research is needed to confirm their usefulness in routine screening. The use of such markers could identify problem drinkers during visits to physicians and thus point out those who might benefit from some level of intervention. The ideal marker would be one that is even more accurate and able to identify gradations of recent alcohol use. Such a precise indicator is not yet available. As markers are found that indicate genetic vulnerability to alcohol abuse (see Chapter 3 and also IOM, 1987), they might also become part of a screening program.

Because screening procedures based on biological, clinical, and verbal report methods all have limitations that affect their sensitivity and specificity, there has been renewed interest in the use of screening procedures that combine these domains. Two such combined screening approaches are the World Health Organization's Alcohol Use Disorders Identification Test (AUDIT) and the Alcohol Clinical Index (Saunders and Aasland, 1987; Skinner et al., 1986). Although these new screening tests have not been sufficiently studied, the use of combined procedures presently offers substantial promise for early identification. The choice of an optimal screening procedure will depend on the resources available, the goals of the screening and intervention, and the nature of the drinking problems within the target population.

One assumption implicit in many screening procedures has been that there is a distinct clinical entity called alcoholism that is either present or absent and can be detected at early stages of development. Although alcohol dependence follows a predictable course in many individuals, evidence of the progressive nature of alcohol-related problems is not compelling when all types of problem drinkers are considered as a heterogeneous group (Babor, Kranzler, and Kadden, 1986). Many problem drinkers appear to mature out of their harmful drinking practices. Early identification should, therefore, assume the less ambitious and more practical task of identifying specific types of alcohol problems within specific groups of problem drinkers, without making undue assumptions about etiology and natural history. This approach suggests the need for screening procedures that are capable of identifying a broad range of alcohol problem dimensions rather than the simple presence or absence of an assumed syndrome. Such dimensions include quantity and frequency of consumption, severity of alcohol dependence, number and intensity of alcohol-related social and health problems, and extent of family history and childhood risk factors for alcohol problems (Babor, Kranzler, and Lauerman, 1989).

The following questions represent opportunities for research questions on screening:

• Which of the many available biochemical, clinical, and self-report screening procedures are best suited to the identification of alcohol problems in primary care clinics, through community surveys, or in employment and criminal justice settings? What are the optimal combinations of such measures?
• Are there biological or biochemical markers, or sets of markers, with sufficient sensitivity and specificity to identify adults and adolescents at risk for future alcohol-related health problems?
• What are the relative validity and cost-effectiveness of verbal report screening methods (interviews, questionnaires, computer-assisted tests) compared with clinical and laboratory procedures? How can the accuracy of such measures be improved? Under what conditions are verbal report methods most or least accurate for the purpose of early identification?
• Can childhood factors that indicate enhanced risk of later alcohol problems (see Chapter 3) provide useful information when incorporated into routine screening tests?

Recruitment

Once individuals at risk have been identified, how can they be engaged in an intervention that is intended to reduce risk? The motivation for, and the involvement of, problem drinkers in the change process pose major challenges (Miller, 1985). The results of the Kristenson et al. (1983) study are encouraging, perhaps because this research group took full advantage of the prestige and resources of the Swedish national health service. The use of coercive recruitment methods by the courts, schools, and industry poses special ethical dilemmas that need to be considered, along with the possibility that "constructive coercion" may yield significant benefits. One procedure that has been found to attract large numbers of heavy drinkers who are likely to be motivated to change is recruitment through the media (Berg and Skutle, 1986; Heather, Whitton, and Robertson, 1986).

The success of media recruitment is apt to be affected by the nature and duration of the interventions that are offered. Programs that require only a brief counseling session and the use of a self-help home study manual may reach a wider (literate) audience than programs that demand regular participation in a series of counseling or educational sessions. The goals of the intervention are likely to affect recruitment as well (Miller, 1987). Almost all of the successful programs reviewed in this chapter recognized the need for flexibility in setting personal goals, with moderation rather than abstinence being the preferred initial option for most individuals. Another common characteristic of early intervention programs to date has been a careful avoidance of labeling. The terms alcoholic and alcoholism are deemphasized in favor of less stigmatizing concepts: heavy drinking, hazardous alcohol use, personal risk, and alcohol-related problems (Miller, 1983).

Recent reports have suggested that the information collected during screening can be used as feedback to motivate an individual's engagement in change programs (Kristenson et al., 1983; Miller, 1985; Miller and Sanchez, in press). Miller, Sovereign, and Krege (1988) reported modest decreases in alcohol use and increased helpseeking among a population of problem drinkers given a "drinker's checkup" that involved feedback regarding personal impairment related to alcohol use.

The following questions represent opportunities for research on recruitment:

• What kinds of recruitment approaches (e.g., voluntary versus coercive; media solicitation versus initiation by a health worker) provide the best chances for engaging high-risk drinkers in an early intervention program?
• What are the characteristics of personnel and procedures that are most optimal for engaging heavy drinkers in intervention programs?
• How can screening information (e.g., lab tests, alcohol consumption estimates, clinical examination findings) be used to increase an individual's motivation for, and engagement in, efforts to change?
• How can public attitudes toward health habits and life-style behavioral risk factors be mobilized to engage more drinkers in intervention programs? Is there a positive relationship among health beliefs, perceptions of risk, fear of harm, and motivation for change?

Implementation

Even when effective screening, recruitment, and intervention strategies have been defined, there remain a number of logistical, technical, and professional issues that must be addressed before promising findings are likely to be applied in clinical practice and public health settings (Miller, 1987). More research attention should be devoted to the evaluation of low-cost, rapid, reliable screening procedures that can be used routinely by primary care practitioners in a variety of health settings. No matter how sophisticated a biochemical test or how reliable a self-report questionnaire, neither may be implemented in routine clinical practice if they lack face validity, ease of use, or affordability. Research is needed to identify common barriers to effective screening that may arise once such technologies have been developed.

One of the reasons alcohol-related problems are ignored or underdiagnosed in primary care settings is that nurses and physicians do not feel responsible for--or competent to intervene in--a situation in which a drinking problem has been identified (Clement, 1986). With the development of screening and early intervention procedures that are effective and easy to use, this reluctance no longer seems warranted. Two areas worthy of research include the training of health care professionals in screening and brief intervention and the development of continuing education materials for health professionals and other groups such as employee assistance program personnel and school counselors. In addition, the reimbursement policies for early intervention should be examined to determine their effect on the delivery of this kind of preventive health service. The Kristenson study indicated that early intervention may have significant long-term effects on morbidity and mortality, which would suggest that remuneration for such services could be highly cost-effective in health care delivery systems.

The following questions represent opportunities for research on program implementation:

- What are the principal barriers to implementation of effective screening, recruitment, and intervention strategies once they have been identified?
- What methods are optimally effective in disseminating and implementing effective brief intervention strategies?
- What are the effects on long-term health care costs of implementing brief interventions for alcohol-related problems? Does reimbursement for such services have a tangible effect on their implementation and consequently on long-term outcomes?

REFERENCES

Alford, G. Alcoholics Anonymous: An empirical study. Addict. Behav. 5:359-370, 1980.

Babor, T. F., and R. Kadden. Screening for alcohol problems: Conceptual issues and practical considerations. Pp. 1-30 in N. C. Chang and H. M. Chao, eds. Early Identification of Alcohol Abuse. NIAAA Research Monograph No. 17. DHHS Publ. No. (ADM)85-1258. Rockville, MD: NIAAA, 1985.

Babor, T. F., H. R. Kranzler, and R. M. Kadden. Issues in the definition and diagnosis of alcoholism: Implications for a reformulation. Progress in Neuropsychopharmacology and Biological Psychiatry 10:113-128, 1986.

Babor, T. F., H. R. Kranzler, and R. J. Lauerman. Social drinking a health and psychosocial risk factor: Anstie's limit revisited. Pp. 373-402 in M. Galanter, ed. Recent Developments in Alcoholism, vol. 50. New York: Plenum, 1987.

Babor, T. F, H. R. Kranzler, and R. J. Lauerman. Early detection of harmful alcohol consumption: A comparison of clinical, laboratory and self-report screening procedures. Addictive Behavior 14(2):139-157, 1989.

Babor, T. F., E. B. Ritson, and R. J. Hodgson. Alcohol-related problems in the primary health care setting: A review of early intervention strategies. Br. J. Addict. 81:23-46, 1986.

Babor, T. F., M. Treffardier, J. Weill et al. The early detection and secondary prevention of alcoholism in France. J. Stud. Alcohol 44:600-616, 1983.

Berg, G., and A. Skutle. Early intervention with problem drinkers. Pp. 205-220 in W. R. Miller and N. Heather, eds. Treating Addictive Behaviors: Processes of Change. New York: Plenum, 1986.

Bernadou, M., P. DeBoucaud, R. Chassin et al. Enquete sur les CHA. Alc. Sante 157:21-24, 1981.

Booth, P. G., B. Dale, and J. Ansari. Problem drinkers' goal choice and treatment outcome: A preliminary study. Addict. Behav. 9:357-364, 1984.

Buck, K. A., and W. R. Miller. Why does bibliotherapy work? A controlled study. Paper presented at the annual meeting of the Association for Advancement of Behavior Therapy, Toronto, 1981.

Chapman, P. L. H., and I. Huygens. An evaluation of three treatment programmes for alcoholism: An experimental study with 6 and 18-month follow-ups. Br. J. Addict. 83:67-81, 1988.

Chick, J. Secondary prevention of alcoholism and the Centres d'Hygiene Alimentaire. Br. J. Addict. 79:221-225, 1984.

Chick, J., G. Lloyd, and E. Crombie. Counselling problem drinkers in medical wards: A controlled study. Br. Med. J. 290:965-967, 1985.

Clement, S. The identification of alcohol-related problems by general practitioners. Br. J. Addict. 81:257-264, 1986.

Edwards, G. A later follow-up of a classic case series: D. L. Davie's 1962 report and its significance for the present. J. Stud. Alcohol 46:181-190, 1985.

Edwards, G., E. Duckitt, E. Oppenheimer et al. What happens to alcoholics? Lancet 2(8344):269-271, 1983.

Elal-Lawrence, G., P. D. Slade, and M. E. Dewey. Predictors of outcome type in treated problem drinkers. J. Stud. Alcohol 47:41-47, 1987a.

Elal-Lawrence, G., P. D. Slade, and M. E. Dewey. Treatment and follow-up variables discriminating abstainers, controlled drinkers and relapsers. J. Stud. Alcohol 48:39-46, 1987b.

Elvy, G. A., J. E. Wells, K. A. Baird et al. Attempted referral as intervention for problem drinking in the general hospital. Br. J. Addict. 83:83-89, 1988.

Finney, J. W., and R. H. Moos. Characteristics and prognoses of alcoholics who become moderate drinkers and abstainers after treatment. J. Stud. Alcohol 42:94-105, 1981.

Foy, D. W., B. L. Nunn, and R. G. Rychtarik. Broad-spectrum behavioral treatment for chronic alcoholics: Effects of training controlled drinking skills. J. Consult. Clin. Psychol. 52:218-230, 1984.

Gottheil, E. C., C. Thornton, T. E. Skoloda et al. Follow-up of abstinent and nonabstinent alcoholics. Am. J. Psychiatry 139:560-565, 1982.

Graber, R. A., and W. R. Miller. Abstinence and controlled drinking goals in behavioral self-control training of problem drinkers: A randomized clinical trial. Psychol. Addict. Behav. 1988.

Heather, N. Change without therapists: The use of self-help manuals by problem drinkers. Pp. 331-359 in W. R. Miller and N. Heather, eds. Treating Addictive Behaviors: Processes of Change. New York: Plenum, 1986.

Heather, N., B. Whitton, and I. Robertson. Evaluation of a self-help manual for media-recruited problem drinkers: Six month follow-up results. Br. J. Clin. Psychol. 25:19-34, 1986.

Helzer, J. E., L. N. Robins, J. R. Taylor et al. The extent of long-term moderate drinking among alcoholics discharged from medical and psychiatric treatment facilities. N. Engl. J. Med. 312:1678-1682, 1985.

Hodgson, R., and P. Miller. Self-Watching. New York: Facts on File, 1982.

Institute of Medicine. Health and Behavior: Frontiers of Research in the Biobehavioral Sciences. D. A. Hamburg, G. R. Elliott, and D. L. Parron, eds. Washington, DC: National Academy Press, 1982.

Institute of Medicine. Causes and Consequences of Alcohol Problems: An Agenda for Research. Washington, DC: National Academy Press, 1987.

Jones, K. L., and D. W. Smith. Recognition of the fetal alcohol syndrome in early infancy. Lancet 2(836):999-1001, 1973.

Jones, K. L., D. W. Smith, C. N. Ulleland, and A. P. Streissguth. Pattern of malformation in offspring of chronic alcoholic mothers. Lancet 1:1267-1271, 1973.

Kristenson, H., E. Trell, and B. Hood. Serum glutamyl-transferase in screening and continuous control of heavy drinking in middle-aged men. Am. J. Epidemiology 114:862-872, 1982.

Kristenson, H., H. Ohlin, M. B. Hulten-Nosslin et al. Identification and intervention of heavy drinking in middle-aged men: Results and follow-up of 24-60 months of long-term study with randomized controls. Alcoholism Clin. Exp. Res. 7:203-209, 1983.

Larsson, G. Prevention of fetal alcohol effects: An antenatal program for early detection of pregnancies at risk. Acta Obstetrica et Gynecologica Scandanavia 62:171-178, 1983.

LeGo, P. M. Le Depitage Precoce et Systematique du Buveur Excessif. Riom, France: Riom Laboratoires, 1977.

Maisto, S. M., M. B. Sobell, and L. C. Sobell. Predictors of treatment outcome for alcoholics treated by individualized behavior therapy. Addict. 16:1247-1254, 1980.

Miller, W. R. Controlled drinking: A history and critical review. J. Stud. Alcohol 44:68-83, 1983.

Miller, W. R. Motivation for treatment: A review with special emphasis on alcoholism. Psychol. Bull. 98:84-107, 1985.

Miller, W. R. Behavioral alcohol treatment research advances: Barriers to utilization. Adv. Behav. Res. Ther. 9:145-164, 1987.

Miller, W. R., and L. M. Baca. Two-year follow-up of bibliotherapy and therapist-directed controlled drinking training for problem drinkers. Behav. Ther. 14:441-448, 1983.

Miller, W. R., and G. R. Caddy. Abstinence and controlled drinking in the treatment of problem drinkers. J. Stud. Alcohol 38:986-1003, 1977.

Miller, W. R., and R. K. Hester. Treating the problem drinker: Modern approaches. In W. R. Miller, ed. The Addictive Behaviors: Treatment of Alcoholism, Drug Abuse, Smoking, and Obesity. Oxford: Pergamon Press, 1980.

Miller, W. R., and R. F. Munoz. How to Control Your Drinking. Albuquerque: University of New Mexico Press, 1982.

Miller, W. R., and V. C. Sanchez. Motivating young adults for treatment and lifestyle change. In G. Howard, ed. Issues in Alcohol Use and Misuse by Young Adults. Notre Dame, IN: University of Notre Dame Press, in press.

Miller, W. R., and C. A. Taylor. Relative effectiveness of bibliotherapy, individual and group self-control training in the treatment of problem drinkers. Addict. Behav. 5:13-24, 1980.

Miller, W. R., C. J. Gribskov, and R. L. Mortell. Effectiveness of a self-control manual for problem drinkers with and without therapist contact. Int. J. Addict. 16:1247-1254, 1981.

Miller, W. R., A. L. Leckman, and M. Tinkcom. Long-term follow-up of controlled drinking therapies. Unpublished manuscripts, University of New Mexico, 1988.

Miller, W. R., T. F. Pechacek, and S. Hamburg. Group behavior therapy for problem drinkers. Int. J. Addict. 16:827-837, 1981.

Miller, W. R., R. G. Sovereign, and B. Krege. Motivational interviewing with problem drinkers. II. The drinker's check-up as a preventive intervention. Behav. Psychother., 1988.

Miller, W. R., C. A. Taylor, and J. C. West. Focused versus broad-spectrum therapy for problem drinkers. J. Consult. Clin. Psychol. 48:590-601, 1980.

Moore, M. H., and D. R. Gerstein, eds. Alcohol and Public Policy: Beyond the Shadow of Prohibition. Washington, DC: National Academy Press, 1981.

Nordstrom, G., and M. Berglund. A prospective study of successful long-term adjustment in alcohol dependence: Social drinking versus abstinence. J. Stud. Alcohol 48:95-103, 1987.

Ogborne, A. C. A note on the characteristics of alcohol abusers with controlled drinking aspirations. Drug Alcohol Depend. 19:159-164, 1987.

Orford, J., and A. Keddie. Abstinence or controlled drinking in clinical practice: Indications at initial assessment. Addict. Behav. 11:71-86, 1986a.

Orford, J., and A. Keddie. Abstinence or controlled drinking in clinical practice: A test of the dependence and persuasion hypotheses. Br. J. Addict. 81:495-504, 1986b.

Peele, S. Why do controlled-drinking outcomes vary by investigator, by country and by era? Cultural conceptions of relapse and remission in alcoholism. Drug Alcohol Depend. 20:173-201, 1987.

Pendery, M. L., I. M. Maltzman, and L. J. West. Controlled drinking by alcoholics? New findings and a reevaluation of a major affirmative study. Science 217:169-175, 1982.

Pfrang, H., and J. Schenk. Controlled drinkers in comparison to abstinents and relapsed drinkers with regard to attitudes and social adjustment. Int. J. Addict. 20:1793-1802, 1985.

Polich, J. M., D. J. Armor, and H. B. Braiker. The Course of Alcoholism: Four Years After Treatment. New York: John Wiley and Sons, 1981.

Rosett, H. L., and L. Weiner. Alcohol and pregnancy: A clinical perspective. Ann. Rev. Med. 36:73-80, 1985.

Rosett, H. L., L. Weiner, A. Lee et al. Patterns of alcohol consumption and fetal development. Obstet. Gynecol. 61:539-546, 1983.

Rychtarik, R. G., D. W. Foy, T. Scott et al. Five-six-year follow-up of broad-spectrum behavioral treatment for alcoholism: Effects of training controlled drinking skills. J. Consult. Clin. Psychol. 55:106-108, 1987.

Sanchez-Craig, M. Random assignment to abstinence or controlled drinking in a cognitive-behavioral program: Short-term effects on drinking behavior. Addict. Behav. 5:35-39, 1980.

Sanchez-Craig, M. Therapist's Manual for Secondary Prevention of Alcohol Problems: Procedures for Teaching Moderate Drinking and Abstinence. Toronto: Addiction Research Foundation, 1984.

Sanchez-Craig, M., H. M. Annis, A. R. Bornet et al. Random assignment to abstinence and controlled drinking: Evaluation of a cognitive-behavioral treatment program for problem drinkers. J. Consult. Clin. Psychol. 52:390-403, 1984.

Saunders, J. B., and O. G. Aasland. WHO collaborative project on identification and treatment of persons with harmful alcohol consumption. Doc. WHO/MNH/DAT/86.3. Geneva: World Health Organization, 1987.

Skinner, H. A., and S. Holt. Early intervention for alcohol problems. Journal of the Royal College of General Practitioners 33:787-791, 1983.

Skinner, H. A., S. Holt, W. J. Sheu, and Y. Israel. Clinical versus laboratory detection of alcohol abuse: The Alcohol Clinical Index. Br. Med. J. 292:1703-1708, 1986.

Stimmel, B., M. Cohen, V. Sturiano et al. Is treatment of alcoholism effective in persons on methadone maintenance? Am. J. Psychiatry 140:862-866, 1983.

Taylor, C., D. Brown, A. Duckitt et al. Patterns of outcome: Drinking histories over ten years among a group of alcoholics. Br. J. Addict. 80:45-50, 1985.

Watson, C. G., L. Jacobs, J. Pucel et al. The relationship of beliefs about controlled drinking to recidivism in alcoholic men. J. Stud. Alcohol 45(2):172-175, 1984.

PATIENT-TREATMENT MATCHING AND OUTCOME IMPROVEMENT
IN ALCOHOL REHABILITATION

In the decade since the Institute of Medicine last reviewed the state of research on the treatment of alcohol problems (IOM, 1980), there has been a substantial amount of work on patient-treatment matching. Perhaps most important has been the recognition that matching patients and treatments is a sophisticated idea with as yet untapped possibilities for improving the effectiveness and efficiency of treatment. In particular, as a result of the work of Glaser (1980), Skinner (1981), and more recently Finney and Moos (1986), it has become accepted that (a) "matching" studies are among the most conceptually, methodologically, and practically complicated of all forms of treatment evaluation research; and (b) appropriate studies of patient-treatment matching can be accomplished only after careful specification of patient and treatment characteristics.

In addition to making conceptual progress, researchers have investigated basic patient characteristics that are generally predictive of outcome across a variety of treatments. Treatment methods have begun to be specified more clearly and to be applied in the manner specified. There has also been progress in the development and utilization of designs appropriate to the study of patient and treatment characteristics that have sufficient power to observe real effects and in the use of statistical treatments that can adequately assess the complexity of various interactions.

Advances in matching over the past decade have occurred primarily in methodological development, patient measurement, and treatment measurement. In the first part of this chapter, progress in each of these areas is summarized, and general suggestions for research opportunities are presented. Review articles by Miller and Hester (1986b), Annis (1987), and Longabaugh (1986) have been particularly helpful, and the reader is encouraged to use these sources for additional information and references.

ADVANCES IN PATIENT-TREATMENT MATCHING RESEARCH, 1978-1988

The developments of the past decade provide a basis for an expectation of additional progress in the matching area. First, after a review of the concepts, methods, and results of existing studies, the committee suggests more focused designs and clearer evaluation questions tailored to the treatments being studied. In the second section of this chapter, the committee discusses potential areas of progress and identifies specific research opportunities.

Advances in Research Methodology

The past decade has seen the increased deployment of rigorous, experimental designs to assess treatment efficacy as well as the development of new and more sophisticated statistical procedures to analyze multiply determined outcomes.

Many patient-treatment matching studies from the 1960s through the late 1970s were retrospective examinations of variables that had been generated at the time of admission to treatment from data taken from patients admitted to two or more different programs or treatments. They were generally analyzed by using a series of t-tests, chi-squares, or simple correlations.

Some of the recent progress in method development is due to the practice developed during the past 10 years of analyzing multiple outcome measures (e.g., amount, duration, and frequency of alcohol consumption; employment; social adjustment; medical services utilization) rather than abstinence or nonabstinence alone when evaluating alcoholism treatment efficacy. This practice has led to the recognition that outcome is not unidimensional and that many aspects of the patient's posttreatment condition (e.g., employment situation or family, psychiatric, and medical status) can have a direct bearing on the likelihood of relapse. The earlier concentration by clinicians and researchers on a unidimensional outcome tended to obscure the complexity of the treatment process and the factors that accounted for treatment failure. The more recent development of measuring multiple outcomes has encouraged researchers to give more thought to determining reasonable goals and expectations from various types of treatments and deciding what types of patients could be expected to show change in each. This trend has resulted in more rigorous designs with better specification of treatments and the patients who should undertake them, as well as testable hypotheses regarding outcome.

Another development that has facilitated matching and is also related to the practice of evaluating multiple outcome measures is the use of multivariate statistics. Current reports rarely contain only two-by-two chi-square distributions of abstinent and nonabstinent frequencies in two treatment programs. It is now recognized (Skinner, 1981; Finney and Moos, 1986) that the number and complexity of the interactions among patient pretreatment characteristics, during-treatment factors, and posttreatment environmental factors cannot be characterized without the sophisticated use of multivariate statistical procedures. The introduction of new statistical procedures has also increased the rigor of measurement, the sophistication of the designs used, and the specificity of the hypotheses tested.

Much progress in our understanding of matching has come from the use of more rigorous methodologies and experimental designs. This usage should be encouraged. However, because randomized controlled trials are not appropriate or possible for all evaluation and treatment matching studies in all clinical settings, it is necessary to develop a range of rigorous, quasi-experimental designs.

There have been few evaluations of patient treatment matching strategies outside of public or institutional settings that treat mainly lower socioeconomic strata patients. Given the importance of social supports and stability in determining outcome across a variety of treatments, it may be that some of the conclusions reached to date apply to only a limited segment of the patient population. In addition, what some researchers have seen as resistance to evaluation on the part of clinics and clinicians may be the result of ethical and financial pressures. Many private clinics that might have liked to participate in evaluations may have been prevented because of design limitations.

Three matching strategies that have been developed within recent years are discussed below.

1. Ewing (1977) proposed a "cafeteria" matching strategy in which patients are offered several alternatives and are permitted to select among them. The major limitation of this strategy is that the attractiveness of a treatment is assessed along with its efficacy, and attractiveness has been shown to be a major factor in determining retention in treatment and acceptance of treatment goals (Luborsky et al., 1984; Miller, 1985).

2. Feedback designs employ early findings to generate testable hypotheses that in turn generate self-correcting further hypotheses (Glaser, 1980; McLellan et al., 1980, 1983a,b). Patients are evaluated pre- and posttreatment within a multiprogram network, with no modification of standard patient-program assignments. Data are analyzed, and patient-program "statistical hunches" are developed on the basis of retrospective data. In the second stage of the project, patients are assigned, based on the hunches, to the programs that may be best for them. Data are again analyzed, and "matched" patients are compared with "mismatched" patients. Limitations include the influence of the self-selection process, the need for adequate variability in program characteristics, and the need for a relatively stable treatment network.

3. Experiments can be designed to test the addition of a critical treatment element to the usual treatment. This strategy can be effective in cases in which there is a minimum standard treatment available. Because no patient is denied the standard treatment and because participation in this type of study can lead to extra care, these designs are often well accepted by both patients and treatment staff. The limitations of this design concern the sample sizes that can reasonably be generated and the types of treatments for which this design can be used.

All three of these designs may allow matching research to be done in settings, treatments, and populations that have not previously been studied. They may also permit the research findings generated thus far to be more easily translated into clinical practice.

The following are opportunities for research on methodology development:

- Ewing's cafeteria matching strategy should be reexamined.
- Statistical models of clinical decision making should be employed. The clinical decision-making process of senior, experienced clinicians can be modeled mathematically by using discriminant function or path analyses. Studies should be performed to examine the data that are used in making treatment assignment decisions (Miller and Hester, 1986b).
- Experiments designed to test the addition of a critical element to the usual treatment should be attempted.
- Studies should be performed using feedback designs.

Advances in Patient Measurement

During the past decade there has been greater recognition of the full range of problems commonly seen among alcoholics who present for treatment. As discussed in Chapter 8, a number of measurement instruments have been developed to assess these problems, both at the time of admission, when such instruments serve as predictors of treatment outcome, and at follow-up points, when they function as outcome criteria. The social, psychological, and economic problems of alcohol-dependent patients may contribute to relapse and therefore should be targets for intervention during alcohol treatment (Finney and Moos, 1986). This realization has broadened the scope and complexity of treatment evaluations.

Several groups have used developments in patient measurement to search for generic patient variables that may be broadly predictive of outcome across several different types and settings of treatment. This rapidly progressing area of research has been reviewed by Longabaugh (1986), Miller and Hester (1986b), and Annis (1987). Four types of measurement appear to be generally predictive of treatment outcome as evidenced by replication in more than one treatment setting and in more than one type of patient population:

1. <u>Social stability/social supports</u>. Fewer supports result in worse treatment response generally but especially in the case of outpatient treatment. This factor appears to be a major generic predictor (McLellan et al., 1983a; Longabaugh and Beattie, 1985).

2. <u>Psychiatric diagnosis including severity/number, duration, and intensity of symptoms</u>. Greater severity indicates generally worse treatment response, especially for outpatient treatments. This measure of overall impairment, irrespective of diagnosis, has been a good predictor across a variety of outcome domains and patient populations (McLellan et al., 1983a,b; Cooney et al., 1987; Rounsaville et al., 1987; Babor et al., 1988). Specific diagnoses (e.g., major or intermittent depressive disorders, panic attacks) have been the symptom patterns usually associated with greater overall severity of psychiatric illness among alcohol-abusing patient populations. These diagnostic entities have received a great deal of attention as predictors of outcome. The differentiation of primary and secondary psychiatric disorders in alcoholics has been emphasized by Schuckit (1984) as a predictor of treatment outcome. As new and more specific treatments develop for psychiatric disorders, these treatments are being provided to patients with concomitant alcohol problems.

3. <u>Severity of alcohol use/severity of alcohol dependence syndrome</u>. Greater severity means worse treatment response generally and, especially for outpatients, more rapid return to drinking and drinking problems. This variable has probably been the best predictor of posttreatment alcohol consumption and alcohol-related problems, although it has been somewhat less effective as a predictor of adjustment in other areas such as employment, medical health, or family relations (Orford, Openheimer, and Edwards, 1976; Polich, Armor, and Braiker, 1980; Lyons et al., 1982; Babor et al., 1988).

4. <u>Antisocial personality (ASP) disorder</u>. The presence of ASP is generally indicative of poor treatment response across all modalities with the possible exception of enforced disulfiram treatment (Schuckit, 1984; Stabenau and Hesselbrock, 1984; Hesselbrock, Meyer, and Keener, 1985; Powell et al., 1985).

Other patient variables have been related to treatment outcome in general, but they have not been examined extensively. These variables include a family history of alcoholism, particularly in a first-degree relative (Schuckit, 1985) and cognitive or information-processing problems (Walker et al., 1983). There is also a large literature on the use of personality tests such as the Minnesota Multiphasic Personality Inventory (MMPI) to develop typologies of clients that would be differentially responsive to treatment; however, thus far no group within these typologies has emerged that has a clear relationship to treatment response. New and promising approaches to the subtyping of patients based on combinations of personality traits, drinking history, and familial variables have been developed by Morey, Skinner, and Blashfield (1984), Zucker (1987), and Cloninger (1987). To the extent that these typologies are found in the future actually to represent homogeneous groups of alcoholics, it will be more efficient to match treatments to patient types defined by multiple characteristics than to patient types defined by individual traits or characteristics.

Although it is encouraging that there has been a great deal of replication of these generic "patient predictor findings," all of which appear to be conceptually sensible and potentially useful clinically, more research should be done on the following areas of patient measurement:

- Parametric work is needed to determine the strength of these variables across a variety of patient mixes and treatment types.

- The extent to which robust predictors covary, especially in selected segments of the population, should be examined. For example, it is possible that a high level of alcohol dependency, ASP, and a history of familial alcoholism may occur together, especially in chronic male alcoholics.

- The American Psychiatric Association's revised edition of the Diagnostic and Statistical Manual of Mental Disorders (DSM-III-R) differs in major ways from DSM-III, and it will be important to determine whether the differences in classification affect patient outcome across a range of treatments.

- With the exception of ASP, there has been very little evidence that the presence of a specific psychiatric disorder is predictive of treatment outcome. Global symptom severity has been more predictive than specific diagnosis. Specific treatments must be developed to address the specific needs of certain diagnostic groups (e.g., depressed alcoholics, alcoholics with panic disorder) before matching can become optimal.

- Additional work is needed to better define and describe the dimensions of ASP (including impulsiveness, learning disorder, childhood aggression, relationship problems, and criminal activity) to determine the particular factors responsible for the observed resistance to treatment for alcohol problems.

- Motivation for change is widely viewed as an important predictor of response to treatment, but there has been little indication that this quality can be measured either reliably or validly. A clear definition of motivation and a means of measuring it would be valuable. Work reported by Prochaska and DiClemente (1983) that describes a method for measuring "readiness for change" should be extended.

ADVANCES IN TREATMENT MEASUREMENT

New treatment models have been developed during the past several years, including the relapse prevention model (Gorski and Miller, 1982; Marlatt and Gordon, 1985) and brief interventions (Sanchez-Craig and Walker, 1982; Sanchez-Craig, 1984; Miller, 1985). There have also been wider use of standard treatments in different settings and experimentation with outpatient detoxification and rehabilitation (Longabaugh et al., 1983; Hayashida et al., 1989). In addition, manual-directed relapse prevention efforts (Marlatt and Gordon, 1985) and self-help treatments (Sanchez-Craig, 1984; Heather, 1986; Miller, 1986) have been developed and implemented. These new models are welcome developments for a variety of reasons. The manuals are an important source of training in theory and practice for clinicians and promote the standardized delivery of treatment. They are also valuable for researchers, enabling the derivation of better measures of treatment goals and processes.

Although there has been progress in treatment process standardization, other areas still require work. New treatments are needed for specific segments of the population such as the cocaine-alcohol-dependent patient, the antisocial personality alcoholic, the alcoholic schizophrenic, and the medical patient with an alcohol-related disorder (e.g., alcohol cardiomyopathy, alcohol hypertension). These new treatments should be conceptually related to the specific problems of the target populations and should use manuals for guidance to ensure the accuracy of treatment application.

It should be noted that patient-treatment matching can occur only when there are clearly different treatments. Many treatments are minor variants in practice. There is no evidence at this time that any single process or approach will work for every patient, and newer methods may succeed where older ones have not. As much attention should be paid to developing instruments that measure characteristics of treatments as has been paid to the development of instruments that measure characteristics of patients.

Although it is frequently said that patient characteristics account for more variability in outcome than do treatment characteristics, this perception could be a function of the lack of available treatment measures (Glaser, 1980). The development of treatment manuals for specific therapies has promoted criterion-based measures of the extent to which treatments are actually delivered as intended, the quantity of treatment provided to a patient, and ratings of its quality. Moreover, evaluation research using these manual-derived process measures has begun (Luborsky et al., 1984). Instruments are now needed to assess the nature and amount of various treatment components across a range of treatment programs and across various stages of the treatment process. This assessment would provide some indication of which training components are most effective as well as suggestions about how to train therapists and improve the delivery of these components. The lack of such instruments has handicapped the study of matching and the accurate evaluation of treatment efficacy.

The following questions represent opportunities for research on treatment measurement:

• What is treatment supposed to do? Many insurance companies and treatment funding agencies have reduced to 28 days the amount of time for which they will reimburse alcohol rehabilitation (formerly, they reimbursed from 90 to 120 days). Have the goals of treatment changed to reflect these time constraints? Are the goals of rehabilitation clearly different from detoxification, or do they complement each other?

• Have patients reached the established goals of treatment by the time they are discharged or released? There are few studies evaluating progress during the course of treatment (as opposed to outcome measures on the completion of treatment).

• How much "treatment" does it take to produce a given level of change for a specified number of patients? It is necessary to develop a more quantified estimate of treatment effects so that more informed decisions can be made regarding how much treatment is necessary and in turn how much treatment should be compensated by insurance companies.

• Does the achievement of during-treatment goals relate to posttreatment success? The work by Finney, Moos, and Mewborn (1980) showing the importance of the posttreatment environment has led to new studies. However, even this excellent research lacks the specificity of measurement necessary to determine if the "treatment" has been applied in the intended manner and to an adequate extent.

• What are the "active ingredients" of treatment? Treatment programs offer many services or interventions. In a study by McLachlan and Stein (1982), patients received a standard treatment package of medical consultation, disulfiram or calcium carbimide, group psychotherapy, education, relaxation training, nutritional counseling, physiotherapy, physical training/exercise, and individual planning for an alcohol-free life-style. Are all of these necessary? Are they all associated with outcome? What are the essential or "active ingredients?" Investigators have been attempting to match people to treatment settings (inpatient and outpatient) or treatment programs without knowing which factors are responsible for observed patient changes.

RESEARCH ON PATIENT-TREATMENT MATCHING:
PERSPECTIVES AND OPPORTUNITIES

Given the advances of the last decade in the areas of methodology development and patient measurement, what can be expected in the future in the area of matching research? The analysis of more discrete and better defined stages of the rehabilitation process offers the greatest potential for progress in refining the process of treatment selection and the provision of specific treatment components during rehabilitation. It can also help to improve the services offered in the posttreatment environment. Just as each of these stages of the rehabilitation process takes place in a different context and requires the patient to set different goals, the clinical possibilities for patient-treatment matching and the potential for matching research will also be different.

In the remainder of this section the committee examines the potential for matching research in each of four areas that correspond to typical treatment situations: (1) matching before treatment starts, (2) matching at the initiation of treatment, (3) matching during the treatment process, and (4) matching following the rehabilitation intervention. Critical commentary is provided regarding the matching research conducted to date, along with suggestions for future methods to be applied and examples of specific types of studies that could be performed.

Matching Before Treatment Starts: Special Populations and Self-Selection

Ideally, the outcome evaluation researcher would like to examine the effects of a representative treatment program, technique, or modality on randomly selected patient samples that proportionally represent the total patient population. However, the population of "alcohol-problemed" individuals is not completely represented by the patients who present for treatment. Moreover, because the nature of the treatment program, including its location, cost, referral network, charter, and preferred modalities, will determine in large part the types of patients who seek treatment, the sample of patients evaluated at a specific treatment program will not be representative of the population of treatment-seeking individuals. Therefore, all outcome studies done to date reflect imperfectly applied treatments in nonrepresentative, generally self-selected patient samples; most often these samples comprise the most severely impaired patients.

Designers of treatment programs have recognized and utilized patient self-selection in their marketing strategies and in their clinical attempts to develop programs tailored to the individual needs of the patient. This process, which can be termed "solicited self-selection," is sensible in that it is not likely that the effects of even conceptually identical and comparably applied treatments would be similar, for example, for both a sample of older, male, lower-socioeconomic, chronic alcoholic veterans treated in a Veterans Administration hospital and a sample of adolescent, middle-class girls referred to treatment at a private facility.

It is apparent that a form of matching takes place prior to the initiation of treatment through the process of specialization as well as the selective marketing and referral of seemingly appropriate patients. This type of marketing has encouraged the development of special programs for special populations such as adolescents, Native Americans, women, abused women, adult children of alcoholics (ACOAs), homeless men, and many others. These specialized programs are by far the most extensive matching work carried out in this country, yet little more than descriptive information is available about outcomes.

Special populations are important for patient-treatment matching (particularly at the level of treatment entry), but they have been difficult to study. It is not easy to discern who constitutes a special population. In a recent seminal report by Saxe and coworkers (1983), the special populations discussed are elderly people, adolescents, women, blacks, Hispanics, Native Americans, drunk drivers, and public inebriates/skid row alcoholics. The problems associated with evaluating treatment options for these groups are numerous and obvious. The three major definitional problems are that (1) these groups have substantial internal variability (e.g., Hispanics include Puerto Ricans, Mexicans, Cubans, etc.); (2) these groups are not mutually exclusive (e.g., a member of the black special population may be elderly, Hispanic, a skid row woman, and convicted of drunk driving); and (3) they are not exhaustive (i.e, more recent designations have added pregnant, physically handicapped, and psychiatrically ill alcoholics to the groups already mentioned).

The matching research that has been done in this area has attempted to determine whether differential outcomes are seen among these groups when they are treated in the same program. To date, the modest amount of research that has been completed has shown no clear indication that these group designations are associated with different outcomes among those patients who have entered treatment (Westermeyer, 1982; Blum, 1987; Blume, 1986). It is quite clear, however, that members of these groups do not enter available "mainstream" treatments in proportions that are representative of the alcohol problems within those groups. For this reason, the major efforts in this area related to patient-treatment matching have been in the development of tailored programs designed and operated by and for selected special population groups. The goal of these efforts has been to attract more alcohol-impaired individuals from these groups into treatment.

Although there has been a marked increase in the number of programs available, it is not yet clear that proportionally more members of these groups have been attracted to treatment or that greater proportions of special populations enter special programs rather than traditional programs. When these programs have offered attractions that were specifically directed toward their target populations (e.g., child care for women's programs, special access for handicapped programs), it is not clear whether or to what extent the actual treatment provided within these programs differed from more mainstream types of treatment or whether they were associated with differential opportunities.

These facts of clinical life do not imply that research in this area is impossible. Matching or the prediction of outcome studies can be performed simultaneously with ongoing treatments as long as the questions addressed and the methodologies employed are suitable in the treatment context. The following questions represent opportunities for research on programs designed with specialized segments of the patient population in mind:

• Do patients with the "right" patient profile stay longer, show more improvement, and remain improved longer than patients with the "wrong" profile?
• Is greater demographic and socioeconomic homogeneity among patients associated with better retention in a specific treatment? How much and what types of diversity can a patient population tolerate and still maintain cohesiveness? This is a particularly relevant question for those treating the increasing numbers of cocaine and alcohol abuse patients who present for treatment at traditional "alcohol-only" programs. Can these patients be treated along with alcohol-only patients? Are treatment goals and methods compatible for these two types of patients? Can women be treated as effectively in mixed male and female settings as in specialized women's facilities? Similar questions could be asked with respect to adolescent alcoholics as well as other significant subgroups in the total patient population.

• Do similar treatment strategies and components (e.g., group therapy, education, Alcoholics Anonymous, disulfiram) have qualitatively similar effects on outcome among programs with different patient profiles?

Matching at the Initiation of Treatment: Levels of Treatment Intensity

There are several different levels of treatment intensity offered in most areas: (a) advice/self-help; (b) brief interventions (usually fewer than five counselor appointments lasting about a week); (c) outpatient care (usually one to three hours per day, three to five days per week); (d) partial hospitalization (usually six to eight hours per day); (e) residential inpatient (nonmedical inpatient setting); and (f) medical inpatient (in a specialized unit in a general or psychiatric hospital).

There now exist a body of valid, replicated data on patient factors in treatment matching and enough understanding of the various levels of treatment that the development of more carefully staged designs is possible. Staged or hierarchical designs refer to the tailoring of matching hypotheses to the treatment goals and patient populations appropriate for different levels of treatment structure (e.g., no treatment, brief treatment, outpatient, inpatient). New work in this area should build on conclusions from previous studies that are sensible and have been replicated. The work of many investigators has been reviewed by Sanchez-Craig (1984) and by Miller and Hester (1986a). These efforts indicate that individuals with less severe and shorter periods of problem drinking, better social supports, and fewer medical or psychological problems can improve without intensive treatment.

The following are opportunities for research on matching at treatment initiation:

• Studies of matching to different levels of treatment intensity should attempt to select patients with approximately the same level of problems and social supports. The results of such studies might then permit a better understanding of the patient factors within the clinically appropriate group that are associated with outcomes from each level of treatment intensity.
• Studies of matching within each level of treatment intensity are needed to evaluate the treatment components (e.g., group therapy, individual therapy, medication, education) and patient characteristics in the clinically appropriate group that are associated with favorable outcome.
• Models of patient assignment to different levels of treatment intensity (e.g., Hoffman et al., 1987) should be evaluated in a series of controlled trials at various sites and with various segments of the patient population.

Matching During the Treatment Process: Role of Treatment Components

There is a fairly discrete set of treatment components that is provided, or at least offered, to most alcohol-dependent patients in treatment, regardless of the treatment modality or setting. These components include (a) group therapy (usually focused on issues of treatment need and denial); (b) individual therapy (usually personal counseling on relationship problems and crises); (c) alcohol or substance abuse education; (d) attendance at Alcoholics Anonymous (AA) meetings; and (e) antidipsotropic medications (usually disulfiram).

Although some research has been conducted to examine matching in treatment settings (e.g., inpatient versus outpatient) and among programs, there has been little matching work done on treatment components (e.g., medication, therapy, education) and even less on therapist or counselor technique. Studies in these areas are potentially important in that the failure to find evidence of differences in efficacy as a result of matching to different programs or settings may be due to the similarity of the therapeutic methods employed in these treatment venues. As has already been emphasized, there is a need for more detailed measurement of the treatment process, as well as a need to identify the active ingredients of treatment. If the active ingredients are identified at the process level and if they are applied fairly similarly across treatment settings and programs, then it would not be surprising if there were not much evidence of differential outcomes from "patient-setting" or "patient-program" matching.

The following are opportunities for research on matching during treatment:

• Random patient assignment methods in controlled experimental trials can be used most effectively used in studies within a treatment setting or program to investigate the value of different combinations of treatment components or the addition of a specific component to the usual treatment. The study by Woody et al. (1984, 1985) of psychotherapy as an adjunct to standard counseling is an example of an approach that can provide clear data on the value of specific treatment components.

• Each of the standard treatment components now used in rehabilitation programs (education, the Twelve Steps, group therapy, etc.) should be evaluated for its contribution to outcome by comparison with programs that have all other aspects of the treatment except the target component.

Matching Following the Rehabilitation Intervention:
Role of the Posttreatment Environment

The work of Finney, Moos, and Mewborn (1980) has shown that the posttreatment environment can profoundly influence the overall outcome for treated alcohol abusers. In the past, the posttreatment environment of patients depended on the patient's personal resources because most programs concentrated on primary treatment and the funds needed to develop individually tailored posttreatment programs were not available. Continuing treatment options offered to patients who had completed primary care were generally restricted to AA meetings and possibly a weekly or monthly continuing care meeting at the primary care site.

Because of recently shortened periods of reimbursed care for primary rehabilitation and some new financial incentives to provide outpatient treatment, clinical programs are now devoting more time to the development of posttreatment continuing care programs and have attempted to bring the family of a patient into the continuing treatment process. The availability of these services provides an opportunity for patient-treatment matching research following the period of primary rehabilitation.

The following are opportunities for research on patient-treatment matching following primary rehabilitation:

• Comparative studies of AA treatment, relapse prevention, individual therapy, or family therapy following the completion of primary rehabilitation might be initiated in a variety of treatment settings and patient populations. Do these interventions add anything beyond primary treatment? What types of patients benefit most from each of these treatments? Ideally, this research should involve parametric studies that investigate the optimum duration and intensity of treatments and should include measures of cost-effectiveness.

• Comparative studies of different posttreatment environments (e.g., halfway houses, quarter-way houses, family treatment centers) should be conducted to determine the overall efficacy of these environments and the types of patients best suited to them.

• Comparative studies of family treatments that are independent of the rest of the patient's treatment program could be used to evaluate the contributions of various forms of family education to the posttreatment adjustment of the patient. For example, during the course of the patient's rehabilitation, families could be assigned to Al-Anon, family therapy, alcohol education, or individual counseling. It should then be determined whether these interventions add anything beyond primary treatment for the affected patient and whether these different approaches can be matched with specific types of families.

PATIENT-TREATMENT MATCHING: SOME CONCLUSIONS AND RESEARCH RECOMMENDATIONS

Work to date on patient-treatment matching leads to three conclusions, which are recapitulated here.

1. Patient factors appear to be more predictive of outcome from treatment than are treatment process factors. Techniques for measuring patient characteristics have shown major development in breadth, reliability, and validity over the past decade. In contrast, treatment processes have been almost unstudied, and there are no available instruments for reliable and valid treatment measurement. The broader range of treatments now available and under development may reveal more potent treatment process factors if treatment is actually provided in an appropriate manner and for an adequate length of time.

2. Of the patient variables that have been studied, psychosocial factors have been shown to be the most important predictors of outcome for different treatment intensities (e.g., inpatient, partial hospitalization, outpatient care). Patients with better social and economic support and fewer psychiatric problems do well in most treatments and seem to benefit equally from inpatient or outpatient interventions. Lower socioeconomic strata patients and those having more serious psychiatric problems do less well in treatment generally and fare particularly poorly in outpatient care. Such patient factors as the severity of alcohol dependence, family history of alcoholism, and presence of antisocial personality disorder have been generally predictive of poorer outcomes from all treatments but are not differentially predictive of response to specific treatments.

3. There have been very few studies in which patients were matched to different treatment components (e.g., group therapy, individual therapy, medication, relapse prevention) within a given level of treatment intensity. There are at this time no clear predictors of differential outcomes from any of these components.

Work on patient-treatment matching offers the potential for significant, practical advances. To achieve this potential, the committee makes the three following recommendations:

1. There is a need for a more specific focusing of matching questions (Longabaugh, 1986; Annis, 1987). Efforts should be made to study well-defined treatments that have clear therapeutic goals for specific segments of the patient population. Matching studies

that employ appropriate designs should be considered at each level of the rehabilitation process. At the levels of referral to the treatment program (primary care) and posttreatment environment (aftercare), experimental designs that employ random patient assignment and nonexperimental designs such as a cafeteria approach (Ewing, 1977) or a feedback system (Glaser, 1980) should be considered. When assigning patients to treatment components or treatment providers within a specific program or environment, experimental designs with random patient assignment are preferable to evaluate the differential efficacy of components of approximately equal attractiveness and comparable intensity.

2. More innovative interventions are needed, as well as programs designed to address specific treatment problems of different groups in the population (e.g., the psychiatrically ill alcoholic, the antisocial alcoholic, the cocaine- and alcohol-dependent patient). Similarly, there is a need to continue evaluation and patient-treatment matching work with recently developed treatments for problem drinkers (Sanchez-Craig, 1984; Miller 1985), for relapse prevention (Gorski and Miller, 1982; Marlatt and Gordon, 1985), and for community reinforcement (Azrin et al., 1982). As discussed in Skinner (1981), it is difficult to study the optimum matching of patients and treatments when there is so little variability in the philosophy, duration, or basic therapeutic components of most treatments.

3. Reliable, valid, practical, and generalizable instruments are needed to measure the types, amounts, and duration of alcohol treatment interventions a patient receives during the course of rehabilitation. These measurements are important both for training therapists and for evaluating of treatment efficacy. If treatments are not applied in an appropriate manner, then it is unreasonable to think that they will work. We do not always know whether a specific intervention (e.g., group therapy for denial), much less a multi-service treatment program, is practiced in the manner originally intended. We do not always know the extent to which different individuals in a single treatment receive the same types, amounts, or duration of treatment components. The often repeated claim that patient factors account for more outcome variation than treatment factors may be simply a function of the unavailability of treatment measurement instruments or the close association between certain client characteristics (e.g., age, marital status, antisocial personality) and the posttreatment environments to which these individuals typically return. The ability to characterize a treatment intervention or program as well as it is now possible to characterize patients should substantially enhance our ability to predict outcomes and assign (match) patients to optimal treatments.

REFERENCES

Annis, H. M. Effective treatment for drug and alcohol problems: What do we know? Paper presented at the annual meeting of the Institute of Medicine, National Academy of Sciences, Washington, DC, October 21, 1987.

Azrin, N. H., R. W. Sisson, R. Meyers et al. Alcoholism treatment by disulfiram and community reinforcement therapy. J. Behav. Ther. Exp. Psychiatry 13:105-112, 1982.

Babor, T. F., Z. S. Dolinsky, B. J. Rounsaville et al. Unitary versus multidimensional models of alcoholism treatment outcome: An empirical study. J. Stud. Alcohol 49:167-177, 1988.

Blum, R. W. Adolescent substance abuse: Diagnostic and treatment issues. Pediatric Clinics of North America 34:523-537, 1987.

Blume, S. B. Women and alcohol: A review. J. Am. Med. Assoc. 256:1467-1469, 1986.

Brandsma, J. M., M. C. Maultsby, and R. J. Welsh. The outpatient treatment of alcoholism: A review and comparative study. Baltimore, MD: University Park Press, 1980.

Cloninger, C. R. Neurogenetic adaptive mechanisms in alcoholism. Science 236:410-416, 1987.

Cooney, N. L., R. M. Kadden, M. D. Litt et al. Alcoholism aftercare treatment matching: Posttreatment results. Paper presented at the Fourth International Conference on Treatment of Addictive Behaviors, Bergen, Norway, 1987.

Ewing, J. A. Matching therapy and patients: The cafeteria plan. Br. J. Addict. 72:13-18, 1977.

Finney, J. W., and R. H. Moos. Matching patients with treatments: Conceptual and methodological issues. J. Stud. Alcohol 7:122-134, 1986.

Finney, J. W., R. H. Moos, and C. R. Mewborn. Post-treatment experiences and treatment outcome of alcoholic patients six months and two years after hospitalization. J. Consult. Clin. Psychol. 48:17-29, 1980.

Glaser, F. B. Anybody got a match? Treatment research and the matching hypothesis. In G. Edwards and M. Grant, eds. Alcoholism Treatment in Transition. London: Crown Helm, 1980.

Gorski, T. T., and M. Miller. Counseling for Relapse Prevention. Independence, MO: Herald House-Independence Press, 1982.

Hayashida, M., A. I. Alterman, A. T. McLellan et al. Comparative effectiveness and costs of inpatient and outpatient medical alcohol detoxification. N. Engl. J. Med. 320(6):358-365, 1989.

Heather, N. Change without therapists: The use of self-help manuals by problem drinkers. Pp. 331-359 in W. R. Miller and N. Heather, eds. Treating Addictive Behaviors: Processes of Change. New York: Plenum Press, 1986.

Hesselbrock, M. N., R. E. Meyer, and J. J. Keener. Psychopathology in hospitalized alcoholics. Arch. Gen. Psychiatry 42:1050-1055, 1985.

Hoffmann, N. G., F. Ninonuevo, J. Mozey et al. Comparison of court-referred DWI arrestees with other outpatients in substance abuse treatment. J. Stud. Alcohol 48:591-594, 1987.

Institute of Medicine (IOM). Alcoholism, Alcohol Abuse, and Related Problems: Opportunities for Research. Washington, DC: National Academy Press, 1980.

Longabaugh, R. The matching hypothesis: Theoretical and empirical status. Paper presented at the Annual Meeting of the American Psychological Association, 1986.

Longabaugh, R., and M. Beattie. Optimizing the cost effectiveness of treatments for alcohol abusers. Pp. 104-136 in B. McGrady, N. E. Noel, and T. D. Nirenberg, eds. Future Directions in Alcohol Abuse Treatment Research. Washington, DC: NIAAA, 1985.

Longabaugh, R., B. McCrady, E. Fink et al. Cost effectiveness of alcoholism treatment in partial versus inpatient settings: Six month outcomes. J. Stud. Alcohol 44:1049-1071, 1983.

Luborsky, L., A. T. McLellan, G. E. Woody et al. Therapist success and its determinants. Arch. Gen. Psychiatry 81:123-130, 1984.

Lyons, J. P., J. Welte, J. Brown et al. Variation in alcoholism treatment orientation: Differential impact upon specific subpopulations. Alcoholism Clin. Exp. Res. 6:333-343, 1982.

Marlatt, G. A., and J. R. Gordon. Relapse Prevention. New York: Guilford Press, 1985.

McLachlan, J. F. C., and R. L. Stein. Evaluation of a day clinic for alcoholics. J. Stud. Alcohol 43:262-272, 1982.

McLellan, A. T., K. A. Druley, C. P. O'Brien et al. Matching substance abuse patients to appropriate treatments. A conceptual and methodological approach. Drug Alcohol Depend. 5(3):189-193, 1980.

McLellan, A. T., L. Luborsky, G. E. Woody et al. Increased effectiveness of substance abuse treatment: A prospective study of patient-treatment "matching." J. Nerv. Ment. Dis. 171(10):597-605, 1983a.

McLellan, A. T., L. Luborsky, G. E. Woody et al. Predicting response to alcohol and drug abuse treatments: Role of psychiatric severity. Arch. Gen. Psychiatry 40:620-625, 1983b.

Miller, W. R. Motivation for treatment: A review with special emphasis on alcoholism. Psychol. Bull. 98:84-107, 1985.

Miller, W. R. Haunted by the Zeitgeist: Reflections on contrasting treatment goals and conceptions of alcoholism in Europe and the United States. In T. F. Babor, ed. Alcohol and Culture: Comparative Perspectives from Europe and America. New York: New York Academy of Sciences, 1986.

Miller, W. R., and R. K. Hester. Inpatient alcoholism treatment: Who benefits? Am. Psychol. 41:794-805, 1986a.

Miller, W. R., and R. K. Hester. Matching problem drinkers with optimal treatments. Pp.175-203 in W. R. Miller and N. Heather, eds. Treating Addictive Behaviors: Processes of Change. New York: Plenum Press, 1986b.

Morey, L. C., H. A. Skinner, and R. K. Blashfield. A typology of alcohol abusers: Correlates and implications. J. Abnormal Psychol. 93:408-417, 1984.

Orford, J., E. Openheimer, and G. Edwards. Abstinence or control: The outcome for excessive drinkers two years after consultation. Behav. Res. Ther. 14:409-418, 1976.

Polich, J. M., D. J. Armor, and H. B. Braiker. Patterns of alcoholism over four years. J. Stud. Alcohol 41:397-416, 1980.

Powell, B. J., E. C. Penick, M. R. Read et al. Comparison of three outpatient treatment interventions: A twelve-month follow-up of men alcoholics. J. Stud. Alcohol 46:309-312, 1985.

Prochaska, J. O., and C. C. DiClemente. Stages and processes of self-change of smoking: Toward an integrated model of change. J. Clin. Consult. Psychol. 51:390-395, 1983.

Rounsaville, B. J., Z. S. Dolinsky, T. F. Babor et al. Psychopathology as a predictor of treatment outcome in alcoholism. Arch. Gen. Psychiatry 44:505-513, 1987.

Sanchez-Craig, M. Therapist's Manual for Secondary Prevention of Alcohol Problems: Procedures for Teaching Moderate Drinking and Abstinence. Toronto: Addiction Research Foundation, 1984.

Sanchez-Craig, M., and K. Walker. Teaching coping skills to chronic alcoholics in a coeducational halfway house. I. Assessment of programme effects. Br. J. Addict. 77:35-50, 1982.

Saxe, L., D. Dougherty, K. Esty et al. Health Technology Case Study 22: The Effectiveness and Costs of Alcoholism Treatment. Washington, DC: U.S. Congress, Office of Technology Assessment, 1983.

Schuckit, M. A. Subjective responses to alcohol in sons of alcoholics and control subjects. Arch. Gen. Psychiatry 41:879-884, 1984.

Schuckit, M. A. The clinical implications of primary diagnostic groups among alcoholics. Arch. Gen. Psychiatry 42:1043-1049, 1985.

Skinner, H. A. Different strokes for different folks. Differential treatment for alcohol abuse. Pp. 349-367 in R. F. Meyer, T. F. Babor, B. C. Glueck et al., eds. Evaluation of the Alcoholic: Implications for Research, Theory and Treatment. NIAAA Research Monograph No. 5. USDHHS Publ. No. (ADM)81-1033. Washington, DC: NIAAA, 1981.

Stabenau, J. R., and V. Hesselbrock. Psychopathology in alcoholics and their families and vulnerability to alcoholism: A review and new findings. Pp. 108-132 in S. M. Mirin, ed. Substance Abuse and Psychopathology. Washington, DC: American Psychiatric Press, 1984.

Walker, R. D., D. M. Donovan, D. R. Kivlahan et al. Length of stay, neuropsychological performance and aftercare: Influences on alcohol treatment outcome. J. Consult. Clin. Psychol. 51:900-911, 1983.

Westermeyer, J. Ethnic factors in treatment. Pp. 709-717 in E. M. Pattison, and E. Kaufman, eds. The American Encyclopedic Handbook of Alcoholism. New York: Gardner Press, 1982.

Woody, G. E., A. T. McLellan, L. Luborsky et al. Psychiatric severity as a predictor of benefits from psychotherapy. Am. J. Psychiatry 141:1171-1177, 1984.

Woody, G. E., A. T. McLellan, L. Luborsky et al. Sociopathy and psychotherapy outcome. Arch. Gen. Psychiatry 42:1081-1086, 1985.

Zucker, R. The four alcoholisms: A developmental account of the etiological process. In P. C. Rivers, ed. Alcohol and Addictive Behavior. Lincoln, NE: University of Nebraska Press, 1987.

12

ADVANCES IN THE TREATMENT OF OTHER
PSYCHOACTIVE SUBSTANCE-USE DISORDERS:
IMPLICATIONS FOR RESEARCH ON TREATMENT OF ALCOHOL PROBLEMS

The alcoholism treatment field has developed largely in isolation from treatments for other addictive disorders, although there are many parallels between alcoholism and other addictive problems. This chapter highlights major advances in the conceptualization and treatment of psychoactive substance-use disorders other than alcoholism; it also considers the implications of this work for research on the treatment of alcohol problems.

SMOKING

The context for smoking cessation research has changed dramatically in the past 25 years. Since the publication of the surgeon general's first report on the issue (U.S. Public Health Service, 1964), evidence has mounted about the detrimental health effects of smoking. The vast majority of smokers are concerned about such effects and would like to quit (Orleans, 1985). In addition, concerns about the health effects of tobacco smoke have led to a strong nonsmokers' rights movement, which has resulted in restrictions on smoking in public places. Smoking has become an increasingly stigmatized behavior.

This climate reflects attitudes that are quite different from attitudes about alcohol use: in the case of alcohol, controversy exists about the beneficial or harmful effects of moderate doses of alcohol, and nondrinkers' rights have become an issue only in relation to drinking and driving. Most persons with drinking problems are not self-identified and are not trying to stop drinking. Thus, research on smoking cessation occurs in a substantially different social climate from alcohol treatment research, which may limit the applicability of some of the smoking research to the alcohol field. However, many of the programs, models, and variables do appear to have relevance. This chapter considers several major areas of smoking research that are relevant to alcoholism treatment research.

There is a very high rate of co-occurrence of alcoholism and smoking, but the recent prominence of the nonsmokers' rights movement and the inclusion of nicotine dependence in the third revised edition of the American Psychiatric Association's Diagnostic and Statistical Manual of Mental Disorders (DSM-III-R) under psychoactive substance-use disorders have increased interest in the promotion of smoking cessation among alcohol patients in treatment. Although no controlled studies have yet been reported, some treatment centers are offering smoking cessation programs, and there are a growing number of nonsmoking meetings available in Alcoholics Anonymous (AA).

Nonetheless, conventional wisdom is that clients should initially focus on changing drinking and other drug-use behaviors and postpone changes in smoking or eating behavior. No data are available to substantiate this belief. The following questions represent opportunities for research on smoking cessation during alcohol treatment:

- What is the impact of concurrent versus consecutive treatment for changing drinking and smoking behavior?
- Are particular types of smoking cessation approaches most effective with alcoholic patients?
- What impact would a smoke-free environment have on inpatient alcohol treatment?

Treatment Process Research

Smoking cessation research has focused on a number of motivational, cognitive, social, environmental, and behavioral processes related to smoking cessation. This section reviews advances in research on several of these variables.

Processes and Stages of Change

Prochaska and DiClemente (1986) have identified five stages in the process of quitting smoking and ten major processes that may characterize change attempts for any personal problem (Prochaska, 1984). Their research suggests that different processes are used at different stages of change. They have recently begun to test treatment and self-change materials that are specifically geared to different stages of change.

Alcoholism treatment research has done little to systematically modify treatment approaches based on different degrees of readiness for change. Although a number of approaches have been developed for the early identification of those with drinking problems (e.g., Lewis and Gordon, 1983; Babor, Ritson, and Hodgson, 1986), techniques that address the unique clinical needs of these populations have not been carefully evaluated, and treatment research has not focused on matching a treatment method to a person's stage of readiness for change. Moreover, alcoholism treatment research has not systematically evaluated the change strategies alcoholics actually use in order to determine which interventions might be effective at different stages in the change process.

The following questions represent opportunities for research on processes of change:

- Do persons with drinking problems go through identifiable stages of change and use unique processes at different stages?
- Can treatment methods be developed to teach clients change techniques that are most relevant for their stage of change and that effectively move clients from one stage of change to the next?
- Do certain types of informational feedback (e.g., health information) have a unique effect in getting people to change their drinking behavior?

Cognitive Predictors of Smoking Cessation

Several investigators have examined the relationships between cognitive variables and smoking cessation. Self-efficacy (see Bandura, 1977) is a cognitive mechanism that is postulated to underlie behavior change. Efficacy expectations, which are situation specific, are believed to determine whether coping behaviors are initiated and sustained, especially in the face of obstacles to change. In contrast, outcome expectancies refer to expectations about the probable consequences of behavior rather than the individual's belief in his or her ability to engage in the behavior. A third cognitive variable, attribution, has also been examined in relation to smoking cessation. Attributions for change (locus of control) may be either internal, in which case the client feels primarily responsible for change, or external--the client attributes change to an external agent (e.g., a drug). These three cognitive variables have been studied as factors that might predict success in initiating or maintaining smoking cessation.

Several research groups have found that higher self-efficacy at the end of treatment is consistently related to positive treatment outcomes at the point of follow-up (DiClemente, 1981; Godding and Glasgow, 1985; Gregory, Etringer, and Lando, unpublished; Velasques et al., unpublished). In addition, a generalized belief in the ability to quit strongly predicted long-term abstinence (Mothersill, McDowell, and Rosser, 1988), even though outcome expectancies have not been found to predict long-term changes in smoking (Godding and Glasgow, 1985).

Studies of attributions for change have found that ex-smokers who have successfully stopped smoking are more likely to attribute the causes of success or failure to internal reasons than are those who have continued smoking (Harackiewicz et al., 1987). Epstein and colleagues (1987) found that 12 months after treatment, those who maintained smoking cessation continued to make more internal attributions for change than did those who had relapsed. This study also demonstrated that attributions could be changed and maintained through therapeutic interventions. It should also be noted that there is a significant difference in the locus of control for change propounded by providers of smoking cessation treatment and by some alcohol treatment providers. Programs that utilize the AA philosophy emphasize the importance of giving responsibility for change to a higher power, an outlook that would appear to be different from the internal attributions for change suggested by the smoking literature.

Cognitive research points to the role of beliefs in smoking cessation. A high level of self-efficacy, a generalized belief in one's ability to change, and internal attributions for change are all positive predictors of the outcomes of smoking cessation attempts. Although none of these variables accounts for the majority of variance in outcomes, all of them contribute to it. Similar variables are beginning to be examined in alcoholism treatment research studies, and specific measures of self-efficacy (Annis, 1988), outcome expectancies for alcohol use (Brown et al., 1980), and drinking-related locus of control (Donovan and O'Leary, 1978) have been developed; however, more research into cognitive variables should be encouraged.

The following questions represent opportunities for research on cognitive variables:

• Do self-efficacy and outcome expectancies predict success in changing and in maintaining changes in drinking behavior?
• If self-efficacy and outcome expectancies predict positive treatment outcome, what treatment techniques or settings can most successfully affect these variables?
• What is the relationship between attributions for change and successful treatment outcome?

Antecedents to Relapse and Coping Skills

In recent years, investigators who study treatment of addictive behaviors have generally shifted their focus from the initiation of change to the maintenance of change. Relapse, the antecedents to relapse, skills for avoiding or coping with relapse, and the mechanisms that underlie relapse have become important research areas (Marlatt and Gordon, 1985). This research has spanned most addictive behaviors. In smoking research, a distinction has been made between the antecedents that lead to full smoking relapse and the antecedents that end with a return to abstinence. Early studies reported that a preponderance of antecedents involved negative affect or withdrawal symptoms (Ossip-Klein et al., 1984; Shiffman, 1985). Full relapsers appear to respond to different kinds of situations than do temporary lapsers or those who experience a temptation to smoke but do not do so (O'Connell and Martin, 1987).

Coping has been conceptualized as a mediating variable between exposure to a potential relapse situation and the choice of relapse or continued abstention. Relapsing smokers do not appear to be deficient in overall coping skills (Abrams et al., 1987), but relapsers evidence higher anxiety in smoking-specific situations and are less skillful in coping with them, especially when they involve interpersonal elements (Abrams et al., 1987). Smoking in response to a potential relapse situation appears to be primarily determined by the coping response used rather than by the type of relapse situation (Shiffman, 1985). Recent research (Glassman et al., 1988) suggests that smokers with a history of depression have lower success rates in quitting smoking. The presence of depression might affect the smoker's ability to use coping responses when confronted with high-risk situations for relapse.

Research on the antecedents to drinking relapse actually preceded research on antecedents to smoking relapse. However, smoking researchers have extended this research in two fruitful directions: (1) the examination of different coping responses and antecedents for those who continue to smoke or those who resume abstinence and (2) studies of the relative effectiveness of different types of coping responses.

The following questions represent opportunities for research on relapse and coping studies:

- Are different types of relapse situations and coping responses associated with different outcomes or drinking episodes?
- Are different types of coping responses utilized at different stages of successful change in drinking?
- Does the presence of a diagnosable depressive disorder affect the alcoholic's ability to use coping responses to avoid relapse?
- What social system variables influence the use of coping responses in potential relapse situations?

Social Support

Higher levels of social support are known to be associated with better physical and psychological functioning. The mechanisms by which social support influences psychological health are not well understood, but a number of investigators have developed partner-involved treatment interventions. Results of the effectiveness of these interventions have been mixed (McCrady, 1986). In the smoking field, early research focused on the relationships between naturally occurring partner behaviors and successful smoking cessation and maintenance. The frequency of social support in itself has not been found to predict successful smoking cessation (Harlow et al., 1986). Positive partner support has been shown to be associated with successful smoking cessation and maintenance, and negative partner behaviors are associated with unsuccessful quit attempts (Mermelstein, Lichtenstein, and McIntyre, 1983; Coppotelli and Orleans, 1985); however, attempts to change partner behaviors to increase support have not yielded improved maintenance of smoking cessation (Lichtenstein, Glasgow, and Abrams, 1986).

Studies have also examined the effectiveness of enhancing other sources of support for smoking cessation and maintenance, for example, coworkers. These studies have also found little evidence for improved long-term maintenance of change as a result of attempts to enhance coworker support (Lichtenstein, Glasgow, and Abrams, 1986); however, higher levels of negative or nonsupportive social interactions have indeed been found to correlate with relapse (Glasgow, Klesges, and O'Neill, 1986). Research has not yet addressed the impact on successful quit attempts of establishing a smoke-free home or workplace.

A number of recent studies (reviewed in Orleans, 1985) have examined the effectiveness of spouse- involved alcoholism treatment. Although most of these studies have yielded promising results, the smoking literature suggests two additional areas of research: (1) studies of types of partner behaviors that are naturally associated with different treatment outcomes and (2) studies of other aspects of the alcoholic's social environment.

The following questions offer opportunities for research on social support studies:

 • Are certain partner behaviors associated with more and less positive alcoholism treatment outcomes? If these behaviors can be reliably identified, can they be taught, and will such a treatment intervention affect treatment outcome positively?
 • What characteristics and behaviors of social support networks outside of the family are associated with more and less positive treatment outcomes?
 • Can effective treatment interventions be designed to enhance the support behaviors of the alcoholic's naturally occurring social environment?

Motivational Factors

A number of motivational factors are associated with successful smoking cessation. Health concerns, expectations of improved future health, and a feeling of personal vulnerability to health risks are strong correlates of successful cessation (Orleans, 1985). Successful quitters report that they desire a greater sense of self-mastery, self-esteem, and self-approval and that they associate these feelings with successful smoking cessation (Orleans, 1987). In contrast to continuing smokers or recidivists, successful quitters report that they expect to succeed, expect quitting to be easier, and expect more benefits from quitting (Orleans, 1985). Some smokers also appear to stop for altruistic motives, such as concerns about the impact of their smoking on others, or because they want to set a positive example for their children (Orleans, 1987).

Smoking researchers have redefined motivation by examining specific components of the desire to quit smoking, including personal beliefs about health, the perceived psychological benefits of quitting, expectations about the quitting process, and concerns about others. Defining motivation in terms of cognitive and affective variables implies that these components of motivation may be amenable to intervention. Similar to Prochaska's work on stages of change, motivational studies suggest particular treatment interventions that could target specific aspects of motivation. In the alcoholism field--with exceptions, such as Miller (1985)--motivation has generally been seen as a global construct rather than as a specific set of factors. Because of the common perception that alcoholics who are actively drinking have high levels of denial of their problems, interventions to affect motivation have usually involved external coercion. Relatively little attention has been given to methods of altering the internal components of an individual's motivation.

The following questions represent opportunities for research on motivation studies:

• Do specific health beliefs or positive expectancies about the benefits of decreasing or stopping drinking positively affect an alcoholic's decision to decrease or stop drinking and to maintain change?
• Do "altruistic motives" (concern for others) predict successful changes in drinking?
• What interventions will successfully affect the motivational factors that are most associated with successful change in drinking?

Treatment Studies on Smoking Cessation

Two recent reviews of the literature on smoking cessation treatment methods offer comprehensive summaries of this literature (Schwartz, 1987; Kamarck and Lichtenstein, in press). The highlights of these reviews are summarized here. Schwartz (1987) described seven approaches to smoking cessation treatment and two innovative large-scale approaches (which are described in the following section on unique, programmatic strategies). For each approach he reviewed the empirical literature and then estimated median success rates at 6 and 12 months. The approaches included self-care, educational and group programs, medications, nicotine chewing gum, hypnosis, acupuncture, and behavioral techniques.

The five methods with the best success rates are noted below.

1. Self-care approaches to smoking cessation have included individually developed cessation approaches, the use of brief instructions or advice, and the utilization of smoking cessation aids (e.g., filters), self-help guides, or "quit kits." Almost a dozen studies in this area find an average success rate of 18 percent one year after attempting to quit (Schwartz, 1987).
2. Educational programs, clinics, and groups have proliferated in the last decade. Such programs are offered commercially and by public service organizations and show median one-year success rates of approximately 25 percent (Schwartz, 1987).
3. Medications to overcome the smoking habit (e.g., clonidine), and medications to minimize withdrawal have both been evaluated. The average rate of successful quitting and maintenance is about 18 percent for medication studies (Schwartz, 1987). However, a recent report (Glassman et al., 1988) found much higher rates of short-term success for clonidine-treated subjects than for placebo-treated subjects (64 versus 29 percent at four weeks), as well as continued higher success rates six months after treatment (29 percent of those on clonidine were still abstinent, compared with 5 percent of those on placebo). This study yielded unusually low abstinence rates in the placebo group, however, and therefore requires replication to increase confidence in the results.

4. Nicotine chewing gum was developed to reduce withdrawal symptoms in the first weeks after smoking cessation and has yielded successful one-year quitting and maintenance rates ranging from 29 to 49 percent, compared with 4 to 37 percent for placebos (Tonnesen et al., 1988). The average success rate after 12 months was 11 percent for nicotine chewing gum treatment, but the rate rose to 29 percent when nicotine chewing gum was combined with behavioral therapy (Schwartz, 1987). A more recent review (Hughes, 1988) updates Schwartz's review, reporting that in three of four new studies nicotine chewing gum in combination with behavior therapy yielded better treatment outcomes than nicotine chewing gum alone.

5. Behavioral methods have been evaluated in studies of individual treatment methods and in studies that combine multiple treatment methods. Aversive smoking procedures have been used in attempts to reduce the reinforcing value of smoking by pairing it with aversive stimuli. Techniques have included rapid smoking, smoke holding, and focused smoking. Rapid smoking alone has produced an average 12-month success rate of 21 percent, smoke holding has yielded a 6-month success rate of 33 percent, and focused smoking has yielded an average 26 percent success rate at one year. When rapid smoking is combined with other behavioral procedures, the average success rate rises to 30.5 percent at the one-year follow-up point (Schwartz, 1987).

Behavioral approaches have also introduced techniques to help people stop smoking and cope with abstinence from cigarettes. Nicotine fading (Foxx and Brown, 1979) is a technique in which the smoker gradually reduces nicotine intake over several weeks by switching to cigarette brands with progressively lower amounts of nicotine. This procedure, when used as a prelude to smoking cessation, has yielded average successful quit rates of 25 percent over six months (Schwartz, 1987). Self-management techniques to cope with abstinence from cigarettes are similar to those used with other behavioral problems and have included self-monitoring, stimulus control, contingency management, desensitization, relaxation, and self-control packages. Recent studies have combined aversive smoking procedures with behavioral self-management techniques, yielding success rates of 32 percent over six months and 40 percent over one year (Schwartz, 1987).

In summary, the highest one-year success rates come from multiple-component, behaviorally based treatment programs that specifically combine rapid smoking with other behavioral treatments and nicotine gum with behavior therapy (Schwartz, 1987).

Several factors differentiate smoking cessation treatment from alcoholism treatment. First, self-help groups have played a more limited role in smoking cessation. Second, smoking researchers show a greater respect for smokers' stated desire to quit "on their own" and have attempted to understand that process and develop materials that will aid the self-change process. In contrast, many clinicians and researchers in the alcoholism field believe that alcoholics experience "loss of control" and "denial" of their problems, which casts doubt on the possibility of self-directed change. Although there are a number of self-change oriented books and tapes for drinkers, this approach has met with limited acceptance. Third, a pharmacologically active but relatively safe alternative to tobacco is now available, and its effectiveness is being evaluated. Fourth, many of the most robust approaches, which are well accepted in the smoking field, have been derived from behavioral approaches to treatment. Although much of the empirical work on the effectiveness of alcoholism treatment has been derived from a behavioral perspective, these techniques have not been widely applied. Fifth, some novel aversive smoking procedures have been developed that appear to have a positive impact on treatment when combined with additional treatment elements. Finally, nicotine fading, an approach to nicotine withdrawal that is radically different from current approaches to alcohol withdrawal, has been introduced and used with success.

The following questions, suggested by smoking treatment studies, represent opportunities for further research:

• What is the effectiveness of currently available self-change materials for drinkers, and for whom are these materials most effective? Would different types of self-change materials be more appropriate for certain types of drinking problems?
• What methods would increase the availability and acceptability of empirically tested self-change materials for drinkers?
• Can a pharmacologically active alternative to alcohol be developed that would decrease the symptoms of a protracted abstinence syndrome without having addictive or other potentially harmful side effects? What would be its role and effectiveness as a treatment agent?
• What would be the outcomes of large-scale clinical trials of multiple-component behavioral programs for alcoholism treatment?

Unique and Programmatic Approaches to Smoking Cessation

Several novel approaches have been used to bring smoking cessation information and materials to the public. These approaches have in common a shift from traditional treatment models, which require clients to seek assistance, to models that make materials accessible in settings with which smokers are already involved. Many of these programs are similar to those described in Chapter 10 on the early identification of brief interventions for alcohol problems.

Physician Counseling

Most physicians feel that it is their responsibility to help their patients quit smoking (Schwartz, 1987). However, only 22 to 25 percent of smokers report that their physician has advised them to quit (Schwartz, 1987). A number of programs have been developed to teach physicians the skills needed to facilitate smoking cessation. The highest reported quit rates (Schwartz, 1987) are for physician interventions with cardiac patients, with a median one-year quit rate of 43 percent. Simple physician advice, taking as little as one minute, will yield median quit rates of 6 percent; physician advice coupled with other interventions (e.g., additional information, questionnaires, feedback about health effects, careful guiding of quit attempts) results in one-year quit rates of 22 percent (Schwartz, 1987).

Formal evaluations of physician interventions to assist patients to change their drinking are relatively few. An increasing amount of medical education on alcoholism (Gottlieb, Mullen, and McAlister, 1987), alcoholism-related training materials (Liepman, Anderson, and Fisher, 1984), and self-directed texts are now available (e.g., from the American Medical Society on Alcohol and Other Drug Dependencies); films directed toward physicians have also been developed (e.g., Kinney et al., 1986). Yet controlled evaluations of the effectiveness of these educational efforts are lacking, and most (with the exception of Kristenson and colleagues, 1983, for example) have focused on alcoholism rather than heavy drinking. In addition, most provide a broad knowledge base about alcoholism but less specific information about how to intervene. An exception to this is the World Health Organization's Amethyst Project (Babor et al., 1987), which is currently developing and evaluating focused interventions for nonalcoholic patients.

The following questions represent opportunities for physician and primary care studies:

- What is the effectiveness of simple physician advice, alone or combined with other interventions, in decreasing drinking in nonalcoholic, heavy-drinking patients? (See Elvy, Wells, and Baird, 1988, for a recent report of such a study.)
- For alcohol-dependent patients, what is the effectiveness of simple physician advice to stop drinking or to seek treatment?
- How effective are physician interventions that are developed uniquely for patients with alcohol-related diseases (e.g., liver disease, pancreatitis)?
- What components are necessary, and what is the most effective sequencing of these components, in physician interventions with alcoholic patients?

Special Populations

The final area of innovation in the delivery of smoking cessation programs is the development of methods for reaching underserved populations. Blacks have the highest smoking rate of any major ethnic or racial group in the United States, along with very high rates of morbidity and mortality from cardiovascular disease and cancer. There are currently several ongoing projects directed at black smokers that include efforts to reach black inner-city smokers through physician advice and quitting aids, televised smoking cessation clinics and in-person classes (which target black women in public housing projects), clinics for Head Start mothers that are led by trained lay counselors, and combined prevention and quit-smoking programs for black communities (U.S. Department of Health and Human Services, 1988). In one of the most innovative programs (U.S. Department of Health and Human Services, 1988), researchers are working with a black-owned insurance company to deliver smoking cessation materials to policyholders. No outcome data are available yet from any of these studies, but they provide unique perspectives on the delivery of services to underserved populations.

The innovative methods described above for the delivery of smoking cessation programs to black smokers could be replicated and evaluated for use in treating drinking problems among blacks and other ethnic/racial minority groups.

The following questions represent opportunities for special population studies:

- What types of alcoholism programs attract and retain the highest proportions of potential subjects who are minority group members?
- What is the relative effectiveness of alcohol treatment materials that are specially tailored to the target population, compared with generic materials?
- What are the outcomes of treatment programs that are uniquely designed to reach the minority group member, compared with existing treatment programs?

OTHER DRUG DEPENDENCIES

There has been a significant increase in the range and quality of treatment studies in the field of drug dependence over the past 10 years similar to the increase seen in smoking research. There has also been a move toward the evaluation of rehabilitation efforts rather than a focus on detoxification procedures. Treatment and research efforts in the field of drug dependence have always been relevant to the field of alcohol dependence. Now, however, the growing group of mixed alcohol- and drug-dependent (particularly alcohol plus cocaine) patients presenting for treatment and the growing reliance among drug dependence treatment providers on methods and procedures similar to those that were traditionally used for alcohol dependence (e.g., AA, relapse prevention, breathalyser screening, disulfiram) bring these two fields even closer and suggest several avenues for future collaborative treatment and research efforts. This section reviews some of the research into drug dependence that is most pertinent for future studies relating to the treatment of alcohol dependence.

Use of Psychotherapy in the Treatment of Drug-Dependent Patients

In a study of cocaine-dependent patients, Siegel (1984) described using frequent supportive psychotherapy sessions, self-control strategies, and liberal use of hospitalization during initial "detoxification." This treatment employs external controls initially to separate the user from the use-fostering environment and then gradually facilitates the internalization of controls through psychotherapy. Half of Siegel's sample of 32 heavy cocaine users dropped out, but 80 percent of those remaining were cocaine free at the nine-month follow-up point. More recently, Rounsaville, Gawin, and Kleber (1985) described their adaptation of interpersonal psychotherapy for ambulatory treatment of cocaine abusers. Gawin and Kleber (1984) reported the outcome for four patients who received a version of this treatment. Although three of these patients completed at least 12 weeks of treatment and cocaine use was reduced, only one patient was entirely abstinent.

Although both of these treatment attempts used professional psychotherapy as an intervention directed primarily at the symptoms of drug use (in these cases, cocaine), other studies have used psychotherapy to address the significant psychiatric problems that are often seen concurrently among substance abusers. This practice reflects the view that "underlying" or coexisting psychiatric problems of these individuals may have fostered the substance use or reduced the efficacy of the primary substance abuse treatment. There has been recognition for some time of the growing population of substance-dependent individuals with significant psychopathology (Rounsaville et al., 1983; Rounsaville, Gawin, and Kleber, 1985) and the limited improvement these patients show in traditional treatment programs (McLellan et al., 1983, 1984; Powell et al., 1985). For this reason, there has been a movement during the last five years toward the use of standard psychiatric interventions with this population.

Two major individual psychotherapy studies were conducted in parallel by groups at Yale (Rounsaville et al., 1983) and at the University of Pennsylvania (Woody et al., 1983). Both studies showed professional psychotherapy to be superior to standard rehabilitation counseling, although this difference was statistically significant only for the University of Pennsylvania subjects. Results from the University of Pennsylvania series of studies showed that two types of psychotherapy significantly reduced drug use and illegal activity and increased employment compared with drug counseling (Woody et al., 1983).

Additional analyses of these data showed that the "psychiatrically severe" opiate addict (current symptoms of depression, anxiety, etc.) was not helped by standard counseling alone but was significantly helped by the additional therapy (Woody, McLellan, and Luborsky, 1984). Finally, additional analyses of patient diagnostic groups within this sample suggested that opiate-dependent patients with a DSM-III diagnosis of antisocial personality disorder were virtually unaffected by the additional treatment (Woody et al., 1985). This failure to find improvement in antisocial patients despite the addition of professional treatment is quite consistent with similar studies from the alcohol literature (Stabenau and Hesselbrock, 1984; Powell et al., 1985).

Group psychotherapy continues to be the most common form of intervention used with alcohol and other substance-dependent patients. Research into the use of individual psychotherapy has demonstrated the value of professional, manual-trained, supervised therapy in producing favorable outcomes among drug-dependent patients. The methods used in these forms of therapy are generally supportive, educational, and insight oriented. By contrast, group therapy, as generally practiced in alcohol dependence treatments, is not manual guided or supervised, may or may not be professionally guided, and often uses a confrontational approach.

The following are opportunities for alcoholism treatment research suggested by psychotherapy research in drug dependence:

- Research is needed to evaluate the role of manual-guided or supervised procedures in the performance and efficacy of group psychotherapy for alcohol-dependent patients.
- Although there have been several studies attempted of psychotherapy with alcoholics, few have used manual-trained and supervised therapists, verification of the integrity of the therapy that was delivered, or examination of multiple outcome measures. Would the generally positive results of psychotherapy with drug-dependent patients be replicated with alcohol-dependent patients if these "quality assurance" procedures were instituted?
- More focused studies are needed in this area to evaluate the role of psychotherapy(ies) as a primary treatment for an alcohol problem (research to date suggests a limited role) as opposed to a treatment for depression, anxiety, or relationship problems that coexist with alcohol problems and often lead to relapse. (Data from the drug dependence field suggest that psychotherapy may play an important role in this context.)
- Modern psychiatric practice commonly combines pharmacologic and psychotherapeutic methods in the treatment of certain disorders. The use of psychotropic medications has sometimes presented philosophic problems for traditional alcohol treatment programs, and for this reason in many studies psychotherapy has been tested against a particular pharmacotherapy. Studies are needed that combine these two types of interventions in alcohol-dependent patients.

Conditioned Factors in Substance Abuse Treatment

The phenomenon of craving is poorly defined and poorly measured but clearly significant in the relapse to alcohol abuse following treatment. Research in both alcohol- and drug-dependent populations indicates that craving for a substance can be elicited reliably by the presentation of stimuli associated with the substance.

In an attempt to understand the persistence of addictive behaviors despite treatment attempts, several investigators have studied the conditioned responses produced by stimuli associated with opioids and other drugs. In particular, stimuli that have been repeatedly paired with drug administration (drug paraphernalia, drug using/buying locations, mood states) can become classically conditioned "reminders" that trigger arousal, drug craving, and sometimes even withdrawal signs and symptoms (Childress, McLellan, and O'Brien, 1984, 1985; McLellan et al., 1986). Conditioned craving and arousal in response to these reminders have been demonstrated in both opiate and cocaine abusers (Childress, McLellan, and O'Brien, 1984, 1985, 1986). An experimental treatment that has been developed based on these findings is designed to reduce the ability of these cues to promote craving and arousal by repeatedly presenting them in laboratory and clinical settings and not following them with drugs. These extinction procedures have been shown to reduce opiate- or cocaine-related arousal and drug craving but only after a long series of exposures, usually 30 sessions (Childress, McLellan, and O'Brien, 1986).

These studies of conditioned factors in drug dependence parallel findings of conditioned physiological responses in alcoholics after the presentation of alcohol-related cues (Ludwig and Stark, 1974; Meyer et al., 1981) and in cigarette smokers when smoking cues are presented (Pomerleau and Pomerleau, 1984). Findings from this research underscore the potential importance of conditioned factors in explaining relapse to drug use and give evidence of the complexity of the application of these factors in a controlled clinical intervention (see Blakey and Baker, 1980).

There is widespread recognition that alcohol-dependent patients often have concomitant marijuana, cocaine, or other substance abuse problems. The prevailing treatment philosophy has been that total abstinence from all such substances is necessary and that even casual use of one substance will rapidly reinstitute use of the other(s). It is possible that the presentation of drug-related cues (e.g., pipes, bags of cocaine-like material) to these patients would result in eliciting a conditioned craving for alcohol. This technique could provide validation and an explanatory mechanism for this clinical observation and could be useful as an educational intervention for these patients.

Much more research is needed to develop treatments for conditioned factors associated with relapse. Evidence from drug-dependence studies indicates that 30 days of inpatient abstinence-oriented treatment does not appreciably affect the strength of conditioned craving and withdrawal phenomena. There is a clear relationship among relapse prevention techniques (cognitive efforts designed to teach alternative responses in the presence of cues associated with alcohol use), extinction techniques (efforts designed to weaken the strength of learned responses to alcohol-associated cues through repeated, nonreinforced exposure), and covert sensitization techniques (efforts designed to change/reduce the reinforcing properties of the cues associated with alcohol) (see Miller and Dougher, in press).

The following are opportunities for research suggested by investigations into conditioned factors associated with drug-dependence relapse:

- More work is needed to identify the physiological parameters of craving and to determine the extent to which it is physiologically and subjectively similar across different substances of abuse, especially alcohol.
- Further work is also needed to determine the conditions under which craving is elicited and the treatment procedures that will reduce or diminish its effects. In addition, studies designed to address conditioned relapse cues through the combination of relapse prevention, extinction, and covert sensitization techniques could be valuable.

Psychopharmacological Treatments for Drug Dependence

The study of pharmacological agents in the treatment of drug dependence has been an especially active field over the past several years. There has been extensive study of medications designed to reduce the immediate and protracted symptoms of withdrawal from drugs of abuse such as nicotine, benzodiazepines, and opiates. These drugs have been evaluated, and the implications for their use in alcohol detoxification are reviewed in Chapter 13.

There are separate types of pharmacological agents that have been developed and tested by drug abuse treatment researchers, each of which has a different therapeutic goal. The first type comprises medications that alter the effects of drug administration. These medications are designed to block reinforcement from drug administration (e.g., naltrexone for opiate dependence) or to attenuate its reinforcing effects; they may also attenuate abstinence symptoms (e.g., desipramine for cocaine dependence). The second type of pharmacological agent includes such medications as anti-depressants, anxiolytics, and antipsychotics, which alleviate the psychiatric symptoms and disorders that are often associated with drug dependence. Although these treatments were developed for drug abuse, it is possible that the medications may have a role to play in the treatment of alcohol dependence (these issues are discussed at length in Chapter 9).

Medications That Treat the Associated Psychiatric Symptoms of Drug-Dependent Individuals

It has been noted that depression is more common among opiate addicts, whether methadone maintained or untreated, than among matched community samples. For this reason, one line of research has focused on evaluating the efficacy of tricyclic antidepressant medications (e.g., doxepin or desipramine) in depressed, methadone-maintained patients (Woody et al., 1983, 1985; Woody, McLellan, and Luborsky, 1984). One study (Woody et al., 1985) compared doxepin with a placebo in methadone-maintained patients just beginning treatment and found that both groups improved but that those receiving doxepin improved more quickly than those receiving the placebo. A follow-up study compared doxepin, desipramine, and a placebo in clinically depressed, methadone maintained addicts who had been stabilized on methadone for at least two weeks. This study showed again that all patients improved but that the doxepin-treated patients improved more quickly than those receiving either the placebo or desipramine. These results indicate that antidepressant medications can be helpful in reducing the intensity of depressive symptoms and the length of the course of depressive illness in methadone-maintained patients.

More recent research by Arndt and her colleagues (1988) with the growing population of cocaine-abusing, methadone-maintained opiate addicts follows the work of a Yale group (Gawin and Kleber, 1984) using the antidepressant desipramine. Although the results are still preliminary, the study's initial findings appear to support the role of this antidepressant medication in reducing cocaine craving and the amount (but thus far not the frequency) of illicit cocaine use in this population. It is uncertain whether the apparent reduction of cocaine craving results from a reduction of anxiety and depression in these patients or whether desipramine has a direct effect on the reinforcing potential of cocaine.

The combination of pharmacological agents with a behavioral or social support program stressing abstinence has regularly produced philosophical problems for alcohol treatment staffs. The availability of seemingly effective medications and the clinical indication for their use in multiproblem populations provide impetus for the study of optimum ways to combine these approaches in the treatment of alcohol dependence.

The following are opportunities for research suggested by studies on agents that treat the associated psychiatric problems of drug-dependent patients:

• There have been few controlled trials of antidepressant medications for depressed alcohol-dependent patients that might reduce symptoms of depression and increase engagement and compliance with other aspects of alcohol rehabilitation. Given the number of depressed alcohol-dependent patients commonly seen in rehabilitation treatment settings, this may be an important area of study.

• Research with cocaine-dependent patients suggests that desipramine can be effective in reducing cocaine craving and use (e.g., Gawin and Kleber, 1984). Desipramine has also been shown to be an effective antidepressant medication irrespective of substance abuse. Desipramine may thus have a role to play in the treatment of the growing population of alcohol-dependent patients who have concurrent problems of depression, cocaine dependence, or both. Further research is needed to evaluate this possibility.

• There is a large and poorly studied population of patients with concurrent problems of schizophrenia and alcohol dependence. Little is known about this group. Treatment, whether pharmacological or psychotherapeutic, has been largely unsuccessful. Research is needed to develop and evaluate combined pharmacological/ psychological interventions that would address both psychiatric and alcohol-use disorders in the context of a complete psychosocial treatment program.

• More research is needed on the efficacy of combined pharmacological and psychotherapeutic treatments for patients with alcohol abuse and psychiatric disorders. Some of the failures of each treatment modality may be due to problems that could be alleviated with the addition of a second modality.

CONCLUSIONS

This review of the psychoactive substance-use treatment research literature points to several common themes across the body of treatment research on addictive behaviors. The review also identifies several areas of major focus in research on other psychoactive substance-use disorders that are different from treatment research in the alcohol field. Five major conclusions can be drawn.

1. There is a significant comorbidity of nicotine dependence and alcohol dependence and a significant comorbidity of other psychoactive drug dependence and alcohol dependence. The high comorbidity rates for these conditions suggest the need for research into the common processes that may underlie these dependence disorders. High comorbidity rates also suggest the need for research on the development of effective approaches to treat multiple psychoactive substance dependencies within the same treatment protocol.

2. Several common theoretical issues are a focus of research across psychoactive substance-use disorders. Research on processes and stages of change, relapse, coping skills, and conditioning factors (especially in craving) have proceeded across the range of psychoactive substance-use disorders.

3. Several treatment approaches are common across different psychoactive substance-use disorders. Approaches that combine pharmacotherapies with psychological treatments, treatments based on social learning principles, brief physician interventions, cue exposure

and extinction procedures, 28-day inpatient treatment programs, and self-help groups have all been applied to the treatment of more than one psychoactive substance-use disorder.

4. Several approaches to change have been used more often in the treatment of other psychoactive substance-use disorders than in the treatment of alcohol problems. These approaches include:

• Self-directed change procedures. Smoking cessation researchers have focused on smokers' expressed desire to quit without formal programs and have developed materials and methods to enhance self-directed quit attempts. Similar work in the alcohol field has been minimal.
• Behavioral approaches. Behavioral methods are among the most commonly applied approaches to smoking cessation and the treatment of other drug dependencies. The use of behavioral approaches has been more limited in the alcohol field.
• Change process research. Smoking cessation researchers have made significant advances in the study of the processes associated with successful smoking cessation. Relatively less emphasis on change processes has characterized alcohol treatment research.
• Psychotherapy. Psychotherapy research, using state-of-the-art methodology and well-specified treatment protocols, has been carried out successfully in a number of drug treatment studies. Comparable research is lacking in the alcohol field.
• Pharmacotherapies. Research on pharmacotherapeutic approaches to treatment has gained wide acceptance in the fields of smoking cessation and treatment of other drug dependencies. Resistance to the use of psychoactive drugs has impeded acceptance of comparable research in the alcohol field.
• Concomitant psychiatric disorders. Active research on the treatment of patients with coexisting psychiatric and drug dependence disorders has yielded important data. Comparable studies in the alcohol field are lacking.

5. The data suggest reasons for optimism. Treatment research studies on other psychoactive substance-use disorders offer reasons to be optimistic in that the differential effects of various treatments have been demonstrated. Overall, formal treatment and other procedures for promoting change appear to make a difference in patient/client rates of successful change.

REFERENCES

Abrams, D. B., P. M. Monti, R. P. Pinto et al. Psychosocial stress and coping in smokers who relapse or quit. Health Psychology 6:289-303, 1987.

Annis, H. M., and C. S. Davis. Alcohol dependence: Cognitive assessment procedures. In G. A. Marlatt, and D. Donovan, eds. Assessment of Addictive Behaviors. New York: Guilford Press, 1988.

Arndt, I. O., L. Dorozynski, A. T. McLellan, and G. E. Woody. Desipramine treatment for cocaine abuse in methadone-maintained patients. In L.S. Harris, ed. Problems of Drug Dependence: Proceedings of the 49th Annual Scientific Meeting, the Committee on Problems of Drug Dependence, Inc., Philadelphia, 1987. NIDA Research Monograph No. 81. Rockville, MD: National Institute on Drug Abuse, 1988.

Babor, T. F., E. B. Ritson, and R. J. Hodgson. Alcohol-related problems in the primary health care setting: A review of early intervention strategies. Br. J. Addict. 81:23-46, 1986.

Babor, T. F., P. Korner, C. Wilbur, and S. P. Good. Screening and early intervention strategies for 3harmful drinkers: Initial lessons from the Amethyst project. Australian Drug and Alcohol Review 6:325-339, 1987.

Bandura, A. Self-efficacy: Toward a unifying theory of behavioral change. Psych. Rev. 84:191-215, 1977.

Blakey, R., and R. Baker. An exposure approach to alcohol abuse. Behav. Res. Ther. 18:319-325, 1980.

Brown, S. A., M. S. Goldman, A. Inn et al. Expectations of reinforcement from alcohol: Their domain and relation to drinking patterns. J. Consult. Clin. Psychol. 48:419-426, 1980.

Childress, A. R., A. T. McLellan, and C. P. O'Brien. Measurement and extinction of conditioned withdrawal-like responses in opiate dependent patients. In Problems of Drug Dependence, 1983. Washington, DC: U.S. Department of Health and Human Services, 1984.

Childress, A. R., A. T. McLellan, and C. P. O'Brien. Assessment and extinction of conditioned opiate withdrawal-like responses. Pp. 202-210 in Problems of Drug Dependence, 1984. NIDA Research Monograph No. 55. Rockville, MD: National Institute on Drug Abuse, 1985.

Childress, A. R., A. T. McLellan, and C. P. O'Brien. Abstinent opiate abusers exhibit conditioned craving, conditioned withdrawal and reductions in both through extinction. Br. J. Addict. 81:655-660, 1986.

Coppotelli, H. C., and C. T. Orleans. Partner support and other determinants of smoking cessation maintenance among women. J. Consult. Clin. Psychol. 53:455-460, 1985.

DiClemente, C. C. Self-efficacy and smoking cessation maintenance: A preliminary report. Cog. Ther. Res. 5:175-187, 1981.

Donovan, D. M., and M. R. O'Leary. The drinking-related locus of control scale: Reliability, factor structure and validity. J. Stud. Alcohol 39:759-784, 1978.

Elvy, G. A., J. E. Wells, and K. A. Baird. Attempted referral as intervention for problem drinking in the general hospital. Br. J. Addict. 83:83-90, 1988.

Epstein, J. A., L. W. Blair, C. Sansone et al. Attributions for long-term maintenance of smoking cessation or relapse. Paper presented at the Annual Meeting of the American Psychological Association, New York, August 1987.

Foxx, R. M., and R. A. Brown. Nicotine fading and self-monitoring for cigarette abstinence or controlled smoking. J. Applied Behav. Anal. 12:111-125, 1979.

Gawin, F. H., and H. D. Kleber. Cocaine abuse treatment: An open pilot trial with lithium and desipramine. Arch. Gen. Psychiatry 41:903-909, 1984.

Glasgow, R. E., R. C. Klesges, and H. K. O'Neill. Programming social support for smoking modification: An extension and replication. Addict. Behav. 11:453-457, 1986.

Glassman, A. H., F. Stetner, B. T. Walsh et al. Heavy smokers, smoking cessation, and clonidine: Results of a double-blind, randomized trial. J. Am. Med. Assoc. 259:2863-2866, 1988.

Godding, P. R., and R. E. Glasgow. Self-efficacy and outcome expectations as predictors of controlled smoking status. Cog. Ther. Res. 9:583-590, 1985.

Gottlieb, N. H., P. D. Mullen, and A. L. McAlister. Patients, substance abuse and the primary care physician: Patterns of practice. Addict. Behav. 12:23-32, 1987.

Gregory, V. R., B. D. Etringer, and H. A. Lando. Preventing relapse in smokers: A comparison of treatments. Unpublished manuscript.

Harackiewicz, J. M., C. Sansone, L. W. Blair et al. Attributional processes in behavior change and maintenance: Smoking cessation and continued abstinence. J. Consult. Clin. Psychol. 55:372-378, 1987.

Harlow, L., J. Rossi, K. Perrin et al. Social support, demoralization, and quitting smoking: A structural model. Paper presented at the Annual Meeting of the American Psychological Association, Washington, DC, August 1986.

Hughes, J. R. Combining pharmacological and psychological treatments. Unpublished manuscript, 1988.

Kamarck, T. W., and E. Lichtenstein. Current trends in clinic-based smoking control. Behav. Med. Abstracts, in press.

Kinney, J., T. R. P. Price, P. C. Whybrow et al. A case study in designing and implementing an alcohol curriculum for medical education. Project Cork Institute, Dartmouth Medical School, Hanover, NH, 1986.

Kristenson, H., H. Ohlin, M. Hulten-Nosslin et al. Identification and intervention of heavy drinking in middle-aged men: Results and follow-up of 24-60 months of long-term study with randomized controls. Alcoholism Clin. Exp. Res. 7:203-209, 1983.

Lewis, D. C., and A. J. Gordon. Alcoholism and the general hospital: The Roger Williams intervention program. Bull. N.Y. Acad. Med. 59:181-197, 1983.

Lichtenstein, E., R. E. Glasgow, and D. B. Abrams. Social support in smoking cessation: In search of effective interventions. Behav. Ther. 17:607-619, 1986.

Liepman, M. R., R. C. Anderson, and J. V. Fisher. Family Medicine Curriculum Guide to Substance Abuse. Kansas City, MO: Society for Teachers of Family Medicine, 1984.

Ludwig, A., and L. H. Stark. Alcohol craving: Subjective and situational aspects. Q. J. Stud. Alcohol 35:899-905, 1974.

Marlatt, G. A., and J. Gordon. Relapse prevention: Maintenance strategies in the treatment of addictive behaviors. New York: Guilford Press, 1985.

McCrady, B. S. The family in the change process. Pp. 305-318 in W. Miller and N. Heather, eds. Treating Addictive Behaviors: Processes of Change. New York: Plenum Press, 1986.

McLellan, A. T., L. Luborsky, G. E. Woody et al. Predicting response to alcohol and drug abuse treatment: Role of psychiatric severity. Arch. Gen. Psychiatry 40:620-625, 1983.

McLellan, A. T., A. R. Childress, J. Griffith et al. The psychiatrically severe drug abuse patient: Methadone maintenance or therapeutic community? Am. J. Drug Alcohol Abuse 10(1):77-95, 1984.

McLellan, A. T., A. R. Childress, C. P. O'Brien et al. Extinguishing conditioned responses during treatment for opioid dependence: Turning laboratory findings into clinical procedures. J. Substance Abuse Treat. 3:33-40, 1986.

Mermelstein, R., E. Lichtenstein, and K. McIntyre. Partner support and relapse in smoking cessation programs. J. Consult. Clin. Psychol. 51:465-466, 1983.

Meyer, R. E., R. Kaplan, C. F. Stroebel et al. Conditioning factors in alcoholism. Paper presented at the annual meeting of the American Psychiatric Association, New Orleans, May 1981.

Miller, W. R. Motivation for treatment: A review with special emphasis on alcoholism. Psych. Bull. 98:504-524, 1985.

Miller, W. R., and M. J. Dougher. Covert sensitization: Alternative treatment procedures for alcoholics. Behav. Psychother., in press.

Mothersill, K. J., I. McDowell, and W. Rosser. Subject characteristics and long term post-program smoking cessation. Addict. Behav. 13:29-36, 1988.

O'Connell, K. A., and E. J. Martin. Highly tempting situations associated with abstinence, temporary lapse, and relapse among participants in smoking cessation programs. J. Consult. Clin. Psychol. 55:367-371, 1987.

Orleans, C. T. Understanding and promoting smoking cessation: Overview and guidelines for physician intervention. Ann. Rev. Med. 36:51-61, 1985.

Orleans, C. T. Research on smoking cessation and treatment. Lecture presented at Rutgers University, November 1987.

Ossip-Klein, D. J., R. Shapiro, R. Ksienski et al. Determinants of relapse for callers to a smoking relapse prevention hotline. Paper presented at the annual meeting of the Association for Advancement of Behavior Therapy, Philadelphia, November 1984.

Pomerleau, O. F., and C. P. Pomerleau. Neuroregulators and the reinforcement of smoking: Towards a biobehavioral explanation. Neurosci. Biobehav. Rev. 8:503-513, 1984.

Powell, B. J., E. C. Penick, M. R. Read et al. Comparison of three outpatient treatment interventions: A twelve-month follow-up of men alcoholics. J. Stud. Alcohol 46:309-312, 1985.

Prochaska, J. O. Systems of Psychotherapy: A Transtheoretical Analysis. Homewood, IL: The Dorsey Press, 1984.

Prochaska, J. O., and C. C. DiClemente. Toward a comprehensive model of change. In W. R. Miller and N. Heather, eds. Treating Addictive Behaviors: Processes of Change. New York: Plenum Press, 1986.

Rounsaville, B. J., F. H. Gawin, and H. D. Kleber. Interpersonal psychotherapy adapted for ambulatory cocaine abusers. Am. J. Drug Alcohol Abuse 11:171-191, 1985.

Rounsaville, B. J., W. Glazer, C. H. Wilber et al. Short-term interpersonal psychotherapy in methadone-maintained opiate addicts. Arch. Gen. Psychiatry 40:629, 1983.

Schwartz, J. L. Review and evaluation of smoking cessation methods: The United States and Canada, 1978-1985. NIH Publ. No. 87-2940. Washington, DC: Division of Cancer Prevention and Control, National Cancer Institute, 1987.

Shiffman, S. Coping with temptations to smoke. Pp. 223-242 in S. Shiffman, ed. Coping and Substance Use. New York: Academic Press, 1985.

Siegel, R. K. Changing patterns of cocaine use: Longitudinal observations, consequences, and treatment. Pp. 92-110 in J. Grabowski, ed. Cocaine: Pharmacology, Effects, and Treatment of Abuse. NIDA Research Monograph No. 50. Washington, DC: National Institute on Drug Abuse, 1984.

Stabenau, J. R., and V. Hesselbrock. Psychopathology in alcoholics and their families and vulnerability to alcoholism: A review and new findings. Pp. 108-132 in S. M. Mirin, ed. Substance Abuse and Psychopathology. Washington, DC: American Psychiatric Press, 1984.

Tonnesen, P., V. Fryd, M. Hansen et al. Two and four mg nicotine chewing gum and group counselling in smoking cessation: An open, randomized, controlled trial with a 22 month follow-up. Addict. Behav. 13:17-27, 1988.

U.S. Department of Health and Human Services. Smoking cessation initiatives for Black Americans. Pp. 509-512 in The Health Consequences of Smoking: Nicotine Addiction. A Report of the Surgeon General. USDHHS Publ. No. 88-8406. Washington, DC: Government Printing Office, 1988.

U.S. Public Health Service, Centers for Disease Control. Smoking and Health: Report of the Advisory Committee to the Surgeon General of the Public Health Service. USDHEW Publ. No. (PHS)1103. Washington, DC: Government Printing Office, 1964.

Velasques, M. L., C. C. DiClemente, A. A. Grossman et al. An analysis of efficacy evaluations in smoking cessation maintenance. Unpublished manuscript.

Woody, G. E., A. T. McLellan, and L. Luborsky. Psychiatric severity as a predictor of benefits from psychotherapy. Am. J. Psychiatry 141:1171-1177, 1984.

Woody, G. E., L. Luborsky, A. T. McLellan et al. Psychotherapy for opiate addiction: Does it help? Arch. Gen. Psychiatry 40:620-625, 1983.

Woody, G. E., A. T. McLellan, L. Luborsky et al. Sociopathy and psychotherapy outcome. Arch. Gen. Psychiatry 42:1081-1086, 1985.

13

HEALTH CONSEQUENCES OF ALCOHOL ABUSE:
OPPORTUNITIES FOR TREATMENT RESEARCH

Alcohol abuse has diverse deleterious effects on health including intoxication, the withdrawal syndrome, and many types of organ damage. The advances in our understanding of how alcohol-related organ damage occurs were reviewed in the IOM report Causes and Consequences of Alcohol Problems (IOM, 1987). This chapter focuses on opportunities for treatment research on alcohol-related illnesses. In terms of mortality, hepatic cirrhosis is probably the most serious alcohol-related disease. In terms of handicapped daily functioning, however, the cognitive impairment induced by alcohol abuse may be more serious. Although advances have been made in treating some alcohol-related illnesses, other disorders have no specific treatment. In general, in the prevention and containment of alcohol-related organ pathology, the paramount concern is to halt the patient's alcohol abuse because abstinence from alcohol in these cases is essential to allow reversibility of organ damage (where possible) and to prevent the progression of cellular and tissue damage.

In considering research approaches to the treatment of alcohol-related health consequences, multisite studies are essential in cases in which the illness occurs with such low frequency that no single site can provide a sufficient number of subjects. Alcoholic hallucinosis, pancreatitis, cardiomyopathy, and certain consequences of cirrhosis of the liver are examples of such disorders. On the other hand, controlled treatment trials for detoxification or for cognitive impairment could be carried out at either single or multiple sites.

INTOXICATION

Work on amethystic agents (agents that reverse intoxication) is in the basic research stage and is not yet ready for treatment evaluation or treatment applications. Liskow and Goodwin (1987) have reported that no single drug reverses all the effects of alcohol. Naloxone reverses the depression of the ventilatory response to hypercapnia that is induced by alcohol, but it does not help as a sobering agent. Lithium may attenuate the subjective sense of intoxication. Zimelidine and ibuprofen appear to reduce several types of alcohol-induced cognitive impairment. None of these effects appears to be pronounced, however, and none of these compounds would qualify as an amethystic agent.

Basic research on the effects of alcohol on membrane proteins, especially the calcium and chloride channels, may lead to the development of new drugs that could block the intoxicating effects of alcohol. Because alcohol intoxication is associated with a wide variety of central nervous system effects including anxiolysis, psychomotor depression, problems of coordination and gait, cognitive impairment, and changes in mood and behavior related to environmental contexts, studies of amethystic agents will have to specify the particular effects of alcohol that are reversed or blocked by the drug. At the present time, certain calcium channel blockers and drugs that serve as partial inverse agonists at the benzodiazepine/GABA chloride channel complex offer promising opportunities for future research on amethystic agents. However, this work is not yet ready for formal study in a treatment research paradigm on the reversal of alcohol intoxication.

ALCOHOL WITHDRAWAL

Pharmacotherapies for Alcohol Withdrawal

A large number of studies, beginning with the work of Kaim, Klett, and Rothfeld (1969), have demonstrated the superiority and safety of benzodiazepines over other drugs (e.g., chlorpromazine and hydroxyzine) in the treatment of alcohol withdrawal. Later studies expanded on this work by evaluating a range of benzodiazepines and concluded that all are efficacious for alcohol withdrawal (Liskow and Goodwin, 1987). The clear establishment of the efficacy of benzodiazepines for alcohol detoxification is a major research accomplishment that emerges from studies conducted during the past 20 years (Moskowitz et al., 1983).

Sellers and coworkers (1983) have exploited diazepam's long duration of action in developing what they call the loading benzodiazepine dose technique. In this method, a 20-milligram (mg) oral dose of diazepam is given at intervals of 1 to 2 hours until clinical improvement occurs or until the patient becomes sedated. In one recent study, all patients treated using this technique successfully completed detoxification, and 50 percent responded within 7.6 hours to an oral dose of 60 mg of diazepam. Only an occasional patient required treatment for more than 24 hours. No patients had serious withdrawal reactions such as seizures, hallucinations, or arrhythmias (Sellers et al., 1983).

Several other nonbenzodiazepine agents have been evaluated, and all seem to reduce many of the peripheral signs of alcohol withdrawal, but they should be used cautiously because they do not work as well as benzodiazepines in suppressing the more serious symptoms of alcohol withdrawal (e.g., seizures, delirium tremens) (Schuckit, 1987). For example, beta blockers attenuate the symptoms of autonomic hyperactivity in alcohol withdrawal, but Liskow and Reed (1986) caution that this effect might disguise the warning signs of more severe symptoms, and they recommend the simultaneous prescription of benzodiazepines. Trials of alpha-2 adrenergic agonists such as lofexidine and clonidine have shown reductions in alcohol withdrawal symptom scores with both agents. However, as with the beta blockers, neither anticonvulsant effects nor the ability to suppress other severe alcohol withdrawal symptoms has been demonstrated with alpha-2 agonists (Schuckit, 1987).

Calcium channel blockers have also been tried. One study compared meprobamate with caroverine (not available in the United States) and found that both helped and were equally efficacious (Koppi et al., 1987). A second study found that several calcium channel blockers reduced seizures and mortality in alcohol-dependent rats (Little, Dolin, and Halsey, 1986). Few human studies have been conducted, but the limited data available suggest that this class of drugs may suppress some of the symptoms of alcohol withdrawal. One problem in using these drugs in a clinical situation is that there is a delay in the time of onset of their action; thus, they must be given several days before alcohol detoxification begins.

In summary, the evidence supports the superiority of benzodiazepines over all other agents used for alcohol withdrawal based on a combination of efficacy, safety, and rapidity of onset. The research agenda for pharmacotherapy of alcohol withdrawal will probably be better served by a shift away from studies of which drug class works best and toward the following issues: how to determine when pharmacotherapy is indicated, how to use it most effectively, whether some treatment settings (e.g., inpatient versus outpatient) are better for detoxification than others, which type and dose of benzodiazepines should be used in specific situations, whether there is any advantage to combining other drugs (such as anticonvulsants) with benzodiazepines, whether to use adjunctive drugs (i.e, antidepressants), and how to increase compliance with rehabilitation after detoxification.

Nonpharmacological Detoxification

Another area of research involves studies of detoxification with psychosocial support alone. In a study done by Whitfield and colleagues (1978), treatment was administered by college graduates with a behavioral science background who were given 8 to 12 hours of classroom training in a series of clearly specified techniques. Trainees had a probationary period of one month during which they worked with an experienced person. Special attention was given to alerting the therapists to clinical signs of severe alcohol withdrawal requiring evaluation by a physician and pharmacotherapy.

All patients were given supportive intervention along with a regular diet and vitamins. Very few required hospitalization or even pharmacotherapy. The average stay in treatment was two to eight days, and only 12 percent left prematurely. A follow-up of two-thirds of the patients at two years indicated that 40 percent had either maintained sobriety or improved. Studies done in other locations have replicated Whitfield's results. One of the largest and best documented of these was the Ontario Detoxication System described by Annis and coworkers (1976), in which only 3 percent of participants needed medical referral.

Withdrawal Scale

A number of scales to measure alcohol withdrawal have been used in many of the studies mentioned above. One of the most commonly mentioned is the Clinical Institute Withdrawal Assessment for Alcohol (CIWA-A). This instrument is a 15-item scale that measures a range of symptoms such as tremor; nausea and vomiting; sweating; tactile, auditory, and visual disturbances; hallucinations; anxiety; agitation; thought disturbances; seizures; headache; and flushing of the face (Shaw et al., 1981). The scale appears to be accurate and reliable (Sellers et al., 1983), and it could be applied on a larger scale to assess the outcome of a range of detoxification techniques that are used in clinical practice.

Recently, a modified version of the CIWA-A was employed in an attempt to measure the severity of alcohol dependence more objectively and to identify patients who needed pharmacotherapy (Foy, March, and Drinkwater, 1988). The patients studied had been admitted to a general hospital for treatment of other medical or surgical problems (e.g., pneumonia, fractures).

The research found, however, that although the CIWA-A was helpful in identifying most patients who needed pharmacotherapy, continuous clinical assessment was required to supplement the initial determination based on the CIWA-A.

Treatment Settings

There is evidence that effective detoxification using pharmacotherapy and other medical services can be delivered in an inpatient, outpatient, or psychosocial setting. A recent study randomly assigned 164 patients with mild to moderate degrees of physical dependence on alcohol to inpatient or outpatient detoxification programs, each of which used oxazepam (Hayashida et al., 1989). The patients selected for participation were required to have no history of recent (past 24 hours) seizures or delirium tremens and no serious medical or psychiatric problems that would require hospitalization. Of the 403 patients requesting "alcohol detox", 29 (7 percent) were excluded for these reasons.

Among those who agreed to participate and were assigned to inpatient treatment, 95 percent completed detoxification, compared with 72 percent of the outpatients, a difference that was statistically significant. Of the 24 outpatients who did not complete detoxification, 7 required referral to inpatient treatment: 6 of these were unable to stop drinking in the outpatient setting, and 1 required hospitalization for acute schizophrenia. In total, 59 percent of the outpatient group and 64 percent of the inpatient group enrolled in a rehabilitation program, a difference that was not significant. All patients improved, and six-month evaluations showed similar outcomes for both groups. The cost of outpatient treatment was about one-tenth that of inpatient treatment.

Other nonrandomized studies of outpatient detoxification have reported similar findings (Feldman et al., 1975; Tennant, 1979; Stinnett, 1982). A close liaison with an inpatient rehabilitation program is necessary if such treatment is to be used. Few studies of combined programs are available.

Special Patient Populations

There are a large number of special patient populations that present unique problems for detoxification and are not well represented in research studies (Cushman, 1988). The uncooperative, obstreperous alcoholic may not tolerate oral medication and often pulls out intravenous lines. Lorazepam, which is the only benzodiazepine that is absorbed well intramuscularly, may be preferable for such patients.

The patient with chronic obstructive pulmonary disease, anemia, or liver disease, or the elderly alcoholic who metabolizes drugs more slowly may need lower doses of benzodiazepines. These patients may be better treated with lorazepam or oxazepam (because these drugs are merely conjugated before excretion), as opposed to chlordiazepoxide or diazepam (which have more complex metabolic pathways).

There is little information available about the effect of other psychiatric problems on the severity of withdrawal symptoms or about interactions between other psychotropic drugs and benzodiazepines during withdrawal treatment. The severity of the alcohol withdrawal syndrome may be accentuated in patients with dual diagnoses if they are not given ancillary psychotropic medication. Many homeless alcoholics suffer from schizophrenia or other major mental disorders (Koegel and Burnam, 1988), and very little information is available about how best to respond to their multiple needs, including the initial step of detoxification (IOM, 1988).

Treatment of Seizures

The treatment of seizures in alcoholics requires the identification of patients with seizures resulting from causes other than alcohol dependence. This group needs long-term treatment with anticonvulsants. Recently, diphenylhydantoin was proposed for use in preventing seizures that result from alcohol withdrawal, but its value is currently uncertain (Liskow and Goodwin, 1987; Simon, 1988). There appears to be agreement that diphenylhydantoin, if used, should be given in combination with a benzodiazepine. Although clear evidence is not available, some clinicians recommend the use of diphenylhydantoin in cases with a history of withdrawal seizures.

Some recent work indicates that an intravenous loading dose of phenobarbital is safe and effective in preventing withdrawal seizures (Young et al., 1987; Simon, 1988). A recent study indicates that a kindling model may apply to alcohol withdrawal syndromes and seizures. Two groups of 25 male alcoholics--one with, and the other without, withdrawal seizures--were evaluated. It was found that the number of detoxifications was an important variable in the predisposition to withdrawal seizures and that this relationship was independent of the amount or duration of alcohol intake (Brown et al., 1988). The authors raise the troubling possibility that benzodiazepines, when used without anticonvulsants, may increase the chances for withdrawal seizures because they do not reduce limbic kindling.

Treatment of Delirium Tremens

Although the literature is clear that benzodiazepines reduce the severity of the alcohol withdrawal syndrome, a few patients develop delirium tremens even though they are treated with apparently adequate doses of benzodiazepines. There is probably considerable variability in blood levels, depending on a range of patient and dietary factors, as has been shown in studies of antidepressant blood levels in patients with major depressive disorders. Some of those who fail to respond to benzodiazepine treatment may be rapid metabolizers; alternatively, they may manifest impaired absorption of benzodiazepines. There may be optimum benzodiazepine blood levels that are associated with the marked suppression of withdrawal symptoms, but little information is currently available in this area. A recent report describes two representative cases from a total of ten who developed benzodiazepine-resistant delirium tremens and who responded to 4 to 6 mg of dexamethasone per day, given parenterally (Fischer et al., 1988).

Engagement in Follow-up Treatment

Although there is a suggestion that treatment completion and engagement in follow-up are better with the longer, medically oriented inpatient programs, these programs are also more expensive. Some indication of these effects is seen in the study by Hayashida and coworkers (1989) in which 95 percent of those completing inpatient detoxification engaged in follow-up treatment versus 72 percent of the outpatient group. In Ontario, Annis found that dropout rates were higher under a nonmedically based detoxification system than they had been under an earlier, medically based system (Annis and Smart, 1978; Annis, 1979). Smart and Gray (1978) studied more than 700 patients treated at five treatment programs in Ontario and also found that patients receiving medically oriented treatment were more likely to remain in the follow-up treatment.

If this difference in engagement rates is characteristic of medical versus nonmedical settings, it may be due to the additional psychiatric or medical treatments that are often applied in medical settings to that proportion of alcoholics who have additional psychiatric or medical problems.

Detoxification of Alcoholics Addicted to Other Substances

Many patients who apply for alcohol treatment are also addicted to cocaine, benzodiazepines, or opiates. Little information is available on the effect of additional drug use on the course of alcoholism. The doses of benzodiazepines required for detoxification may be altered by additional drug use. Inpatient treatment may often be necessary for these patients. Diazepam may be a very poor choice for detoxification with this subgroup because of its liability to abuse, especially among those who have used opiates or who have been socialized into "street" drug use (Woody, O'Brien, and Greenstein, 1975).

Alcoholic Hallucinosis and Paranoia

Few studies have been done on the treatment of alcoholic hallucinosis and paranoia, but haloperidol appears to be useful in patients with severe agitation, thought disorders, and hallucinations. Because haloperidol lowers the seizure threshold, it should be used in combination with a benzodiazepine, an anticonvulsant, or both.

The following are opportunities for research on the treatment of alcohol withdrawal:

- Research is needed to determine whether there are advantages to combining other drugs (e.g., anticonvulsants, beta blockers, calcium channel blockers, alpha-2 adrenergic agonists) with benzodiazepines in the treatment of alcohol withdrawal.
- Further studies are needed to develop better criteria to identify appropriate patients for nonpharmacological detoxification in nonmedical settings. Additional research is also needed to identify criteria for assigning patients appropriately to inpatient, outpatient, or psychosocial settings for supervised detoxification.
- Further research is needed to study the detoxification of specific patient populations such as the elderly or those with complicated medical or psychiatric disorders.
- Controlled studies should be performed on the pharmacological treatment of alcoholic hallucinosis. This research is best carried out as cooperative, multisite studies.
- There is a need for a multicenter study of the treatment of delirium tremens to examine the relationship between benzodiazepine blood levels and treatment response. The recently reported study using dexamethasone in the treatment of benzodiazepine-resistant delirium tremens needs to be examined in other settings.
- There is a need to examine the relationship of detoxification setting, the use of pharmacotherapy, and the ability to engage patients in follow-up treatment and aftercare. In these studies, patients should be characterized in terms of presence or absence of psychopathology and comorbid medical disorders, as well as severity of alcohol dependence and withdrawal.
- Studies of the treatment of alcohol withdrawal that is complicated by other drug abuse or dependence are indicated across drug classes. This type of effort may require a multisite study.

Treatment of Postwithdrawal Symptoms

Alcohol withdrawal is associated with a generalized hyperexcitability of the central nervous system (Hemmingsen et al., 1988), which persists for days, weeks, or longer following detoxification (Begleiter and Porjesz, 1979). Clinical symptoms are usually associated with anxiety, restlessness, emotional lability, and insomnia. The duration of postwithdrawal symptoms and their relationship to patient age, amount and duration of alcohol intake, and presence of associated psychiatric or medical problems are not known. It is possible that the type, duration, and amount of pharmacotherapy or psychotherapy/social support used during detoxification can influence the duration and severity of postwithdrawal symptoms. This question needs to be examined.

The following are opportunities for research on postwithdrawal symptoms:

• Studies should be initiated on the following topics: (a) the natural course of postwithdrawal symptoms in appropriately defined subgroups of alcoholics; (b) the efficacy of pharmacological and psychosocial treatments for postwithdrawal symptoms (e.g., see Meyer, 1986); and (c) the relationship between postwithdrawal symptoms and treatment outcome.

Insomnia in Alcoholics

Effects of Alcohol on Sleep

Insomnia is a common problem in alcoholics during periods of drinking and abstinence. Among both social drinkers and alcoholics, a moderate dose of alcohol initially produces sedation characterized by rapid sleep onset, decreased rapid eye movement (REM) sleep, and enhanced delta or slow-wave sleep. Later in the night, as the blood alcohol concentration declines, the sedative effects diminish, and signs of alcohol withdrawal occur. These signs of withdrawal are usually more pronounced in alcoholics than in social drinkers. They are noted on the electroencephalogram by decreased slow-wave sleep, frequent arousals, more rapid shifts of sleep stage, and increased frequency of REM sleep and REM disruptions.

With continued heavy drinking, such as occurs in alcoholics, the sedative effects diminish, and increased amounts of alcohol are required to attain the original levels of sedation. Similarly, withdrawal signs become more pronounced (Yules, Freidman, and Chandler, 1966; Knowles, Laverty, and Kuechler, 1968; Gross et al., 1972, 1973; Rundell et al., 1972; Gross and Hastey, 1976). Gross and Hastey (1976) interpreted these effects as indicating increased tolerance and physical dependence. Thus, alcoholics when drinking have disrupted sleep, especially during the second half of the night.

Sleep During Acute Alcohol Withdrawal

Almost all investigators have found marked increases in REM sleep time associated with alcohol withdrawal. These increases are characterized by more rapid REM sleep onset and reduced inter-REM intervals. Williams and Rundell (1981) found that the most striking characteristic of this sleep was its fragmentation. Sleep onset is usually not delayed, but it is constantly disrupted by restless bodily movement and brief arousals. These interruptions are especially prominent during REM sleep.

The increases in REM time and restless sleep associated with acute alcohol withdrawal diminish rapidly, and by the sixth or eighth day after detoxification is completed, the total amount of REM time has returned to normal (Allen et al., 1971). However, the overall pattern of sleep remains abnormal and is characterized by increases in stage 1 and decreases in stage 4 sleep. The fragmented sleep noted above continues, although to a lesser degree, and sleep is characterized by delays in onset, more rapid changes between stages, and a decrease in the total amount of sleep time.

Improvement with Abstinence

Several researchers have followed abstinent alcoholics over extended periods of time to see if and when these abnormalities disappear. Most have found evidence of gradual improvement over a period of years; some have found persistent disturbances (Adamson and Burdick, 1973; Wagman and Allen, 1975; Williams and Rundell, 1981; Imatoh et al., 1986). There may be an alteration in the circadian rhythm of REM sleep in abstinent alcoholics. Most studies have found prolonged sleep disturbances, with the most severe disruptions diminishing within days to weeks after detoxification. There are no clear data on what percentage of alcoholics eventually develops normal sleep (and how long it takes) or on the causes of sleep disturbances. One might predict that alcoholics with sleep disturbances would be more likely to drop out of treatment and return to drinking earlier than those who do not have them; however, whether this trend in fact occurs is unclear because few data are available in this area. Moreover, although the kinds of sleep problems that generally occur are highly suggestive of toxic effects secondary to excessive and prolonged alcohol consumption, the studies do not exclude the possibility that some of the observed sleep problems predate the alcoholism and are contributors to its onset and maintenance.

Influence of Detoxification Procedures on Sleep Disorders

There is little information available about the influence of detoxification procedures on sleep disturbances. The most severe disorders are limited to the few days after detoxification, and many advise a conservative approach with only general supportive and educational measures. One study compared detoxification using low doses of alcohol versus chlordiazepoxide (CDP) and found that the CDP group experienced marked suppression of REM sleep along with virtual elimination of stage 3 and stage 4 sleep, whereas patients in the low-dose alcohol group had significantly less disruption of sleep (Funderburk, Allen, and Wagman, 1978). All 18 subjects studied completed treatment, indicating no obvious problems while using alcohol for detoxification in a hospital setting. Long-term follow-up was not available; thus, it is uncertain if any delayed adverse effects occurred in the alcohol-treated group.

This study is especially interesting because there is so little available information about the effects of detoxification procedures on such postwithdrawal symptoms as insomnia. It would be useful to examine the effect of several pharmacotherapies on sleep and also to see if there are differences in the type, severity, or prevalence of sleep disturbances in those who are detoxified with supportive care only versus those given pharmacotherapy. Similarly, studies could evaluate the efficacy of behavioral treatments, that have been shown to reduce insomnia in a substantial proportion of nonalcoholics (IOM, 1979).

The following are opportunities for research on sleep disorders:

• Studies could be conducted to determine if sleep disturbance predisposes individuals to alcoholism. This type of research might be possible by following the careers of people who have been treated for primary sleep disorders.

• Another promising route of investigation might be to determine how long sleep disturbances last in groups that differ on such important variables as age, psychopathology, years of drinking, medical status, and level of physiologic dependence.

• The influence of sleep disturbances on outcome after rehabilitation could be studied.

• Studies could be performed using pharmacotherapies and behavior therapies for postdetoxification insomnia.

NERVOUS SYSTEM EFFECTS

Cognitive Impairment in Alcoholism

Types of Impairments

The two most prominent cognitive impairments in alcoholism are alcoholic amnestic disorder (Wernicke-Korsakoff syndrome) and alcoholic dementia. Wernicke-Korsakoff's syndrome is associated with prolonged and heavy use of alcohol and often follows an acute episode of Wernicke's encephalopathy. It is characterized by clear consciousness and severe anterograde and retrograde amnesia. Memory problems are so pronounced that disorientation may occur. Confabulation, which tends to disappear over time, is often seen. Although its exact etiology is unclear, alcoholic amnestic disorder is felt to be largely preventable by proper diet and administration of vitamins, including thiamine. It is seen infrequently in current medical practice, but it generally is incurable once it has developed: 80 percent of all Korsakoff patients show no improvement and have a lifelong disability. Recently, Martin and coworkers (1989) reported some improvement in cognitive function in Korsakoff patients treated with fluvoxamine.

Alcoholic dementia has a gradual onset and thus presents with varying degrees of impairment. It is characterized by difficulties in short- and long-term memory, abstract thinking, and judgment and by other disturbances of higher cortical function (e.g., apraxia, constructional difficulties--the inability to assemble blocks or arrange sticks in specific designs), and reductions in problem-solving ability. It is associated with poor performance on tests of psychomotor speed and with impaired control of impulses. Verbal I.Q. is less affected and usually remains within the normal range (Grant, 1987; see also Graff-Redford et al., 1982). Although alcoholic dementia is a common problem, as many as 25 percent of alcoholics have no measurable cognitive deficits (Goldstein and Shelly, 1980). Alcohol-related central nervous system pathology is discussed at greater length in Causes and Consequences of Alcohol Problems (IOM, 1987).

From the perspective of opportunities for treatment research, it is important to note that many cognitive deficits improve with abstinence, although often not completely (McCrady and Smith, 1986). Most of the improvement occurs within the first two to three weeks, but there also appears to be a more gradual and continuing recovery with prolonged abstinence (Brandt et al., 1983). Short-term memory and psychomotor skills are usually the first to recover; visual-spatial learning, long-term memory, and abstraction are most resistant to improvement. For example, Brandt and colleagues (1983) studied cognitive loss and its recovery in long-term alcohol abusers. They found that both young and old alcoholics displayed impairments on tasks that required the learning of new associations and their long-term retention. These deficits were apparent in alcoholics who had been abstinent for as long as seven years.

Another important finding is that there may be an interaction between age and the recovery of cognitive function. One study found that alcoholics under 40 years of age recovered from most of their cognitive deficits within three weeks; however, those over 40 had not substantially recovered even after three months (Goldman, Williams, and Klisz, 1983).

Relationship Between Cognitive Impairment and Treatment Outcome

The literature provides some indication that alcoholics with impaired neuropsychological function have poorer outcomes. Abbott and Gregson (1981) found a significant relationship between impaired cognitive function and poor treatment outcome at three months and at one year after treatment. Leber, Parsons, and Nichols (1985) asked experienced clinicians to rate alcoholic patients according to how they were progressing in therapy; they then compared the ratings with the results of neuropsychological testing. The patients who were rated as making the least progress were also those with the most impairment.

Other studies have found weaker or absent relationships. Goldstein and Shelly (1971) found no relationship between cognitive function and ratings of adjustment one year after discharge; McLachlan and Levinson (1974) found no relationship between cognitive functioning and drinking/abstinence at one year. Walker and coworkers (1983) found a very modest relationship between cognitive impairment and outcome, but the strongest correlate of outcome was involvement in aftercare. Recent studies by Donovan, Walker, and Kivlahan (1987) have shown that the relationship between cognitive functioning and treatment outcome in alcoholics is complex. In general, Donovan's studies showed that cognitive functioning did not significantly predict alcohol consumption but did predict employment status. Similar findings showing a weak or absent relationship between cognitive functioning and outcome have been reported by Eckhardt et al. (1988).

In summary, although there is evidence that impaired cognition has a negative influence on outcome, this relationship is probably of varying strength, perhaps depending on such factors as the severity of impairment, the area assessed, and demographic or educational levels of the population studied. There are few available studies that attempt to relate cognitive status to a wide range of outcome measures. It would not be surprising to find that cognitively impaired patients do poorly in complex vocational or social situations, as noted by Donovan and colleagues (1987), whereas such patients perform similarly to those who are not impaired in less complex vocational situations. This entire area is one in which considerably more treatment research could be done.

Treatment Programs and Cognitively Impaired Patients

The overall structure of the treatment program may have an important interaction with cognitive function. Some work indicates that cognitively impaired alcoholics do best in a highly structured program, whereas nonimpaired patients do better in a less structured

environment (McLachlan and Levinson, 1974). Although these findings are intuitively sensible, few studies have examined this area of patient-treatment matching in detail.
Most residential rehabilitation programs last 28 days and include a significant amount of educational material, the dissemination of which begins early in treatment. This type of program may be inappropriate for some patients. Becker and Jaffe (1984) showed that alcoholics could not remember the information from a 55-minute film about alcoholism when it was shown during the first week of treatment. They suggested presenting information in small, easily assimilated chunks and in several different contexts within the treatment environment. They also believed that their results raised serious questions about the trend toward shortening the period of residential care. Similarly, Goldman and Rosenbaum (1977) argued strongly that new information should not be presented to alcoholics during the first several weeks following detoxification because of their impaired ability to remember and use the information.

Very little information is available about how programs manage cognitively impaired alcoholics. For example, it is not known whether there are systematic differences between the ways cognitively impaired patients are managed in medically/psychiatrically oriented programs as opposed to freestanding programs. There is little information about the kinds of interventions or strategies most commonly used, and there is no information available about specific follow-up programs for cognitively impaired patients. Moreover, little is known about the use of formal cognitive assessment procedures by alcohol treatment programs. This area offers numerous treatment research opportunities.

The following are opportunities for research on treatment and cognitive impairment:

• Further studies are needed on the relationship between cognitive status and treatment outcome. Do cognitively impaired alcoholics acquire new information and skills that help in their rehabilitation? Are they more likely to attend and benefit from Alcoholics Anonymous, a program in which simple, direct messages are constantly repeated?
• Studies are needed on how alcohol treatment programs deal with cognitively impaired patients. Are there treatment programs or techniques that do better (or worse) with cognitively impaired patients? Do programs that screen for cognitive impairment and then modify treatment accordingly do better with these patients than programs that do not? Does program structure make a difference?

Cognitive Retraining

If there are negative outcomes associated with impaired cognitive performance, treatment may be improved by techniques that can hasten or extend the normal recovery process. There is a considerable literature on cognitive rehabilitation techniques for head injury (Rimmelle and Hester, 1987). A detailed review of these studies is beyond the scope of this section, but there is good evidence that a variety of specific techniques can be used to improve cognitive deficits.

A few researchers have applied these techniques to cognitively impaired alcoholics with encouraging results. Godfrey, Spittle, and Knight (1985) found evidence that a memory training program increased the chances for a regular discharge in cognitively impaired chronic alcoholics. However, Yohman, Schaeffer, and Parsons (1988) found no significant changes in response to memory training except in younger subjects. In other studies, Parsons (1987) found improvement in memory and problem solving in alcoholics who were given specific techniques designed for these problems.

Goldman (1987) has summarized much of the literature in this area and has performed a series of studies which indicate that cognitive retraining techniques can result in gains greater than those to be expected from the normal recovery processes that accompany abstinence. He suggests that certain cognitive functions may not recover unless specific techniques are applied and that the recovery may be related to structural changes (e.g., dendritic arborization) that are stimulated by retraining techniques.

The following questions represent opportunities for research on cognitive retraining:

• How effective are cognitive retraining techniques for cognitively impaired alcoholics? If these techniques are effective, how do they influence outcome?

Nootropic Drugs

Although not available at present, a new class of drugs to improve cognitive function (termed "nootropic" drugs) is now under development. Much of this work is being done to find pharmacotherapies for Alzheimer's disease. Drugs that act on the serotonin system may be important for alcohol clinical research, as indicated by studies showing that zimelidine can improve cognitive performance and that tryptophan can reverse certain kinds of alcohol-induced memory impairment (Westrick et al., 1988; see also Linnoila et al., 1987). Nootropic drugs could be used alone or in combination with retraining techniques, as has been done in studies with psychotherapy and pharmacotherapy. No promising candidates for clinical trials stand out at this time, but some drugs may emerge from the research on Alzheimer's disease.

The following opportunities exist for research on nootropic drugs:

• As new drugs to enhance cognitive function become available, they should be studied in context with alcohol-induced cognitive impairments (including Korsakoff's disease).

CARDIOVASCULAR EFFECTS

Chronic alcohol consumption adversely affects the cardiovascular system in three ways: (1) alcohol abuse is associated with hypertension and stroke; (2) alcohol ingestion can cause arrhythmias; and (3) chronic alcohol abuse can result in cardiomyopathy. However, it should also be recalled that epidemiological evidence suggests that people who have two drinks per day may have less coronary artery disease than nondrinkers (Rohan, 1984).

Hypertension

In a large number of cross-sectional population studies, an independent association between alcohol consumption and blood pressure has been reported (MacMahon and Norton, 1986). A Kaiser-Permanente study of 84,000 persons (Klatsky et al., 1977) reported that the consumption of three or more drinks per day was associated with higher blood pressure:

blood pressure increased with increasing alcohol intake. At the level of six drinks per day, there was a twofold increase in the number of whites with hypertension and a 50 percent increase in hypertension in blacks. A small number of prospective, randomized controlled studies have evaluated the blood pressure effects of eliminating alcohol consumption (MacMahon and Norton, 1986). Potter and Beevers (1984) studied 16 hypertensive men who drank up to 80 grams of alcohol daily. When alcohol consumption ceased, diastolic and systolic blood pressures decreased significantly. The reintroduction of alcohol resulted in significant increases in systolic and diastolic pressures.

Alcohol-induced hypertension is probably partly responsible for the increase in stroke in heavy drinkers (Kozararevic et al., 1980; Donahue et al., 1986; Gill et al., 1986). Gill and colleagues (1986) found that the relative risk of stroke, when adjusted for hypertension, cigarette smoking, and medication, was four times higher in heavy drinkers than in nondrinkers.

Major advances have occurred in the past several years in the treatment of hypertension. Angiotensin converting enzyme (ACE) antagonists have been added to the therapeutic armamentarium of diuretics and beta blockers. The ACE inhibitors have an advantage over diuretics and beta blockers in that they usually have fewer side effects. The calcium channel blockers are not currently approved for treating hypertension, but they are effective for this purpose and will be approved shortly. Like the ACE inhibitors, they have relatively few side effects.

The following are opportunities for research on hypertension:

• Studies should be pursued to determine the best treatments (and combinations of treatments) for hypertension associated with heavy drinking and alcohol dependence.

Arrhythmias

Alcohol is an arrhythmogenic agent. Acute alcohol ingestion can cause ventricular fibrillation (Singer and Lundberg, 1972) and a syndrome called the "holiday heart" syndrome, which is characterized by transient tachyarrhythmias occurring in individuals otherwise free of overt heart disease after periods of excessive alcohol ingestion. Electrophysiological studies have shown that the administration of alcohol can prolong conduction times (Engel and Luck, 1983) and sinus recovery time (Greenspon and Schaal, 1983). Similar cardiac effects can occur during alcohol withdrawal (Van Thiel and Gavaler, 1985). The ingestion of only 3 ounces of 80-proof whiskey caused atrial and ventricular tachyarrhythmias in 14 patients with a history of chronic alcohol consumption and palpitations or light-headedness (Greenspon and Schaal, 1983). It is likely that alcohol-induced arrhythmias are due to the direct toxic effects of alcohol on the myocardium and on the conduction system (Van Thiel and Gavaler, 1985).

Advances have been made in the development of new antiarrhythmic agents (e.g., calcium channel blockers for atrial flutter, and encainide or flecainide for ventricular ectopy). Encainide is 5 to 10 times more potent than previous antiarrhythmic agents, and effective doses have no untoward effects on blood pressure, heart rate, or intracardiac conduction (Woosley, Wood, and Roden, 1988). Although antiarrhythmic drugs can suppress ventricular ectopy, any evidence that these agents improve survival in many of these types of patients is lacking (Woosley, 1988). Those who are symptomatic probably do benefit, but suppressive therapy is of unknown benefit in asymptomatic patients. The important factor in preventing alcohol-related arrhythmias, however, is abstinence. Because with many patients abstinence cannot be ensured, there is a need to identify medication that would mitigate alcohol-related arrythmias.

The following are opportunities for research on cardiovascular disorders:

• Electrophysiological monitoring studies could be used to precipitate arrhythmias with the administration of alcohol in a sample of individuals who are known to experience alcohol-induced arrhythmias. Studies could then be conducted to determine which antiarrhythmic drugs abolish the arrhythmia.

LIVER EFFECTS

Alcohol abuse results in three histologic types of liver disease: (1) fatty liver, (2) alcoholic hepatitis, and (3) cirrhosis. As described in the companion volume to this report (IOM, 1987), alcoholic liver disease is the most common cause of chronic illness and death from alcoholism. Approximately 8 to 15 percent of chronic abusers of alcohol develop liver cirrhosis, and most people who die from alcoholic liver disease have cirrhosis.

The pathogenic mechanisms responsible for alcoholic hepatitis, fibrosis, and cirrhosis are presently unknown. Alcoholic hepatitis is a precursor (but not a prerequisite) in the development of cirrhosis. The current, generally accepted treatment for alcoholic hepatitis is supportive care, but research to identify effective treatment agents is in progress. One promising direction comes from evidence that alcohol consumption may induce pathological changes in the centrilobular area of the liver as a consequence of hypoxia (Israel et al., 1975). As a result of increased hepatic oxygen consumption in other areas of the liver, Israel and coworkers (1975) found that propylthiouracil (PTU) rendered the centrilobular area more resistant to hypoxia and cell necrosis. Based on these findings, Orrego and colleagues (1987) evaluated PTU in patients with alcoholic liver disease. This study is important, not only because of reported benefits from PTU but also because the authors employed a rigorous research design that enabled them to separate the effect of the drug from the effect of abstinence or reduced alcohol consumption. The rigor of this research design should serve as a model for other studies in which experimental treatments are applied to alcohol-related pathology. For this reason, several important aspects of this study are described below.

Patients were well characterized in terms of the presence of hepatitis, with or without cirrhosis. All patients were seen in a liver clinic in which compliance with drug treatment was measured by using a urinary drug marker (riboflavin). Among the 310 compliant patients (positive for riboflavin), the cumulative mortality in the PTU group was significantly lower (13 percent) than in the placebo group (25 percent). This reduction represented a 48 percent decrease in mortality in patients with moderate to severe liver disease. There was no significant difference in those with mild disease. Although patients were followed for up to two years, favorable survival was only seen early in this period. After 12 weeks, approximately the same number of deaths occurred in the drug and placebo groups. There was no significant difference in cumulative mortality between noncompliant patients in the drug and placebo groups.

Of special importance is the finding of Orrego et al. (1987) that continued heavy drinking negated the beneficial effects of PTU. Drinking was monitored by testing daily urine specimens for alcohol. The ability of these investigators to obtain daily urine samples sets a new standard for treatment in trials of alcohol-related disorders. These findings demonstrate the importance of assessing both compliance with drug treatment and alcohol consumption in evaluations of drug treatments for alcohol-related pathology. It is also of interest that PTU was effective only in patients with a moderate degree of illness. An earlier study by this group (Orrego et al., 1979) found accelerated recovery with PTU treatment in hospitalized patients but no significant improvement in survival. Halle and colleagues (1982) failed to find any benefit from PTU in hospitalized patients. Thus, PTU is most effective in patients with mild disease or in those who are not ill enough to be hospitalized.

There is no effective treatment for cirrhosis of the liver apart from abstinence from alcohol. Almost all studies examining the effects of abstinence on survival have found abstinence to be associated with longer life. What is of great significance is that these studies also report a greater likelihood of long-term abstinence or reduced alcohol consumption in patients with cirrhosis compared with those alcoholic individuals of similar socioeconomic background who do not have this life-threatening illness. This pattern suggests that the development of a major complication of alcoholism may have a profound effect on drinking behavior.

Liver Transplantation

Liver transplantation has become an accepted treatment for end-stage liver disease, and the number of centers that perform hepatic transplantation is increasing. The timing of surgery is critical because transplantation should be reserved for those who are otherwise likely to live less than a year. Liver transplantation has not been done often in patients with alcoholic cirrhosis for two primary reasons. One concern was that patients with alcoholic cirrhosis had higher operative and postoperative mortality than patients with other forms of cirrhosis. The other reason was a fear that those with alcoholic cirrhosis would resume drinking and destroy the transplanted liver. These concerns may be unjustified. Starzl and coworkers (1988) have presented data that indicate that operative mortality is the same regardless of the type of cirrhosis and that this group has a very high abstinence rate.

The following are opportunities for research on liver transplantation for alcoholic cirrhosis:

• What percentage of cirrhotic alcoholics who have received transplants return to drinking?
• What characteristics predict posttransplantation sobriety?

Complications of Cirrhosis

The four most serious complications from hepatic cirrhosis in terms of mortality and morbidity are (1) hemorrhage from esophageal varices, (2) hepatic encephalopathy, (3) ascites, and (4) hepatorenal syndrome. At this writing, there are no specific treatment research opportunities that might be considered for a multicenter trial. Clearly, future treatment trials in these disorders should be designed by following the rigorous standards established by Orrego and coworkers (1987).

OTHER HEALTH CONSEQUENCES OF ALCOHOL ABUSE

As described in the companion volume to this report (IOM, 1987), excessive alcohol ingestion adversely affects a number of other organs and organ systems including (1) the pancreas, (2) the heart, (3) the hematopoietic system, (4) muscle, (5) peripheral nerves, (6) bone, (7) stomach and esophagus, and (8) endocrine organs. It can also lead to impaired nutrition and is a major risk factor in injury-related deaths (see Chapter 2 on the epidemiology of alcohol-related problems). Heavy drinking is associated with acute and chronic pancreatitis; cardiomyopathy; abnormal gonadal function; impaired immunity; cancer of the mouth, pharynx, and esophagus; and other disorders. Advances in our understanding of the mechanisms for the deleterious effects of alcohol on these organs are well summarized in Causes and Consequences of Alcohol Problems (IOM, 1987). Unfortunately, advances in treatment in these areas have not kept pace with knowledge about the role of alcohol as a critical risk factor. Abstinence remains the single most important goal in the prevention of these disorders. This emphasis underscores the importance of improving both the prevention and the treatment of alcohol dependence and problem drinking behavior.

REFERENCES

Abbott, M. W., and R. A. M. Gregson. Cognitive dysfunction in the prediction of relapse in alcoholics. J. Stud. Alcohol 42(1):230-243, 1981.

Adamson, J., and J. A. Burdick. Sleep of dry alcoholics. Arch. Gen. Psychiatry 28:146-149, 1973.

Allen, R. P., A. Wagman, L. A. Faillace et al. Electroencephalographic (EEG) sleep recovery following prolonged alcohol intoxication in alcoholics. J. Nerv. Ment. Dis. 153:424-431, 1971.

Annis, H. M. The detoxification alternative to the handling of public inebriates: The Ontario experience. J. Stud. Alcohol 40(3):196-210, 1979.

Annis, H. M., and R. G. Smart. Arrests, readmissions and treatment following release from detoxification centers. J. Stud. Alcohol 39(7):1276-1283, 1978.

Annis, H. M., N. Giesbrecht, A. Ogborne et al. Task Force II Report on the Operation and Effectiveness of the Ontario Detoxication System. Toronto: Addiction Research Foundation of Ontario, 1976.

Becker, J. T., and J. H. Jaffe. Impaired memory for treatment-relevant information in inpatient men alcoholics. J. Stud. Alcohol 45:339-343, 1984.

Begleiter, H., and B. Porjesz. Persistence of a "subacute withdrawal syndrome" following chronic ethanol intake. Drug Alcohol Depend. 4:353-357, 1979.

Brandt, J., N. Butters, C. Ryan et al. Cognitive loss and recovery in long-term alcohol abusers. Arch. Gen. Psych. 40:435-442, 1983.

Brown, M. E., R. F. Anton, R. Malcolm, and M. Ballenger. Alcohol detoxification and withdrawal seizures: Clinical support for a kindling hypothesis. Biol. Psychiatry 23(5):507-514, 1988.

Cushman, P. Alcohol withdrawal: A look at recent research. Report to the NIAAA Advisory Council. Washington, DC: NIAAA, May 1988.

Donahue, R. P., R. D. Abbott, D. M. Reed et al. Alcohol and hemorrhagic stroke: The Honolulu Heart Program. J. Am. Med. Assoc. 255:2311-2314, 1986.

Donovan, D. M., R. D. Walker, and D. R. Kivlahan. Recovery and remediation of neuropsychological functions: Implications for alcoholism rehabilitation process and outcome. Pp. 337-360 in O. A. Parsons, V. Butters, and P. Nathan, eds. Neuropsychology of Alcoholism: Implications for Diagnosis and Treatment. New York: Guilford Press, 1987.

Eckhardt, M. J., R. R. Rawlings, B. I. Graubard et al. Neuropsychological performance and treatment outcome in male alcoholics. Alcoholism Clin. Exp. Res. 12(1):88-93, 1988.

Engel, T. R., and J. C. Luck. Effect of whiskey on atrial vulnerability and "holiday" heart. J. Am. Coll. Cardiol. 1:816-818, 1983.

Feldman, D. J., E. M. Pattison, L. C. Sobell et al. Outpatient alcohol detoxification: Initial findings on 564 patients. Am. J. Psychiatry 132:407-412, 1975.

Fischer, D. K., R. K. Simpson, F. A. Smith et al. Efficacy of dexamethasone in benzodiazepine-resistant delirium tremens. Lancet 1(8598): 1340-1341, 1988.

Foy, A., S. March, and V. Drinkwater. Use of an objective clinical scale in the assessment and management of alcohol withdrawal in a large general hospital. Alcoholism Clin. Exp. Res. 12(3):360-364, 1988.

Funderburk, M. A., R. P. Allen, and A. M. I. Wagman. Residual effects of ethanol and chlordiazepoxide treatments for alcohol withdrawal. J. Nerv. Ment. Dis. 166(3):195-203, 1978.

Gill, J., A. V. Zezulka, M. J. Shipley et al. Stroke and alcohol consumption. N. Engl. J. Med. 315:1041-1046, 1986.

Godfrey, H. P., B. J. Spittle, and R. G. Knight. Cognitive rehabilitation of amnesic alcoholics: A twelve month follow-up study. N.Z. Med. J. 784(98):650-651, 1985.

Goldman, M. S. The role of time and practice in recovery of function in alcoholics. Pp. 291-321 in O. A. Parsons, N. Butters, and P. E. Nathan, eds. Neuropsychology of Alcoholism: Implications for Diagnosis and Treatment. New York: Guilford Press, 1987.

Goldman, M. S. and G. Rosenbaum. Psychological recoverability following chronic alcohol abuse. In J. F. Seixas, ed. Currents in Alcoholism, vol. 2. New York: Grune and Stratton, 1977.

Goldman, M. S., D. L. Williams, and D. K. Klisz. Recoverability of psychological functioning following alcohol abuse: Prolonged visual-spatial dysfunction in older alcoholics. J. Consult. Clin. Psychol. 51:370-378, 1983.

Goldstein, G., and C. H. Shelly. Field dependence and cognitive, perceptual and motor skills in alcoholics: A factor analytic study. Q. J. Stud. Alcohol 32:29-40, 1971.

Goldstein, G., and C. H. Shelly. Neuropsychological investigation of brain lesion localization in alcoholism. Adv. Exp. Med. Biol. 126:731-743, 1980.

Graff-Radford, N. R., R. K. Heaton, M. P. Earnest et al. Brain atrophy and neuropsychological impairment in young alcoholics. J. Stud. Alcohol 43(9):859-868, 1982.

Grant, I. Alcohol and the brain: Neuropsychological correlates. J. Consult. Clin. Psychol. 55(3):310-324, 1987.

Greenspon, A. J., and S. F. Schaal. The "holiday heart": Electrophysiological studies of alcohol effects in alcoholics. Ann. Intern. Med. 98:135-139, 1983.

Gross, M. M., and J. M. Hastey. Sleep disturbances in alcoholism. In R. G. Tarter and A. A. Sugerman, eds. Alcoholism: Interdisciplinary Approaches to an Enduring Problem. Reading, MA: Addison-Wesley, 1976.

Gross, M. M., D. R. Goodenough, J. M. Hastey et al. Sleep disturbances in alcoholic intoxication and withdrawal. In N. K. Mello, ed. Recent Advances in Studies of Alcoholism. Washington, DC: Government Printing Office, 1972.

Gross, M. M., D. R. Goodenough, M. Nagaragan et al. Sleep changes induced by experimental alcoholization. Pp. 291-304 in M. M. Gross, ed. Alcohol Intoxication and Withdrawal: Experimental Studies. New York: Plenum Press, 1973.

Halle, P., P. Pare, E. Kaptein et al. Double-blind controlled trial of propylthiouracil in patients with severe alcoholic hepatitis. Gastroenterology 82:925-931, 1982.

Hayashida, M., A. I. Alterman, A. T. McLellan et al. Comparative effectiveness and costs of inpatient and outpatient detoxification of patients with mild-to-moderate alcohol withdrawal syndrome. N. Engl. J. Med. 320(6):358-365, 1989.

Hemmingsen, R., S. Vorstrup, L. Clemesen, S. Holm et al. Cerebral blood flow during delerium tremens and related clinical states studied with xenon-133 inhalation tomography. Am. J. Psychiatry 145:1384-1390, 1988.

Imatoh, N., Y. Nakazawa, H. Ohshima et al. Circadian rhythm of REM sleep of chronic alcoholics during alcohol withdrawal. Drug Alcohol Depend. 18:77-85, 1986.

Institute of Medicine. Sleeping Pills, Insomnia and Medical Practice. Washington, DC: National Academy Press, 1979.

Institute of Medicine. Causes and Consequences of Alcohol Problems: An Agenda for Research. Washington, DC: National Academy Press, 1987.

Institute of Medicine. Homelessness, Health and Human Needs. Washington, DC: National Academy Press, 1988.

Israel, Y., H. Kalant, H. Orrego et al. Experimental alcohol-induced hepatic necrosis: Suppression by propylthiouracil. Proc. Natl. Acad. Sci. U.S.A. 72:1137-1141, 1975.

Kaim, S. C., C. J. Klett, and B. Rothfeld. Treatment of acute alcohol withdrawal state: A comparison of four drugs. Am. J. Psychiatry 125:1640-1646, 1969.

Klatsky, A. L., G. D. Friedman, A. B. Siegelaub et al. Alcohol consumption and blood pressure. Kaiser-Permanente multiphasic health examination data. N. Engl. J. Med. 296:1194-1200, 1977.

Knowles, J. B., S. G. Laverty, and H. A. Kuechler. Effects of alcohol on REM sleep. Q. J. Stud. Alcohol 29:342-349, 1968.

Koegel, P., and A. Burnam. Alcoholism among homeless adults in the inner city of Los Angeles. Arch. Gen. Psych. 45:1011-1018, 1988.

Koppi, S., G. Eberhardt, R. Haller et al. Calcium-channel blocking agent in the treatment of acute alcohol withdrawal: Caroverine versus meprobamate in a randomized double-blind study. Neuropsychobiology 17:49-52, 1987.

Kozararevic, D., D. McGee, N. Vojvodic et al. Frequency of alcohol consumption and morbidity and mortality: The Yugoslavia Cardiovascular Disease Study. Lancet 1:613-616, 1980.

Leber, W. R., O. A. Parsons, and N. Nichols. Neuropsychological test results are related to ratings of men alcoholics' therapeutic progress: A replicated study. J. Stud. Alcohol 46(2):116-121, 1985.

Linnoila, M., M. Eckardt, M. Durcan et al. Interactions of serotonin with ethanol: Clinical and animal studies. Psychopharm. Bull. 23:452-457, 1987.

Liskow, B. I., and D. W. Goodwin. Pharmacological treatment of alcohol intoxication, withdrawal and dependence: A critical review. J. Stud. Alcohol 48(4):356-370, 1987.

Liskow, B., and J. Reed. Atenolol for alcohol withdrawal. N. Engl. J. Med. 314:783, 1986.

Little, H. J., S. J. Dolin, and M. J. Halsey. Calcium channel antagonists decrease the ethanol withdrawal syndrome. Life Sci. 39:2059-2065, 1986.

MacMahon, S. W., and R. N. Norton. Alcohol and hypertension: Implications for prevention and treatment (editorial). Annals of Internal Medicine 105(1):124-126, 1986.

McCrady, B. S., and D. E. Smith. Implications of cognitive impairment for the treatment of alcoholism. Alcoholism Clin. Exp. Res. 10(2):145-149, 1986.

McLachlan, J. F. C., and T. Levinson. Improvement in WAIS block design performance as a function of recovery from alcoholism. J. Clin. Psychol. 30:65-66, 1974.

Martin, P. R., Adinoff, B., Eckardt, M. J. et al. Effective pharmacotherapy of alcohol amnestic disorder with fluvoxamine: preliminary findings. Arch. Gen. Psychiat., 46:617-621, 1989.

Meyer, R. E. Anxiolytics and the alcoholic patient. J. Stud. Alcohol 47(4):269-273, 1986.

Moskowitz, G., T. C. Chalmers, H. S. Sacks et al. Deficiencies of clinical trials of alcohol withdrawal. Alcoholism Clin. Exp. Res. 7:42-46, 1983.

Orrego, H., K. Kalant, Y. Israel et al. Effect of short-term therapy with propylthiouracil in patients with alcoholic liver disease. Gastroenterology 76:105-115, 1979.

Orrego, H., J. E. Blake, L. M. Blendis et al. Long-term treatment of alcoholic liver disease with propylthiouracil. N. Engl. J. Med. 317:1421-1426, 1987.

Parsons, O. A. Do neuropsychological deficits predict alcoholics' treatment course and posttreatment recovery? Pp. 273-290 in O. A. Parsons, N. Butters, and P. E. Nathan, eds. Neuropsychology of Alcoholism: Implications for Diagnosis and Treatment. New York: Guilford Press, 1987.

Potter, J. F., and D. G. Beevers. Pressor effect of alcohol in hypertension. Lancet 1:119-122, 1984.

Rimmelle, C. T., and R. K. Hester. Cognitive rehabilitation after traumatic head injury. Arch. Clin. Neuropsychol. 2:353-354, 1987.

Rohan, T. E. Alcohol and ischematic heart disease: A review. Australian and New Zealand J. Med. 14:75-80, 1984.

Rundell, O. H., B. K. Lester, W. J. Griffiths et al. Alcohol and sleep in young adults. Psychopharmacologia 26:201-218, 1972.

Schuckit, M. A. Guidelines for treatment of alcoholic withdrawal. Fair Oaks Hospital Psychiatry Letter 5(4):13-20, 1987.

Sellers, E. M., C. A. Naranjo, M. Harrison et al. Diazepam loading: Simplified treatment of alcohol withdrawal. Clin. Pharmacol. Ther. 34:822-826, 1983.

Shaw, J. M., G. S. Kolesar, E. M. Sellers et al. Development of optimal treatment tactics for alcohol withdrawal. I. Assessment and effectiveness of supportive care. J. Clin. Psychopharmacol. 1:382-383, 1981.

Simon, R. P. Alcohol and seizures. N. Engl. J. Med. 319:715-716, 1988.

Singer, K., and W. B. Lundberg. Ventricular arrhythmias associated with the ingestion of alcohol. Ann. Intern. Med. 77:247-248, 1972.

Smart, R. G., and G. Gray. Multiple predictors of dropout from alcoholism treatment. Q. J. Stud. Alcohol 35:363-367, 1978.

Starzl, T. E., D. Van Thiel, A. G. Tzakis et al. Orthotopic liver transplantation for alcoholic cirrhosis. J. Am. Med. Assoc. 260:2542-2544, 1988.

Stinnett, J. L. Outpatient detoxification of the alcoholic. Int. J. Addict. 17:1031-1046, 1982.

Tennant, F. S. Ambulatory alcohol withdrawal. J. Family Practice 8:621-623, 1979.

Van Thiel, D. G., and J. S. Gavaler. Myocardial effects of alcohol abuse: Clinical and physiological consequences. Recent Dev. Alcohol 3:181-187, 1985.

Wagman, A. M. I., and R. P. Allen. Effects of alcohol ingestion and abstinence on slow wave sleep of alcoholics. Pp. 453-465 in M. M. Gross, ed. Alcohol Intoxication and Withdrawal: Experimental Studies. II. Advances in Experimental Medicine and Biology. New York: Plenum Press, 1975.

Walker, R. D., D. M. Donovan, D. R. Kivlahan et al. Length of stay, neuropsychological performance, and aftercare: Influences on alcohol treatment outcome. J. Consult. Clin. Psychol. 51:900-911, 1983.

Westrick, E. R., A. P. Shapiro, P. E. Nathan et al. Dietary tryptophan reverses alcohol-induced impairment of facial recognition but not verbal recall. Alcoholism Clin. Exp. Res. 12(4):531-535, 1988.

Whitfield, C. L., G. Thompson, A. Lamb et al. Detoxification of 1,024 alcoholic patients without psychoactive drugs. J. Am. Med. Assoc. 239(14):1409-1410, 1978.

Williams, H. L., and O. H. Rundell. Altered sleep physiology in chronic alcoholics: Reversal with abstinence. Alcoholism Clin. Exp. Res. 5(2):318-325, 1981.

Woody, G. E., C. P. O'Brien, and R. A. Greenstein. Misuse and abuse of diazepam: An increasingly common medical problem. Int. J. Addict. 10(5):843-848, 1975.

Woosley, R. L. Indications for antiarrhythmic therapy: A wealth of controversy, a dearth of data. Ann. Intern. Med. 108:450-452, 1988.

Woosley, R. L., A. J. J. Wood, and D. M. Roden. Encainide. N. Engl. J. Med. 318:1107-1115, 1988.

Yohman, J. R., K. W. Schaeffer, and O. A. Parsons. Cognitive training in alcoholic men. J. Consult. Clin. Psychol. 56:67-72, 1988.

Young, G. P., C. Rores, C. Murphy, and R. H. Dailey. Intravenous phenobarbital for alcoholic withdrawal and convulsions. Ann. Emergency Med. 16(8):847-850, 1987.

Yules, R. B., D. X. Freidman, and K. A. Chandler. The effect of ethyl alcohol on man's electroencephalic sleep cycle. Electroencephalogr. Clin. Neurophysiol. 20:109-111, 1966.

14

TREATMENT COSTS, BENEFITS, AND COST OFFSETS: PUBLIC POLICY CONSIDERATIONS

The purpose of this chapter is to assess the current state of research in the area of costs and cost-benefit analysis of alcoholism treatment. The chapter also deals with associated public policy issues such as insurance coverage for alcohol treatment. These issues have implications for a number of public health policy concerns including cost containment, appropriate utilization of medical care services, and efficient resource allocation.

The criteria most commonly used to analyze health policy issues have been those that measured changes in the potential of the system to cure disease. In the last 20 years, however, a counterinfluence has developed that embodies an equally single-minded perspective in health policy analysis: the exclusive use of economic criteria. Neither of these approaches is sufficient to deal with the complexities of most relevant issues and especially with the policy questions that surround the costs of insurance coverage for alcohol treatment.

Distinctions can be made among treatment effects, benefits, and efficiency. The committee presents here an approach originally proposed by Freeborn and Greenlick (1973), which requires the simultaneous assessment of treatment effectiveness and efficiency (Greenlick and Colombo, 1977).

TREATMENT EFFECTIVENESS, BENEFITS, AND EFFICIENCY

Effectiveness (sometimes referred to as treatment outcome or quality of care) requires measurement against stated goals, or possibly against generally accepted goals. This measurement has two dimensions because goals may be defined from the viewpoint of the system or of the client or provider. Technical effectiveness measures the extent to which the technical goals of the system are met; determining technical effectiveness involves measuring how well different treatment modalities achieve treatment goals. Several examples of research issues that relate to technical effectiveness are whether adequate numbers of patients are treated, given the resources available; whether inpatient treatment "works" better than outpatient treatment; and which specific ingredients of treatment improve outcome.

How well a particular treatment meets the psychological or social needs of the patient population involves an assessment of psychosocial effectiveness. In assessing such effectiveness, it is necessary to consider not only patients and their satisfaction but questions of equity (i.e., fairness in the receipt of care) and access.

Traditionally, cost-effectiveness analyses "are used to evaluate the relative cost of alternative treatments per unit of effectiveness" (Saxe et al., 1983). They have addressed such issues as how many dollars per unit of outcome change the treatment costs, or how costly one treatment modality is in comparison with another. Cost-benefit analyses consider the number of dollars' worth of benefit created per dollar of program cost or per dollar of investment made to create the benefits. Benefits are primarily defined in terms of monetary values placed on indicators of reduced alcohol impairment, for example, job performance or earnings, or reduced numbers of catastrophic events (e.g., motor vehicle crashes and

-289-

arrests). <u>Costs</u> are economic and are limited mainly to medical care costs, a limitation that produces underestimation of the true expense of alcohol abuse and the cost savings of reducing it (Fein, 1984).

<u>Efficiency</u> involves the assessment of costs for the total input needed to produce the required services for a population of given characteristics. In this way, costs can be assessed for health care systems under alternative conditions. In evaluating the relative efficiency of health care alternatives, the production function (the relationship between output and factor inputs) is examined, at least implicitly. An estimate of the production and cost function may permit the identification of a more efficient mix of services and resources.

This method of examining treatment effectiveness and efficiency has at least two advantages. First, it indicates interrelationships among criteria. For example, a policy alternative, such as mandating health insurance coverage for alcoholism treatment, could be assessed as having a positive effect on one dimension and a negative effect on another. Second, this approach allows decision makers to identify possible trade-offs when other parties are presenting subjective analyses or are failing to identify problems in other dimensions of care.

The following represent opportunities for research on treatment effectiveness:

• How do questions of effectiveness, including patient satisfaction and efficiency, interact in alternative treatment modalities and treatment programs? There is a particular need for studies that provide simultaneous measurement of effectiveness, satisfaction, and efficiency.

METHODOLOGICAL APPROACHES TO POLICY ANALYSIS

Public policy research can take a variety of forms. For the purposes of this review, the committee distinguishes among policy analysis, meta-analysis, demonstrations, and clinical trials.

Policy analysis entails a review of what is known about a particular area in order to consider systematically all policy alternatives. Fein's 1984 monograph, which uses data from a variety of sources to assess the usefulness of insurance coverage for alcohol treatment, is an example of policy analysis in the alcohol field. Fein concludes that enhancing insurance coverage is an appropriate public policy solution. Several large cost-of-illness studies of alcohol abuse have been conducted (Berry and Boland, 1977; Parker et al., 1987), yet good cost-benefit analyses of alcoholism treatment have been rare. Two exceptions are the Air Force study (Orvis et al., 1981) and the JWK Corporation study of NIAAA-funded alcoholism treatment centers (ATCs) (NIAAA, 1976).

These two studies offer a comprehensive look at a range of costs and benefits of treatment. They provide guides to the assumptions and estimation methods used in evaluating treatments. More studies like these are needed to answer questions such as the following: What other costs besides total health care costs are reduced by successful alcoholism treatment? What other benefits accrue besides benefits to the third-party insurer, health maintenance organization (HMO), or provider in the forum of reduced utilization costs? Of particular importance is the study of the costs of alcoholism to other family members, work, neighbors, and communities.

Meta-analysis is a form of scientific inquiry that is useful in fields in which more classical research approaches have been unable to provide answers. A study by Tobler (1986) of the outcome of 143 adolescent drug prevention programs indicates how meta-analysis can be used in formulating alcohol policy. Meta-analysis weights differentially the information produced by imperfect studies so that each study influences the policy debate in proportion to the scientific value of its findings. Scientific value is quantitatively defined on a prior basis according to methodological considerations. Although meta-analysis can be useful when properly applied to a series of studies with common outcome measures, the lack of commonly accepted and standardized measures of outcome makes its use somewhat problematic in cost-effectiveness analyses of treatment for alcohol abuse. The use of professional judgments to rate individual studies and to make assessments (even by using explicit criteria) for a meta-analysis may introduce the same bias as the use of more qualitative assessment techniques. Traditional reviews of the scientific literature require a succession of subjective decisions, each of which may be hidden from the reader and each of which affects conclusions. Meta-analysis makes this process more accessible but is also subject to bias.

Clinical trials are the traditional tool for evaluating treatment in biomedical science. In the area of alcohol treatment policy, clinical trials are difficult because they require the random selection of patients and their random assignment to treatment and nontreatment groups. Ethical and legal concerns may obviate their use. However, a number of well-controlled quasi-experimental studies have been conducted to evaluate treatment outcome. These studies explicitly ask what types, durations, and combinations of treatment produce a better outcome. The types of clients that are best served by a particular treatment are also examined (McCrady et al., 1986).

Most studies do not include data on the costs of treatment, but those that do indicate that outpatient care or partial hospitalization is less expensive than extended inpatient treatment, at least over the short term (see the research summaries by Miller and Hester, 1986; Holder, 1987). These reviews suggest that the cost-effectiveness of treatment can be maximized if less costly treatment is used, provided patients are appropriately matched or selected (Longabaugh et al., 1983; Longabaugh and Beattie, 1985; McCrady et al., 1986). A burden-of-proof argument has been suggested for more costly treatment alternatives. This argument states that, given equal effectiveness, a higher cost treatment should be used only with specific justification.

A major methodological issue is determining which component of treatment works best and whether observed outcome changes are indeed treatment effects, especially after several years have elapsed. Naturalistic studies offer a contrast to studies that randomly assign subjects to different types of treatment. Both types of research are meritorious if designed carefully. Typically, naturalistic studies report high success rates, but the samples in such studies are highly selective. On the other hand, random assignment does not solve the problem of selectivity because refusals and dropouts affect the randomness of the treatment effects that are seen. The attrition rates (cases lost to follow-up) are frequently high enough in these studies (averaging 30 to 50 percent) to cause problems in the interpretation of posttreatment changes (McCrady et al., 1986). Study designs need to incorporate efforts to account for, locate, and obtain outcome data on subjects who are lost through refusal, mortality, and migration. Separating the effects of different treatment modalities is a major challenge, as is the inclusion of the cost of treatment as a central variable in alcoholism treatment evaluations.

The following are opportunities for research in the methodology of policy analysis:

- Systematic policy analyses are needed in the area of costs and cost-effectiveness of alcohol treatment. Study designs that include cost of treatment as a central variable should be encouraged.
- More evaluation of the meta-analysis approach is needed.
- Study designs that include sustained efforts to locate lost subjects should be encouraged.

THE COST OFFSET EFFECT

Cost offset is defined as "the reduction in total health care costs adjusting for the costs of alcoholism treatment attributed to the treatment" (Holder and Shachtman, 1987). The costs here are confined to treatment costs, and the effects are limited to reduced medical care utilization, which is sometimes measured in terms of cost savings (Holder, 1987). Cost offset ideally involves a process whereby the total posttreatment health care costs (including alcoholism treatment) incurred by treated alcoholics are subtracted from the total health care costs the same group would have incurred if no alcoholism treatment had been received. However, estimates of costs in the absence of treatment are difficult to obtain.

A question of critical interest is the extent to which coverage for alcoholism treatment stimulates the use of such treatment services, thereby improving the patient's condition and reducing the patient's overall use of other medical services. This question outlines both an effectiveness and an efficiency issue in the health insurance field because the cost per unit input is reduced if there are offsetting savings in other treatment areas. If sufficient cost offset can be documented, the opposition to including coverage for alcoholism treatment among insurance benefits will be less justified.

The results of cost offset studies suggest, with some exceptions, that (1) overall medical care costs of alcoholic patients are significantly higher than those of matched nonalcoholic controls or comparison populations; (2) medical care utilization and costs incurred by alcoholic patients do decline between the pre- and posttreatment periods; (3) most of the cost savings or reductions in service utilization are the result of decreases in general medical hospitalization (frequency, length of stay, or both); and (4) groups with the highest pretreatment costs experience the largest declines in costs in the posttreatment period (Jones and Vischi, 1979; Holder, 1987).

Cost offset studies of alcoholism treatment can be divided into studies that use units of services as proxies for costs, studies that use cost data alone, and studies that include both service utilization and cost data. Most of the early work on offset effects was done in HMOs (Wersigner et al., 1978; Sherman, Reiff, and Forsythe, 1979; Boyajy and Adams, 1980; Plotnick et al., 1982; Putnam, 1982). This emphasis occurred because of the ability of HMOs to furnish longitudinal data from medical records on utilization of their services. Most of these studies contain no cost data, although they are unique in permitting detailed examination of the effects of treatment on the illness and utilization experience of alcoholics, their family members, and comparison groups.

Assessing costs for outpatient care (in contrast to inpatient care) is difficult, as indicated by the few HMO studies that attempt to compare costs for care before and after alcoholism treatment (Forsythe, Griffiths, and Keiff, 1982; Holder and Hallan, 1986). In these studies, medical costs are based on fee schedules, and alcoholics are found to be higher cost users than nonalcoholics. The results for family members are similar; however, data for adult and child family members are rarely disaggregated. Differences between studies can result from differences in sample composition or utilization levels.

Cost considerations cover a variety of issues, including the charge to patients for service, the payments (if any) on behalf of a patient by an insurance program, and out-of-pocket expenses for the patient. The use of fee or charge data rather than cost data is nearly universal in the few existing studies of cost offset or cost-effectiveness. One study of cost offset effects illustrates the use of claims data for federal employees with Aetna coverage in a fee-for-service context (Holder and Blose, 1986; Holder and Shachtman, 1987). Charges are seen as surrogate but fairly comprehensive indicators of utilization. However, a measurement problem that may be encountered when using health insurance claims data is unreported medical costs (i.e., claims that are not submitted for insurance payments).

Most of the studies reviewed by Holder (1987) used pretreatment/posttreatment or longitudinal designs in which the criteria for including subjects were carefully specified and efforts were made to control for confounding variables. Only one study had fewer than 50 subjects, and most had study groups numbering in the hundreds. None of the studies, however, was a clinical trial with comparison groups randomly selected from the same population as the treated population. The studies used relatively long pretrial periods (generally more than 12 months) but usually short posttreatment periods (12 months).

In none of the reviewed studies was there a nontreatment control group. In the studies in which there was randomization to different forms of treatment, no significant difference in medical care cost reduction could be discerned. Holder concluded that different alcohol treatment settings may be equally associated with reductions in total health care costs.

Cost offset studies suffer from the absence of an explanatory model and from methodological problems similar to those in other health care research. The first relevant question is whether reduced demand for care following treatment is real or artificial, that is, whether the decline can be attributed to the treatment rather than to regression to the mean as has been observed for high utilizers of medical services. The tendency for crisis-oriented medical care visits to peak around intake falsely inflates pretreatment rates and makes posttreatment declines easier to achieve. Adequate statistical control should be employed for regression to the mean.

The "washout" of offset effects over time is also a possibility. Studies of psychiatric offset that have found no overall effect of treatment on utilization have used quarterly intervals and relatively long follow-up periods (Kogan et al., 1975), suggesting that the longer the posttreatment interval, the more the offset effect washes out (Goldberg, Krantz, and Locke, 1970). This issue is not yet resolved in the alcoholism treatment literature; indeed, some studies suggest greater offset with time (Holder and Hallan, 1986; Longabaugh, 1988).

The issue of substitution is rarely explored in the alcoholism literature, but it has been covered in the psychiatric treatment offset effect literature (Follette and Cummings, 1967; Goldberg, Krantz, and Locke, 1970; Hankin and Oktay, 1979; Kessler, Steinwachs, and Hankin, 1982; Schlesinger et al., 1983; see also Parron and Solomon, 1980). This substitution is an important area for further research and raises a number of interesting questions. To what can the decline in medical care utilization or in the costs of medical care after alcoholism treatment be attributed? Are alcoholics substituting mental health or counseling services for medical care services that were used inappropriately before treatment? Are they substituting outpatient for inpatient services? Are demand and need for care simply shifting into different categories and not declining overall? Is the reduced utilization of ambulatory medical care services after treatment simply a result of reductions in certain diagnostic categories (e.g., emotional and psychosomatic disorders, injuries, and other acute conditions)?

Similarly, it is necessary to ask whether reduced demand for care among adult and child family members is accompanied by reduced need, that is, greater health. Are family members deferring needs for care to accommodate the alcoholic's crisis and need for attention? Reduced utilization and costs thus may not be an altogether laudable goal if such reductions involve postponed or foregone care in the face of need for care. Appropriate utilization may be the preferred goal.

Clearly, an essential question concerns the relative mix of inpatient and ambulatory services (both scheduled and emergency) that constitutes the overall posttreatment decline in utilization for alcoholics and family members. To the extent that posttreatment declines occur in ambulatory utilization, which is largely discretionary for patients, they reflect changes in actual need or in patients' perceptions of the need for care and may, indeed, be indicative of treatment effects. Insofar as such declines are confined to inpatient services, which are largely under the control of physicians or other providers who act as "gatekeepers" to the system, changes may reflect differences over time in HMO or provider policies rather than changes in the need for care from the patient's perspective. Declines in inpatient rates could reflect secular trends rather than treatment effects if calendar dates are used (Putnam, 1982); however, many cost offset studies use point-of-treatment utilization (Holder and Blose, 1986). The perspective of medical sociologists who have developed models to predict how, why, and when people use medical and psychiatric services would be valuable in attempting to explain complex changes in utilization across time and subgroups (Andersen, 1968; McKinlay, 1972; Wan and Soifer, 1974; Tessler and Mechanic, 1978; Wolinsky, 1978; Andersen and Anderson, 1979; Mechanic, 1979).

Cost offset studies, like treatment effect studies, are vulnerable to dropouts from the study population, a problem that increases for longer study periods. Well-controlled cost offset studies utilize only those cases for whom there are continuous data over the study period and examine differences between continuous and noncontinuous (dropout) subjects. Putnam (1982), who compared treatment dropouts with patients who have remained in treatment in terms of utilization effects, found that the acceptance of alcoholism treatment was associated with reduced medical care utilization, whereas a lack of acceptance was associated with increased medical care utilization, especially for injuries and other "acute" conditions. Benefit-to-cost ratios for dropouts and those who have remained in treatment were studied by the Orvis research team (1981); the utilization, cost, and demographics of both groups were studied by Holder and Blose (1986).

Actual recovery status in the posttreatment period is a critical variable in cost offset studies. Unfortunately, only one offset study (Hayami and Freeborn, 1981) includes measures of treatment outcome (abstinence measures). A remaining question is whether changes in drinking behavior and alcohol impairment can be linked directly to changes in utilization or costs of services. A related question is whether a small proportion of alcoholics with very high utilization rates account for all of the observed decline in utilization in the posttreatment period. It is in this respect that cost offset studies require cost effectiveness studies.

Holder (1987) concluded that the studies reported in the last decade were characterized by significant methodological improvement compared with earlier studies. He concluded further that the existing methodological shortcomings do not "prevent reasonable (but perhaps cautious) policy statements about alcoholism treatment and health care costs." He reported that "as a group, the studies reviewed confirm the potential of alcoholism treatment to contribute to sustained reductions in total health care utilization and costs." Clearly, much research remains to be done, and several areas for such research are suggested by Holder (1987). The feeling persists that the ideal study would include no-treatment controls. The legal, ethical, and methodological difficulties of locating a randomly selected group of alcoholics from a defined general population and randomly assigning them to treatment and no-treatment conditions are considerable. Yet despite these formidable problems, it is important to develop research that moves as close as possible to true experimental strategies in this area.

Several fruitful research possibilities include the need for more information about total health care costs and utilization associated with a variety of sociodemographic factors and the interaction of these factors with alcoholism treatment. As yet no studies have had a sufficient sample size or a sufficiently long follow-up period to permit the complex analyses that are needed to guide public policy. Longer periods of follow-up and better matching designs are required.

A methodological problem in longitudinal studies of health care cost offset is the absence of an adequate baseline for comparison. There is a need to match alcoholic patients with nonalcoholic patients on the basis of medical care utilization. Some research compares treatment utilization across a variety of diseases to allow some assessment of the range of pre- and postutilization changes that could be expected. However, using this research may establish a baseline bias in which posttreatment costs for alcoholics are likely to be lower (possibly as a result of regression to the mean) than costs for the comparison group. An alternative strategy would be to develop reliable baseline measures for the age/gender cohort of treated alcoholics.

Some researchers argue that the random assignment of patients to treatment is adequate for this purpose (Miller and Hester, 1986). Unfortunately, some patients' refusal to cooperate with a randomized design, group differentials in dropout rates, and the lack of approximation to an untreated group remain as selectivity biases. Finally, more cost offset studies including both cost and utilization data are needed. Such studies may provide an empirical basis for modeling differences in demands for care in prepaid versus fee-for-service carriers and with various levels of coverage.

The following are opportunities for research on cost offset:

 • Research designs should approximate the use of nontreatment controls, moving as close as possible to experimental strategies.
 • Studies need to be undertaken to assess the health status of patients after treatment and to determine the relationship between health status and utilization after treatment.
 • Models must be developed to explain the determinants of medical care utilization so that changes in utilization across time can be better understood.

• Changes in actual drinking behavior and alcohol impairment need to be linked to changes in medical care utilization.

• Studies need to include better baseline measures of comparisons of alcoholic versus nonalcoholic samples on prior medical care utilization to allow a clearer assessment of posttreatment change.

• Studies should include both cost and utilization data to provide an empirical basis for modeling the utilization phenomena.

MANAGED CARE AND PREFERRED PROVIDER RESEARCH ISSUES

A new dimension that has increasingly been added to health care benefits is managed care. These cost containment programs have been established by payers (e.g., insurance companies) in direct response to reports claiming that insured persons are subjected to medically unnecessary surgery, psychiatric treatment, and hospitalization. In general, managed care programs provide information to assist in the selection of treatment options, typically through review procedures that scrutinize and specify the conditions under which treatment is to be delivered. Managed care helps to reduce costs to payers by eliminating presumably unnecessary care.

Review procedures include a hospital preadmission review, continued-stay review, mandated second opinion programs, discharge planning, major case management, and alternate service recommendations. The procedures may be managed by a peer review organization, a health insurance company staff, or private case management companies.

Although managed care providers have now begun to organize these specialized cost containment services, no research is available to evaluate the effectiveness of these procedures in achieving the goals of providing quality care at reduced costs. Because of this gap, the committee points out several research opportunities.

The following are opportunities for research on managed care:

• Research should be undertaken to evaluate managed care alternatives in treatment for alcohol problems. One approach is to make available specific alternatives (e.g., preadmission review, case management, second opinion programs) to insured populations by using randomized clinical trial methodology with appropriate measures of costs, charges, and outcome.

• Research should be encouraged to develop and evaluate scientifically based criteria for assigning clients to appropriate levels and intensities of treatment services. These criteria should be consistent with current scientific evidence and available technologies of assessment, giving appropriate emphasis to the severity of alcohol dependence, medical and psychiatric complications, psychosocial functions, demographic characteristics, and access to treatment (see Chapter 11).

OTHER INSURANCE ISSUES

There remain a variety of additional insurance and cost-related research issues. Almost no research has been conducted on the effect of different insurance benefits on entry into treatment, on the selection of a specific treatment modality, on the satisfaction of consumers, and on the ultimate costs of the system.

The cost savings of alternative reimbursement policies for alcoholism treatment services have been studied very little and less successfully than the cost savings reported in the psychiatric offset literature (Follette and Cummings, 1967; Goldberg, Krantz, and Locke, 1970; Goldberg, Regier, and Burns, 1980; Schlesinger, Mumford, and Glass, 1983). The question of whether broader insurance coverage for alcoholism treatment will reduce medical care spending has led to some comparisons of fee-for-service systems with prepaid systems, but these comparisons have rarely been based on costs (Edwards et al., 1977; Hayami and Freeborn, 1981; NIAAA, 1981). Evidence suggests that utilization is higher under a plan with full coverage and no copayment requirement (Hayami and Freeborn, 1981).

There is a great need for research that compares payment sources. Obstacles to this type of research are related to differences in the organization and delivery of care in different systems. Problems involved in estimating units of prepaid service comprise how much overhead and other indirect costs to include, differential costs of treatment by physicians versus nonphysicians, and substantial differences in economic incentives for hospitalization compared with ambulatory care. Prepaid plans are known to be oriented toward short-term, outpatient alcoholism treatment, compared with an orientation toward hospitalization in other systems (Miller and Hester, 1986). One study of the effects of psychiatric care on medical care utilization finds no differences between fee-for-service and prepaid groups that can be attributed to the method of payment; rather, differences are attributed to selection criteria for fee-for-service coverage (Kogan et al., 1975). Studies of alcoholism treatment effects using this kind of model are needed. Studies with extended pretreatment and posttreatment periods are difficult to conduct in a fee-for-service setting, except in relation to problems severe enough to require hospitalization. This difficulty is largely due to the openness of the system and problems of access to records. Data on family members' utilization are even more difficult to collect.

Employer research is a promising area for studies comparing the effects of treatment on utilization by payment source. Companies, especially large ones, represent the kind of relatively closed system needed for such research. Employee assistance programs provide an opportunity to answer research questions on the costs and effectiveness of certain treatments. Cost-saving measures that can be studied, particularly in instances in which the company has a medical department, include the causes of absenteeism for sickness (or injury), average sickness or accident benefits paid, wage and salary information on job retention and earnings, and personnel record data for monitoring changes in work performance (Kurtz, Googins, and Howard, 1984).

Insurance coverage for alcoholism services can be structured in many ways. An assortment of services can be covered under insurance, including inpatient detoxification, residential treatment, partial hospitalization, extended or long-term care, and outpatient care. However, in the past, alcoholism treatment services have generally been excluded from coverage or covered under sharply limited mental health treatment services. As these services have been added more recently to health insurance coverage, different combinations of services have been included in different circumstances. Much research is needed to determine the effectiveness and particularly the cost-effectiveness of the structure of insurance coverage, especially when the benefit package is mandated. Controlled assessment of state-mandated health insurance coverage for alcoholism treatment is essential because this issue is currently a significant policy concern, with strong positions being taken by health insurance carriers and alcoholism treatment providers.

An important research question is the extent to which alcoholism coverage induces people to accept needed services that would not otherwise have been utilized. Epidemiological catchment area studies (Shapiro et al., 1984) show that the prevalence of alcohol, drug, and mental disorders is considerably greater than the number of people who seek care for these problems. In general, people who use privately insured alcoholism treatment programs tend to be white, middle-aged males of higher than average social stability, educational attainment, and occupational status. Critical research questions include the identification of barriers to care and the cost factors that affect the nature of the population that is served. These questions bear on efficiency, technical effectiveness, and psychosocial effectiveness, as well as on the issue of equity.

The effect of differential insurance coverage has been the subject of two studies. A 1981 HMO study at Kaiser-Permanente in Portland, Oregon (Hayami and Freeborn, 1981), examined the effect of coverage on the use of alcoholism treatment services. The study used a randomized design in which employee groups with a total of 110,000 members were randomly assigned to two categories. One group was given a new benefit package that included total coverage for detoxification and outpatient treatment services. The other group retained the coverage they had, a 50 percent copayment benefit for alcoholism treatment services. The full coverage group was significantly more likely to use alcoholism treatment services than the 50 percent copay group, but there was no difference between the groups in the utilization of medical care services in the posttreatment period. The full benefit group tended to be slightly more improved than the 50 percent copay group. The study supports the feasibility of adding outpatient detoxification and outpatient treatment services to an HMO coverage package.

The most recent study of how cost sharing affects the utilization of specialized treatment services was the Rand health insurance study (Manning et al., 1986). This study, which dealt only with mental health and not with alcoholism treatment services, used a randomized design and enrolled more than 5,800 people. The study found that subjects who needed to pay a large portion of the first-dollar costs of services had less than half the probability of using mental health services than those whose insurance coverage paid for the total costs of the services. However, this study cannot easily be generalized to alcoholism treatment. What is needed is research that focuses on coverage, utilization, and costs, carefully correlating these with outcomes and the nature of the population using the services. Hornbrook (1988), among others who have reviewed the equity implications of differential coverage of services for alcohol, drug, and mental (ADM) conditions compared with coverage for other conditions, has suggested that this differential represents discrimination against persons who need care for ADM disorders. Research on the potential effects of this discrimination is in order.

The following are additional opportunities for research concerning health insurance:

• Studies are needed to investigate the relationship between payment source and type and the effectiveness of the treatment received.
• Studies examining differences between treatment patterns in fee-for-service systems and in managed care systems need to be expanded. These studies should have relatively long follow-up periods and use sophisticated follow-up techniques.
• Employee assistance programs provide an excellent opportunity to study alcohol insurance effects. With appropriate safeguards, the records of such programs should be made available for objective research.

• Priority should be assigned to studies of groups that are frequently excluded in this area, in particular, the uninsured, the unemployed, youth, women, and minorities.

• State-mandated health insurance coverage for alcoholism treatment should be carefully analyzed.

• More systematic studies are needed of the effect of insurance coverage and cost factors on the utilization of alcoholism treatment services.

OTHER COST-RELATED RESEARCH AREAS

One important policy question concerns the role that should be played by public and private financing for alcoholism treatment. Increased private expenditures for treatment (either through insurance or through direct pay mechanisms) may result not in private but rather in public cost offsets. These offsets could be seen as increased productivity, which affects taxes, and decreased public expenditures for criminal justice and motor vehicle accidents. This type of research differs from previous research efforts in that it is closer to cost-benefit studies than to cost offset studies.

Two types of research are appropriate. First, systematic policy analysis can help illuminate many public policy questions. Second, it is necessary to initiate long-term, population-based studies. Extending research support beyond catchment area studies to long-term work in other populations (e.g., employees and insured populations) would be quite useful.

Little has been done to determine the relative efficiency of alternative modes of treatment or to link formative work on the technical effectiveness of treatment modes with the costs of these treatments. The only way that the efficiency of alternative treatment modes can be assessed is by determining the relative success rate of different treatments and by linking costs of treatment to success rates. This may require a series of microanalyses.

COST, INSURANCE, AND PUBLIC POLICY
RESEARCH NEEDS SPECIFIC TO ADOLESCENTS

Adolescent alcohol and drug abuse problems are receiving increasing attention from policymakers. These problems result in extensive individual and social costs and have a significant impact on the medical care system. The abuse of alcohol or drugs may affect physical health and the development of coping abilities. The use of alcohol is correlated with the abuse of other substances as well as with behavioral problems. The leading causes of death among persons aged 15 to 24 years are accidents, homicides, and suicides. Many of these deaths are related to alcohol and drug abuse.

Health insurance plans, including HMOs, are under increasing pressure to expand benefits and services for the treatment of alcohol and drug abuse among adolescents. Unfortunately, there is little or no information on which to base decisions about coverage or the types of services that should be provided. This is partly because data are not available on utilization and costs because most plans do not provide coverage for an appropriate array of services for adolescents (e.g., outpatient, intensive outpatient, partial hospitalization, inpatient). Only a few studies have examined the effectiveness of treatment.

The literature contains little on the effectiveness of treatment for adolescents with drug and alcohol abuse problems (Jones and Vischi, 1979; Friedman and Beschner, 1985), but it does provide some insight into the treatment needs of these young people (Sells and Simpson,

1979) and their response to treatment. Most of these studies are descriptive and do not address the relative effectiveness of different approaches to treatment (Jellinek, 1960; Vollmer, 1982; Vaillant et al., 1983; Westermeyer and Peake, 1983).

Using data from a sample of 27,000 drug-abusing youth who participated in publicly funded programs, Sells and Simpson (1979) reported significant life-functioning improvements four to six years after treatment. Klinge, Lennox, and Vaziri (1977-1978) questioned two groups of adolescents six months after discharge from a psychiatric ward and attempted to measure differences in functioning. One group consisted of adolescents with emotional problems but without drug involvement; the other group consisted of those with substance abuse problems. The substance-abusing group was found to be using drugs more than the first group, but both groups were functioning better after discharge.

Herrington, Riordan, and Jacobson (1981) conducted one of the few studies that compared two different types of treatments. One adolescent group was treated in a mixed (adolescent/adult) chemical dependency unit and was selected retrospectively for research purposes. The other group was prospectively chosen for a newly designed chemical dependency treatment unit that only treated adolescents. Both treatments were residential. It was concluded that the adolescent-only group setting was more effective in terms of certain outcomes (participating in Alcoholics Anonymous or Narcotics Anonymous, returning to school, association with non-drug-using peers) and diminished likelihood of arrest, but that there was little association between the specialized adolescent program and improved quality of life or use of alcohol or drugs.

These adolescent treatment studies use outcome measures that are different from those used in studies of adults. School attendance, legal problems, and other age-specific measures were the outcomes most frequently considered. However, there are some adolescent developmental issues that need to be examined and that require a longitudinal approach. For example, Donovan, Jessor, and Jessor (1982) conducted a 10-year follow-up of youthful drug abusers. They reported that a majority of the adolescents reverted without treatment to a lower level of involvement with drugs and alcohol. Such studies have been used to raise many questions regarding appropriate and cost-effective treatment approaches for the chemically abusing, dependent adolescent. Type and length of treatment, matching client to treatment, involvement of the family, and the best ways to keep patients in some form of aftercare are all important issues (Spiegel and Mock, 1978; Filstead and Anderson, 1983). Finally, as reviewed in Chapter 10, results based on samples of adults indicate that a less intensive approach to treatment (e.g., outpatient) may often be as effective as a more intensive approach (e.g., residential). This type of information does not exist for samples of adolescents (Jones and Vischi, 1979).

The following are opportunities for research on issues in the utilization of adolescent treatment for alcohol problems:

• The factors that may influence adolescents' use of treatment services for alcohol and drug abuse should be studied, as should the relationship between the utilization of treatment services and the need for care.
• The insurance issues relative to adolescent care should be studied; for example, how does variation in copayment rates and levels of benefits affect the utilization of treatment services?
• The extent to which treatment for alcohol and drug abuse affects subsequent general medical care utilization and costs for adolescents and their families must be adequately investigated.

OTHER PUBLIC POLICY RESEARCH NEEDS

The above discussion leads into the final area of research needed in public policy. Very little research has been conducted in the area of consumer and patient attitudes toward alcoholism treatment and the relationship of these attitudes to the probability of accepting and completing treatment. This research is necessary not only to allow proper understanding of the dynamics of the treatment process but also to provide the proper alternatives in policy debates. For example, it is not understood how much the availability of a full range of alternative modes of treatment affects the probability that a patient will accept any treatment. There is also insufficient information on how different modes of treatment are selected by the patient (Finney, Moos, and Mewborn, 1980). Knowledge of patient attitudes and desires cannot be ignored if program planners are to design interventions that are both effective and efficient.

The following are opportunities for research on public policy:

• Long-term population-based studies should be developed. Cohorts from employee and insured populations should be found to allow studies of the population dynamics of alcoholism treatment and costs.
• Studies should be undertaken to explore consumer attitudes toward alcoholism treatment and the relationship between these attitudes and the probability of completing treatment.

REFERENCES

Andersen, R. A Behavioral Model of Families' Use of Health Services. Research Series No. 25. Chicago: Center for Health Administration Studies, University of Chicago, 1968.

Andersen, R., and O. W. Anderson. Trends in the use of health services. Pp. 371-397 in H. E. Freeman, S. Levine, and L. G. Reeder, eds. Handbook of Medical Sociology. Englewood Cliffs, NJ: Prentice-Hall, 1979.

Berry, R. E., Jr., and J. P. Boland. The Economic Cost of Alcohol Abuse. New York: The Free Press, 1977.

Boyajy, T. G., and K. M. Adams. Alcoholism treatment programs within prepaid group practice HMOs: An update. Washington, DC: Group Health Association of America, 1980.

Collins, T., and M. Lutz. An evaluation of the Fairview Deaconess Hospital Adolescent Chemical Dependency Program. Unpublished manuscript, Fairview Deaconess Hospital, Minneapolis, MN, 1983.

Donovan, J. E., R. Jessor, and L. Jessor. Problem Drinking in Adolescence and Young Adulthood: A Follow-up Study. Publ. No. 184. Boulder, CO: Institute of Behavioral Science, University of Colorado, 1982.

Edwards, D., S. Bucky, P. Cohen et al. Primary and secondary benefits from treatment for alcoholism. Am. J. Psychiatry 134(6):682-683, 1977.

Fein, R. Alcohol in America: The Price We Pay. Newport Beach, CA: Care Institute, 1984.

Filstead, W. J., and C. L. Anderson. Conceptual and clinical issues in the treatment of adolescent alcohol and substance mis-users. Child and Youth Services 6(1-2):103-116, 1983.

Finney, J. W., R. H. Moos, and C. R. Mewborn. Posttreatment experiences and treatment outcome of alcoholic patients six months and two years after hospitalization. J. Consult. Clin. Psychol. 48:17-29, 1980.

Follette, W., and W. A. Cummings. Psychiatric services and medical care utilization in a prepaid health plan setting. Med. Care 5:25-35, 1967.

Forsythe, A. B., B. Griffiths, and S. Keiff. Comparison of utilization of medical services by alcoholics and non-alcoholics. Am. J. Public Health 72(6):600-602, 1982.

Freeborn, D. K., and M. R. Greenlick. Evaluation of the performance of ambulatory care systems: Research requirements and opportunities. Med. Care 11:68-75, 1973.

Friedman, A., and G. Beschner. Treatment Services for Adolescent Substance Abusers. Washington, DC: National Institute on Drug Abuse, 1985.

Goldberg, I. D., G. Krantz, and B. Z. Locke. Effect of a short-term outpatient psychiatric therapy benefit on the utilization of medical services in a prepaid group practice medical program. Med. Care 8:419-428, 1970.

Goldberg, I. D., D. A. Regier, and B. J. Burns, eds. Use of health and mental health outpatient services in four organized health care settings. In Mental Health Service System Reporter. USDHHS Publ. No. (ADM)80-859. Rockville, MD: National Institute of Mental Health, 1980.

Greenlick, M. R., and T. J. Colombo. A framework for assessing the impact of health policy alternatives. Pp. 53-59 in Papers on the National Health Guidelines: Conditions for Change in the Health Care System. Washington, DC: U.S. Government Printing Office, 1977.

Hankin, J., and J. S. Oktay. Mental Disorder and Primary Medical Care: An Analytical Review of the Literature. NIMH Series D, USDHEW Publ. No. (ADM)78-661. Washington, DC: National Institute of Mental Health, 1979.

Hayami, D. E., and D. K. Freeborn. Effect of coverage on use of an HMO alcoholism treatment program, outcome, and medical care utilization. Am. J. Public Health 71(10):1133-1143, 1981.

Herrington, R. E., P. R. Riordan, and G. R. Jacobson. Alcohol and other drug dependence in adolescence: Characteristics of those who seek treatment, and outcome of treatment. Currents in Alcoholism 8:253-267, 1981.

Holder, H. D. Alcoholism treatment and potential health care cost savings. Med. Care 25(1):52-71, 1987.

Holder, H. D., and J. O. Blose. Alcoholism treatment and total health care utilization and costs: A four-year longitudinal analysis of federal employees. J. Am. Med. Assoc. 256(11):1456-1460, 1986.

Holder, H. D., and J. B. Hallan. Impact of alcoholism treatment on total health care costs: A six-year study. Advances in Alcohol and Substance Abuse 6(1):1-15, 1986.

Holder, H. D., and R. H. Shachtman. Estimating health care savings associated with alcoholism. Alcoholism Clin. Exp. Res. 11(1):66-72, 1987.

Hornbrook, M. C. Mental health services in HMOs: An oxymoron? Administration in Mental Health. 15(4):236-245, 1988.

Jellinek, E. M. The Disease Concept of Alcoholism. New Haven, CT: College and University Press, 1960.

Jones, K. R., and T. R. Vischi. Impact of alcohol, drug abuse and mental health treatment on medical care utilization: A review of the research literature. Med. Care 17:1-82, 1979.

Kessler, L. G., D. M. Steinwachs, and J. R. Hankin. Episodes of psychiatric care and medical utilization. Med. Care 20(12):1209-1221, 1982.

Klinge, V., K. Lennox, and H. Vaziri. Follow-up of adolescent drug abusers and nonusers previously hospitalized in an inpatient psychiatric facility. Drug Forum 6(2):143-151, 1977-1978.

Kogan, W. S., D. J. Thompson, J. R. Brown et al. Impact of integration of mental health service and comprehensive medical care. Med. Care 13:934-942, 1975.

Kurtz, N. R., B. Googins, and W. C. Howard. Measuring the success of occupational alcoholism programs. J. Stud. Alcohol 45(1):33-45, 1984.

Longabaugh, R. Longitudinal outcome studies. Pp. 267-280 in R. M. Rose and J. E. Barrett, eds. Alcoholism: Origins and Outcome. New York: Raven Press, 1988.

Longabaugh, R., and M. Beattie. Optimizing the cost effectiveness of treatment for alcohol abusers. Pp. 104-136 in B. McCrady, N. E. Noel, and T. D. Nirenberg, eds. Future Directions in Alcohol Abuse Treatment Research. Washington, DC: NIAAA, 1985.

Longabaugh, R., B. McCrady, E. Fink et al. Cost effectiveness of alcoholism treatment in partial vs. inpatient settings: Six-month outcomes. J. Stud. Alcohol 44(6):1049-1071, 1983.

Manning, W. G., K. B. Wells, N. Duan et al. How cost sharing affects the use of ambulatory mental health services. J. Am. Med. Assoc. 256:1930-1934, 1986.

McCrady, B., R. Longabaugh, E. Fink et al. Cost-effectiveness of alcoholism treatment in partial versus inpatient settings after brief inpatient treatment: 12-month outcomes. J. Consult. Clin. Psychol. 54(5):708-713, 1986.

McKinlay, J. Some approaches and problems in the study of the use of services: An overview. J. Health Soc. Behav. 13:115-152, 1972.

Mechanic, D. Correlates of physician utilization: Why do major multivariate studies of physician utilization find trivial psychosocial and organizational effects? J. Health Soc. Behav. 20(4):387-396, 1979.

Miller, W. R., and R. K. Hester. Inpatient alcoholism treatment: Who benefits? Am. Psychologist 41(7):794-805, 1986.

National Institute on Alcohol Abuse and Alcoholism. Benefit-Cost Analysis of Alcoholism Treatment Centers, vols. 1 and 2. Prepared for NIAAA by the JWK International Corporation. NTIS (PB-253419). Springfield, VA: National Technical Information Service, 1976.

National Institute on Alcohol Abuse and Alcoholism. Health insurance coverage for alcoholism treatment. USDHHS Special Selection. Alcohol Health Res. World 5(4):2-41, 1981.

Orvis, B. R., D. Armor, C. Williams et al. Effectiveness and Cost of Alcohol Rehabilitation in the United States Air Force. A Project Air Force Report (R-2813-AF). Santa Monica, CA: Rand Corporation, 1981.

Parron, D. L., and F. Solomon, eds. Mental Health Services in Primary Care Settings. DHHS Publ. No. (ADM)80-995. Washington, DC: Government Printing Office, 1980.

Parker, D. L., J. M. Schultz, L. Gertz et al. The social and economic costs of alcohol abuse in Minnesota, 1983. Am. J. Public Health 77(8):982-986, 1987.

Plotnick, D. E., K. M. Adams, K. R. Hunter et al. Alcoholism Treatment Programs Within Prepaid Group Practice HMOs: A Final Report. Washington, DC: Group Health Association of America, 1982.

Putnam, S. Short-term effects of treating alcoholics for alcoholism on their utilization of medical care services in a health maintenance organization. Group Health J. 3(1):19-30, 1982.

Saxe, L., D. Dougherty, K. Esty et al. The Effectiveness and Costs of Alcoholism Treatment. Health Technology Case Study No. 22, Washington, DC: U.S. Congress, Office of Technology Assessment, 1983.

Schlesinger, H. J., E. Mumford, V. Glass et al. Mental health treatment and medical care utilization in a fee-for-service system: Outpatient mental health treatment following the onset of a chronic disease. Am. J. Public Health 73(4):422-429, 1983.

Sells, S. B., and D. O. Simpson. Evaluation of treatment outcome for youths in the Drug Abuse Reporting Program (DARP): A follow-up study. Pp. 571-628 in G. M. Beschner and A. S. Friedman, eds. Youth Drug Abuse. Lexington, MA: D.C. Heath, 1979.

Shapiro, S., E. Skinner, L. Kessler et al. Utilization of health and mental health services. Arch. Gen. Psychiatry 41:971-978, 1984.

Sherman, R. M., S. Reiff, and A. B. Forsythe. Utilization of medical services by alcoholics participating in an outpatient treatment program. Alcoholism Clin. Exp. Res. 3:115-120, 1979.

Spiegel, R., and W. L. Mock. A model for a family systems theory approach to prevention and treatment of alcohol abusing youth. Presented at the National Council on Alcoholism conference in St. Louis, MO, May 1978.

Tessler, R., and D. Mechanic. Factors affecting children's use of physician services in a prepaid group practice. Med. Care 16(1):33-46, 1978.

Tobler, N. S. Meta-analysis of 143 adolescent drug prevention programs: Quantitative outcome results of program participants compared to a control or comparison group. J. Drug Issues 16(4):537-567, 1986.

Vaillant, G. E., W. Clark, C. Cyrus et al. Prospective study of alcoholism treatment: Eight year follow-up. Am. J. Med. 75:455-463, 1983.

Vollmer, H. Pp. 417-434 in P. Golding, ed. Alcoholism, A Modern Perspective. Richmond, NJ: G. A. Bogden, 1982.

Wan, T., and J. S. Soifer. Determinants of physician utilization: A causal analysis. J. Health Soc. Behav. 15(2):100-108, 1974.

Wersinger, R., J. Roberts, K. Roghmann et al. The inpatient hospital and ambulatory utilization experience of an alcoholic population compared to a matched control group within an HMO. In Proceedings of the 28th Annual Group Health Institute, New York, June 18-21, 1978. Washington, DC: Group Health Association of America, 1978.

Westermeyer, J., and E. Peake. A ten-year follow-up of alcoholic Native Americans in Minnesota. Am. J. Psychiatry 140(2):189-194, 1983.

Wolinsky, F. D. Assessing the effects of predisposing, enabling and illness morbidity characteristics on health services utilization. J. Health Soc. Behav. 19(4):384-396, 1978.

III

SUPPORT FOR SCIENTIFIC PROGRESS IN THE PREVENTION AND TREATMENT OF ALCOHOL-RELATED PROBLEMS

INTRODUCTION

Exploiting the opportunities delineated in the preceding pages requires a scientific infrastructure adequate to the task. Part III concludes the committee's discussion of research opportunities in the prevention and treatment of alcohol problems with a consideration of the infrastructural elements necessary to support such efforts. Chapter 15 examines federal support for the scientific infrastructure for prevention research, and Chapter 16 explores similar issues for treatment research.

15

SUPPORTING THE SCIENTIFIC INFRASTRUCTURE
FOR PREVENTION RESEARCH

The National Institute on Alcohol Abuse and Alcoholism now allocates $5.5 million, approximately 9 percent of its total budget for extramural research and research training, to prevention research (including research on safety and trauma). The most common form of research support is the investigator-initiated (RO1) project grant. The kinds of research topics that are investigated under this mechanism include early intervention, risk precursors, high-risk groups, health promotion, prevention modalities, the influence of law and policies, and other miscellaneous topics. One of NIAAA's 12 alcohol research centers is devoted exclusively to prevention. Almost all of the prevention research projects currently funded by the institute are devoted either to basic or to applied research in the early hypothesis-testing stages.

In the 1970s, NIAAA supported several community-based intervention programs through its Division of Prevention; however, the Prevention Demonstration and Education Program was discontinued when funding for community treatment and prevention programs became part of the block grants for the states. Funding decisions on the community-based prevention research grants that NIAAA did fund were primarily based on the perceived quality of the proposed intervention components, with little effort made to ensure sound evaluation. Consequently, information about outcomes or intervention efficacy was limited. Since then, however, much has been learned about outcome evaluation. The experience and sophistication gained through the demonstration and education research grants programs funded by the National Heart, Lung, and Blood Institute (NHLBI) and by the National Cancer Institute (NCI) have provided new insights into the way future alcohol problem prevention programs might be designed, implemented, and evaluated.

Federally directed funding for community prevention programs again became available after the passage of the Omnibus Anti-Drug Abuse Act of 1986. Under this act, $24 million was appropriated for demonstration projects administered by the Office of Substance Abuse Prevention (OSAP) working directly under the administrator of the Alcohol, Drug Abuse and Mental Health Administration (ADAMHA). To date, 131 demonstration projects have been initiated. Program evaluation, however, was not included as a requirement in the initial announcement. These demonstration projects are sponsored mainly by local community organizations (55 percent) and by state and county agencies (22 percent). University-based programs account for only 12 percent of the total. Although there has been an effort on the part of OSAP to institute outcome evaluation through contract mechanisms, at this time it is unclear whether such remedial after-the-fact action will be sufficient. There may not be enough expertise in the contract
research community to meet this challenge. Should the federal government decide to continue this prevention demonstration program on substance abuse (both alcohol and drug), it should specify an outcome evaluation component as necessary for every funded site.

The existing OSAP demonstration programs are in the early stages of applied research (i.e., "component" research) and are heavily targeted toward special populations. Yet without outcome evaluation, intervention effectiveness cannot be assessed; in addition, the testing of hypotheses, if it is assumed that the programs were conceived according to existing theory and basic research knowledge, will not be possible. Prevention trials should become an established tradition at NIAAA, as they are at the National Institutes of Health (NIH). A significant opportunity now exists for NIAAA, the National Institute on Drug Abuse (NIDA), and OSAP to conduct controlled prevention demonstration projects with well-designed evaluation components. Future funding of prevention demonstration projects under federal anti-drug abuse initiatives should include at least a 5 to 20 percent set-aside for the joint design and evaluation of prevention trials by NIAAA, NIDA, and OSAP. Such controlled prevention demonstration projects require participation by both program design and outcome evaluation researchers. A central position for researchers in developing the total program has been a key factor in the success of NHLBI and NCI community trials.

Mechanisms of Support for Prevention Research

The traditional mechanisms of federal research funding (investigator-initiated "RO1s," center grants, etc.) are appropriate for funding basic research and much of the applied research in prevention. The kinds of needed studies that can be supported readily in these ways include pilot projects, prototype studies, controlled intervention trials, and studies of defined populations. Although NIH also uses traditional mechanisms for the support of community-based demonstration and education research projects, the cost of such projects relative to the total research budget of NIAAA might make these funding mechanisms somewhat unrealistic.

The committee recommends the following:

• Major preventive trials involving comprehensive, multiyear research efforts at several sites are necessary to establish the effectiveness and generalizability of interventions aimed at preventing alcohol problems. Funding such trials through a separate budget line, for both new and recurring initiatives, would be preferable to traditional mechanisms of support.
• Outcome evaluation should be specified as an integral part of any program.
• Cooperative agreements of the type suggested for treatment research (see Chapter 16) would help to standardize methodology and coordinate research directions.
• There is often a need for rapid review of a prevention research proposal. For example, obtaining baseline data when new laws are passed is difficult, given the time allotted for proposal review. Response to changes in the legal environment (e.g., tax hikes or labeling laws) also requires rapid response. The committee proposes the development of a mechanism to expedite the review of proposals for the study of rapidly implemented legal and regulatory interventions.

Infrastructure Needs

A network of expertise in outcome evaluation is needed to help NIAAA and scientists interested in alcohol prevention research. The expertise and experience developed through the Planned Approach to Community Health (PATCH) program of the Centers for Disease Control (CDC), the Stanford Center for Research in Disease Prevention, and other research teams that have conducted successful research demonstration programs should be marshaled in this effort.

The committee recommends the following:

- A successful program should develop a research team that includes scientists with expertise in alcohol-specific issues, research design and evaluation, and implementation. The training of personnel in all of these areas is needed. The communications and community assistance divisions of OSAP might also be directed toward these areas of expertise.
- NIAAA should take the lead in coordinating alcohol prevention/intervention research efforts in collaboration with other federal agencies including the Veterans Administration, the Department of Defense, the Department of Transportation, the Department of Education, and other branches of the Department of Health and Human Services.
- Prevention demonstration and education research projects similar to the Stanford University Three-Community/Five-City projects could be developed through the Department of Defense.
- Research on the effects of changes in regulation and policy might be jointly sponsored by NIAAA and the Department of Transportation.

Community Initiatives

A support mechanism is needed that can respond to prevention efforts arising from community initiatives that represent new or unique research opportunities. Existing research funding mechanisms may not be suitable for these novel initiatives. Programs and activities that communities develop themselves are more likely to utilize available resources and may have a greater chance of long-term survival than programs initiated in response to outside funding, utilizing researchers who are not part of the community.

- It is proposed that initial funding be made available to communities for planning and development if the local initiative is judged to be a worthwhile research opportunity. This initial support could be followed by funding for assistance with implementation, data collection, and outcome evaluation. In all of these efforts, the community would be provided with help from collaborating researchers. The initial planning and development phase could have a fixed cost but need not be time limited. In this way the community would not be compelled to apply for funds to implement a program before adequate community support existed. The cooperative efforts of OSAP and NIAAA could be especially helpful in this regard.
- The provision of technical expertise to prevention programs that are already under way would enable a community to undertake program evaluation and outcome data collection. This kind of funding would ensure that outcome evaluation is performed and, consequently, that what is learned from a given initiative is transferable to other communities. Such a support mechanism for community initiatives in prevention research does not presently exist. However, if it were instituted, it would substantially increase the benefits obtained from prevention research and would stimulate the initiation of local prevention activities. Most of this opportunity is now missed. Again, close cooperation between OSAP and NIAAA could be critically helpful to committees and prevention researchers.

Cooperative Studies

A research strategy that ultimately leads to prevention programming will require a collaborative design and highly coordinated analyses. Collaborative studies involving several research laboratories have been successful. An example is the multihospital studies of the phenothiazine treatment of schizophrenia in the early 1960s.

A system is needed that will connect research groups in cooperative studies that combine individual strengths, and support strong theoretical and methodological integration, while allowing for continued independence as appropriate. It is necessary to determine with what degree of success this has been accomplished in other research areas. For example, in recent years, foundations have supported small networks or consortia of selected research teams with longitudinal interests in factors relating to mental health. In the alcohol field, federal support is needed on a larger scale than is likely to be provided by private sources. Therefore, various mechanisms (consortia, cooperative agreements, etc.) should be explored as NIAAA seeks to provide leadership in this area. With such leadership, a structure should emerge that fosters the exchange of information among research groups in the early and intermediate stages of their preventive research activities and perhaps lead to the planning of joint research projects.

NIAAA is to be commended for the organizational steps it has taken to foster cross-fertilization from different investigative areas. It should continue in this endeavor. Indeed, prevention research could not proceed if it were isolated from other research areas. The fragmentation of different aspects of NIAAA's mission could result in lost or delayed research opportunities--a risk shared by other research agencies. The committee also commends NIAAA for the steps it has taken, and should continue to take, in the direction of integrating biobehavioral, biomedical, psychosocial, and prevention research categories. The committee recommends that NIAAA continue to work actively to promote collaborative strategies and new prevention research initiatives.

In addition, the committee makes the following recommendations for a collaborative prevention research strategy:

   • Collaborative examination is required of existing longitudinal data bases. Analyses are needed in which a laboratory would attempt to replicate specifically chosen findings from other laboratories.
   • Collaborative design of new studies should be undertaken, and this process should specify the population samples from which the data are to be collected. Planning should include the possibility of extending existing longitudinal data bases to allow for additional follow-up.
   • Experimental interventions can be analyzed by taking known predictors of substance use into account. In addition, some existing data can be reanalyzed, and new preventive intervention trials can be designed which are directed at early antecedents that have not yet been addressed. The purpose of these experimental interventions is to understand the function of the specific predictors in the causal paths leading to heavy alcohol use and other outcomes. After preventive intervention evaluation studies, researchers will be in a position to recommend a national policy on alcohol abuse and to help design and implement prevention interventions aimed at specific antecedents.

16

SUPPORTING THE SCIENTIFIC INFRASTRUCTURE
FOR TREATMENT RESEARCH

Steady progress has been made over the last decade in increasing the alcohol research budget. In 1980, NIAAA's research support was $22.2 million, which included 167 research projects. By fiscal year 1989, the institute's total research funding had grown to $107.1 million with 485 grants supported. Linked to this growth has been a significant improvement in the knowledge base dealing with the biomedical and psychosocial aspects of alcohol problems (IOM, 1987). NIAAA supports programs of intramural and extramural research that span basic, clinical, and epidemiological studies. Unfortunately, not until 1988, when NIAAA created its new Division of Clinical and Prevention Research, was treatment research given a prominent place in the research portfolio. This previous lack of support is reflected in the relatively small portions of the intramural (14 percent) and extramural (12 percent) research budgets that are devoted to treatment-related research.

Until now NIAAA has relied on two mechanisms to fund treatment research: the investigator-initiated (R01) grant and the research center. NIAAA funds a treatment research center at the University of Connecticut Health Center in Farmington. The Veterans Administration (VA) also funds a clinical research center at the San Diego VA Hospital and has provided some support for treatment trials through its Merit Review Program and through two multicenter collaborative studies. The NIAAA and VA research support mechanisms have together led to improvements in methodology and theory and to a slowly expanding pool of researchers and facilities.

However, one recent development that provokes serious concern is the cutback in the fiscal year 1989 budget for VA health care programs. This cutback has already resulted in the closing of alcohol treatment programs that were linked to important NIAAA- and VA-funded research. Moreover, the new impediments that have been raised to the admission to VA hospitals of non-service-connected or indigent veterans will have a disastrous effect on a number of major clinical and basic alcohol research programs.

Recently, the ADAMHA Office of Substance Abuse Prevention (OSAP) initiated support through large-scale grants for a high-risk-youth demonstration project and community-based programs, but these funding mechanisms have not provided adequate support for systematic evaluation. For the federal government to begin to exploit the opportunities in treatment research described in this report, it must address the need within the alcohol field to develop a scientific infrastructure appropriate to the task. It is a challenge whose dimensions have been previously charted by treatment and prevention research efforts at the National Institutes of Health (NIH)--particularly the National Cancer Institute; the National Heart, Lung, and Blood Institute; and the National Institute on Allergy and Infectious Diseases in its program of AIDS research. Maintaining support for agencies and programs that provide this infrastructure is essential.

Recent reviews of treatment efficacy (Saxe et al., 1983; Lettieri, Sayers, and Nelson, 1984; Tims and Ludford, 1984; Miller and Hester, 1986) identified approximately 200 controlled studies. Few of these studies, however, employed advanced clinical assessment methodologies (e.g., assessments of comorbid psychopathology or severity of dependence). Similarly, although 150 random assignment trials have been conducted, few have been devoted to comparisons of treatment modalities or settings in relation to outcome. Studies of treatment efficacy are needed to define the dimensions of treatment outcome in relation to the expected effects of treatment. Research should be designed and funded in such a way that treatment effects can be examined not only at the termination of treatment but (at least) one year beyond in order to investigate the potential enduring benefits of certain treatment modalities and settings.

Although clinical trials were introduced as a method of scientific investigation before 1945 and have been used extensively in psychiatry and medicine since then, it is only recently that large-scale clinical trials have been conducted in alcoholism treatment research (Fuller et al., 1986). The relative dearth of controlled trials and treatment matching research (see, for example, Skinner, 1981) is in part a result of the lack of funding in this area and the formidable practical and methodological challenges to researchers.

In the early development of new treatment modalities (e.g., a new pharmacotherapy for the treatment of alcohol withdrawal), the investigator-initiated grant application (R01) can be utilized effectively to compare the new modality with established treatment practice. Random assignment to treatment is highly desirable in this type of study. The investigator-initiated grant may also be the mechanism of choice for studies of well-specified treatment populations (e.g., minorities, women, military personnel, specific age cohorts) in which the investigator has special access to the particular patient or client group. One major disadvantage of the R01 application for these types of studies has been the traditional limited funding period associated with this grant. Three years of funding may not be adequate to initiate a study, collect a cohort of clients/patients who meet the research criteria, and conduct adequate follow-up of a sufficient number of subjects at least 12 months after the treatment intervention. Treatment research grant announcements should strongly encourage four- and five-year awards, with the requirement that the proposal include adequate follow-up of a sufficient number of subjects for at least one year after the treatment intervention.

Treatment research methods are often shaped by the requirements of the treatment program, a factor that may limit the rigor of the research design. These studies are of necessity scientifically less exact and more complex and difficult than other projects reviewed by the existing grant review committees. There is a need to increase the number of qualified treatment researchers through increased support for postdoctoral training in relevant specialities (e.g., psychiatry, psychology, internal medicine, family medicine, epidemiology, sociology, health care economics). The Scientist Development Award for Clinicians appears to be an excellent vehicle for the career development of young investigators interested in treatment (and prevention) research, but the present maximum stipend of $45,000 per year is not adequate salary support for young physicians.

Center grants offer another vehicle for studying treatment research. For example, the National Institute on Drug Abuse (NIDA) recently established three treatment research centers with the stated goal of "systematically test[ing] existing and new treatment strategies in well-controlled designs." Because of the need to develop large subject samples, NIDA urged applicants to "consider the advantages of coordination between related studies, and between Centers doing similar work." NIDA emphasized its interest in developing treatment process as well as outcome data; it also urged the funded centers to develop research training opportunities. In some respects, the new NIDA program is modeled after NIAAA's highly successful, but more broadly based, alcohol research centers program.

Only one of 12 NIAAA centers conducts alcohol treatment research. The latter program includes studies at three sites: a VA hospital, a treatment program within a university hospital, and a large outpatient program within a mental health center at a neighboring university. Affiliations with several other institutions in the area have been essential to this center in its efforts to maintain an adequate and diverse patient base for its treatment research programs. (A postdoctoral research training program is also part of the core activities of that center.) The committee suggests that NIAAA consider funding one or more additional centers devoted to treatment research in collaboration with another federal agency (e.g., the VA or the Department of Defense) or in conjunction with one of the state-funded alcohol research centers.

A significant proportion of the alcohol treatment in this country takes place in freestanding inpatient units that are generally not affiliated with major academic and research centers. The rapid growth in the number of inpatient beds in proprietary and nonprofit facilities over the past 15 years (Yahr, 1988) has stimulated a strong interest in research on treatment settings and the matching of patient subtypes to specific treatments. This interest has been expressed in many quarters: the Congress, the executive branch of the federal government, the insurance industry, and the treatment community. Since the introduction of the block grant program, NIAAA has lost its ability to evaluate community-based treatment programs as it did in the 1970s through contracts with the Rand Corporation (Armor, Polich, and Stambul, 1978; Polich, Armor, and Braiker, 1981). The Rand studies were generally limited by the sparseness of patient assessments, but the large number of subjects who were studied across a wide variety of treatment settings provided important information on differential routes to recovery among patients/clients who differed in the severity of their alcohol dependence.

The committee commends the recent policy decision to set aside 5 to 15 percent of funds within block grants to evaluate alcohol and drug abuse treatment programs and to determine the quality and appropriateness of various forms of treatment (including the effect of living in the types of housing provided in these programs). The evaluations are to be funded through grants, contracts, or cooperative agreements provided to public and nonprofit private entities. This policy could well encourage linkages among university-affiliated researchers, state agencies, and not-for-profit treatment facilities.

A potentially important initiative was launched recently by a programmatic decision by the leadership at NIAAA and NIDA to utilize the funds appropriated through Section 1923 of the Public Health Service Act (an amendment added by the Anti-Drug Abuse Act of 1986) to fund grants for up to five years to evaluate alcohol and cocaine treatments. Unfortunately, the conditions of the appropriation mandated annual awards, with continuation contingent on the availability of funds "and progress achieved." New grant money in the amount of $2.3 million was made available for this purpose in fiscal year 1988. This program could be limited in achieving its stated goals because of uncertainties regarding long-term funding and a failure to address the need to develop treatment research networks of adequate size and diversity. This uncertainty about long-term support could have a negative impact on the scientific dimensions of these evaluations and will also make it more difficult to attract competent investigators to this important research area.

To systematically examine questions that relate to treatment setting and treatment matching, it is essential to develop an adequate number of treatment facilities willing to participate in controlled treatment trials. In this context, specific funds must be set aside for thorough patient assessments at intake and at the follow-up point. These assessments must be conducted with a high degree of reliability within and between sites. The optimal mechanisms for this type of study would appear to be the "cooperative agreement" within the Public Health Service and the "collaborative study" within the VA. As an example of the latter, the conduct of the VA collaborative study on disulfiram (Fuller et al., 1986) has been especially instructive. This study involved nine sites and 14 investigators. Out of an initial pool of 6,629, researchers recruited 605 subjects. The small pool of eligible subjects for this study highlights the formidable logistical problems involved in well-controlled treatment research. The results also highlight the importance of rigorous experimental design in these studies (Fuller et al., 1986).

Table 16-1 compares regular research grants with cooperative agreements. Under a cooperative agreement, institute staff work with the scientific community in a cooperative venture. Institute staff and consultants assist colleagues in the scientific community in the design of the study, project coordination, and the dissemination of research results. As a mechanism for ensuring close cooperation between treatment facilities and investigators, and as a means of securing large treatment samples from multiple sites, the cooperative agreement is preferable to investigator-initiated grants.

Experience at NIH suggests that the cooperative agreement is an especially useful instrument for the rapid transfer of knowledge from research to clinical practice. Examples of cooperative agreements include the new network of AIDS clinical studies being funded by the National Institute on Allergy and Infectious Disease and the Clinical Trials Cooperative Groups supported by the National Cancer Institute (NCI). In the NCI program, each project typically includes physicians from multiple medical centers who cooperatively design and conduct clinical trials to evaluate treatment of various types and stages of cancer. The data are collected and analyzed in a coordinating center. Most of the participants are located at major medical centers in urban areas. The program was further extended in 1976 to include the participation of physicians at community hospitals and in private practice.

Similarly, the National Heart, Lung, and Blood Institute has funded placebo-controlled trials in a multicenter program for the treatment of cardiac arrhythmia. Cooperative agreements have also been utilized to test new diagnostic instruments. The National Institute of Mental Health (NIMH), an ADAMHA institute, has used the cooperative agreement mechanism to fund a multicenter collaborative study of depression to determine whether different aspects of the disorder respond to different treatments (pharmacotherapy versus psychotherapy). NIAAA is initiating cooperative agreements in fiscal year 1989, including a multisite trial of alcoholism treatment that involves patient-treatment matching.

The use of the cooperative agreement to fund large-scale alcohol treatment research should be encouraged. Similar to the VA collaborative study of disulfiram (Fuller et al., 1986), the data from such treatment studies will benefit both the research and the clinical communities. NIAAA staff could play a critical role in bringing together a network of investigators and a variety of treatment facilities from the public and private sectors. In this context, the requirements both of research design and of clinical practice can be considered. NIAAA, the VA, the Health Care Financing Administration, and the Department of Defense should also consider developing cost-sharing arrangements with interested states, universities, service providers, and third-party payers.

Table 16-1. Distinguishing Between Grants and Cooperative Agreements

Element	Grant	Cooperative Agreement
Intent	Support or stimulation to accomplish a public purpose	Support or stimulation to accomplish a public purpose
Scope of work	Any program activity eligible under NIH/ADAMHA legistation	Any program activity eligible under NIH/ADAMHA legislation
Initiation	Applicant initiated; may be in response to an RFA or PA	Awarding a component initiated through an RFA or PA
NIH/ADAMHA role	Normal programmatic and administrative stewardship responsibilities; no substantial programmatic involvement	Normal stewardship responsibilities plus substantial programmatic involvement during performance of award
Examples of staff participation	Providing technical assistance at the recipient's request	Participating in the design of activities
	Close monitoring of an external organization	Advising in the selection of contractors, trainees, staff, etc.
	Ensuring compliance with policy requirements and terms of award	Coordinating or participating in the collection and/or analysis of data
	Evaluating performance through progress reports and site visits	Advising in training and selection of project staff
		Reviewing and approving each stage of a clinical trial
		Advising on management and technical performance
		Participation in the preparation of publications
		Participation in all responsibilities required by grants

It should be recognized that multisite clinical trials are difficult to implement. Problems in this type of research include control over the therapies being delivered, quality control over the selection and training of therapists, and developing an effective means of monitoring day-to-day implementation of the research and clinical protocols. Cooperative studies are best carried out after smaller, single-site studies have been conducted; such smaller-scale research allows for careful specification and testing of procedures. Cooperative efforts are easiest to implement in drug and assessment studies; they are most feasible when the treatments under investigation are well specified, time limited, and relatively easily taught.

Finally, in any consideration of scientific infrastructure, the federal government needs to consider the personnel requirements that are essential to the conduct of treatment research. In 1986, NIAAA supported four postdoctoral and two career development stipends that could be classified as treatment research. In conjunction with the centers program and the proposed cooperative agreements, NIAAA should target funding for additional scientists in treatment research careers including epidemiologists, social and behavioral psychologists, physicians (psychiatrists, internists, family physicians), health services researchers, and biostatisticians.

Within the institute, new initiatives in the area of treatment research should be complemented by the active use of outside consultants, planning panels, and other mechanisms, such as the proposed Clinical Staff Program for Prevention and Treatment Research. This program is designed to provide greater interaction among the intramural research program, the extramural research program, and clinicians/researchers in the field. This mechanism should also be used to attract visiting scientists to the institute for one- or two-year periods.

Over the years NIAAA has developed a number of programs and activities that are capable of stimulating research, facilitating technology transfer, and providing expert advice to the field. These include not only research grants, training grants, the Alcohol Research Centers program, and cooperative agreements but also planning panels, expert committee meetings, research conferences, technical reviews, bilateral international agreements, interagency agreements, contracts, and the intramural research program. NIAAA is also using a developmental grant mechanism (R21) that offers up to two years of support ($40,000 in direct costs per year) to assist institutions in building their capacity to do alcoholism treatment research; conducting pilot studies that lead to expansion, enhancement, or modification of existing treatment research programs; and planning and conducting pilot research that can lead to the development of clinical trials. Projects aimed at the treatment of alcoholism in special groups such as women, minorities, and defined age groups (e.g., adolescents and the elderly) have been encouraged under this mechanism.

There appears to be sufficient flexibility in NIAAA's operational mechanisms to permit the implementation of the treatment research opportunities outlined in Part II of this report. As new funding and funding mechanisms are brought into play, NIAAA should evaluate the experience of other agencies that have been involved in clinical trials and large-scale collaborative studies. For instance, NIDA has devoted a substantial proportion of its research budget to treatment grants and has supported a longitudinal evaluation of drug treatment programs (called the Treatment Outcome Perspective Study) since 1978. NIMH has sponsored the NIMH Treatment of Depression Collaborative Research Program through cooperative agreements with seven participating sites. The VA supports investigator-initiated treatment grants through its Merit Review System and has sponsored the VA collaborative study of disulfiram.

International research may also offer some guidance. The alcohol research program of the World Health Organization (WHO) has initiated international collaborative projects in the areas of screening, early intervention, community responses to alcohol problems, and the comparison of alcoholism treatment systems. These projects are typically funded through cooperative agreements among collaborating research centers and health ministries. One WHO program that has been beneficial to treatment research in the United States is the WHO/ADAMHA program on nomenclature and classification of mental disorders and alcohol- or drug-related problems. This program has facilitated the standardization of nomenclature and diagnostic procedures with respect to alcohol-use disorders. It has also led to the development of new diagnostic instruments that promise to assist treatment planning and epidemiological research.

These programs not only serve as models for achieving some of NIAAA's goals for treatment research, they also indicate that there may be large areas of common interest among the various national and international agencies engaged in treatment research. These indications take on added vitality in light of the growing participation of state and private agencies in alcohol treatment research and program evaluation. A number of state agencies now engage in treatment evaluation through their own information systems or in cooperation with state-supported research centers. In addition, several private hospital groups have established treatment evaluation components. What is needed is for NIAAA to coordinate activities, divide responsibilities, and share data among the agencies and organizations involved in similar pursuits. Given the recognized leadership position that NIAAA has achieved in the field of treatment, the institute is in a unique position to form a network of mutually beneficial partnerships among various agencies and organizations that are involved in similar activities. By coordinating activities among such interest groups as research centers, pharmaceutical companies, hospital chains, insurance companies, single state agencies, and federal agencies, NIAAA may be able to guide the field toward a more coherent course of action.

The committee makes the following recommendations for funding treatment research:

• The present research program of investigator-initiated grants should be enhanced to encourage the funding of treatment research for periods up to five years. This expansion will allow for start-up work and at least one year of posttreatment evaluation.
• There is a need to increase the pool of treatment research investigators. This goal can be achieved by a variety of mechanisms including support of M.D./Ph.D. programs in medical schools targeted toward clinical investigators in alcoholism. The newly initiated Scientist Development Award for Clinicians should help to create a pool of young investigators interested in treatment research.
• NIAAA should play a leadership role in bringing interested groups together to support treatment research in the alcohol field. The National Heart, Lung, and Blood Institute is interested in the effects of abstinence or reduced drinking on hypertension secondary to excessive alcohol use. NIDA is interested in the treatment of polysubstance abuse including cocaine, opiates, and alcohol. NIMH is interested in the comorbidity of psychotic disorders and substance abuse. The VA and the Department of Defense have a strong interest in alcoholism treatment. The Department of Transportation also has an interest in alcoholism treatment because excessive alcohol use can affect safety on roads and railroads, in sea lanes and rivers, and in the air. Insurance companies and state, not-for-profit, and proprietary alcoholism treatment programs all have a stake in treatment outcome research.

• Recent actions by the VA to curtail the availability of alcoholism treatment will have a devastating impact on treatment research in the alcohol field. Given the high percentage of veterans with alcohol-related pathology who are hospitalized on medical/surgical units in VA hospitals, the committee recommends that the VA reverse these actions and renew its commitment to alcohol treatment and treatment research.

• The program to use funds appropriated in the 1986 Anti-Drug Abuse Act to support controlled trials of alcohol and cocaine treatment should be stabilized, extended, and used as a model for the evaluation of all federally supported treatment initiatives. Similarly, the recent decision to allocate a percentage of block grant funds to evaluation provides an opportunity to advance carefully designed process and outcome evaluation as an integral component of treatment programs supported by the federal government and implemented at the state level. This initiative should be used to encourage cooperation between academic and research institutions on the one hand and publicly supported treatment programs on the other.

• Cooperative agreements should be implemented as a mechanism for funding complex, multisite treatment outcome studies and clinical trials. NIAAA should be provided with the personnel resources to provide proper staffing of these initiatives.

• NIAAA should encourage the inclusion of salary support on grants for clinical facility personnel involved in treatment evaluation research as a means of encouraging the participation of such facilities in treatment trials. Salary support should be identified on individual grant proposals and within cooperative agreements.

• NIAAA should continue to highlight the state of the art in treatment research studies by establishing and upgrading guidelines for quality designs and methods of treatment research.

REFERENCES

Armor, D. J., J. M. Polich, and H. B. Stambul. Alcoholism and Treatment. New York: John Wiley and Sons, 1978.

Fuller, R. K., L. Branchey, D. R. Brightwell et al. Disulfiram treatment of alcoholism. A Veterans Administration cooperative study. J. Am. Med. Assoc. 256:1449-1255, 1986.

Institute of Medicine. Causes and Consequences of Alcohol Problems: An Agenda for Research. Washington, DC: National Academy Press, 1987.

Lettieri, D., M. Sayers, and J. Nelson. Summaries of Alcoholism Treatment Assessment Research. NIAAA Treatment Handbook Series, vol. 1. Washington, DC: Government Printing Office, 1984.

Miller, W. R., and R. K. Hester. Inpatient alcoholism treatment: Who benefits? Am. Psychol. 41(7):794-805, 1986.

Polich, J. M., D. J. Armor, and H. B. Braiker. The Course of Alcoholism: Four Years After Treatment. New York: John Wiley and Sons, 1981.

Saxe, L., D. Dougherty, K. Esty, and M. Fine. The effectiveness and costs of alcoholism treatment. Health Technology Case Study 22. Office of Technology Assessment, U.S. Congress. Washington, DC: Government Printing Office, 1983.

Skinner, H. A. Different strokes for different folks: Differential treatment for alcohol abuse. Pp. 349-368 in Evaluation of the Alcoholic: Implications for Research, Theory, and Treatment. NIAAA Research Monograph No. 5. Rockville, MD: NIAAA, 1981.

Tims, F., and J. Ludford. Drug Abuse Treatment Evaluation: Strategies, Progress and Prospects. National Institute on Drug Abuse Monograph Series, vol. 51. Washington, DC: Government Printing Office, 1984.

Yahr, H. T. A national comparison of public and private-sector alcoholism treatment delivery system characteristics. J. Stud. Alcohol 49:233-239, 1988.

ACKNOWLEDGMENTS

Steering committee members, panelists, and Institute of Medicine staff officers gratefully acknowledge the contributions of a number of persons who helped significantly in reviewing material that eventually was synthesized into this committee report. Special recognition is due Sandra Putnam, of the Rhode Island Department of Health, for her major contributions to Chapter 14, "Treatment Costs, Benefits and Cost Offsets." Similarly, Robert Saltz, of the Pacific Institute for Research and Evaluation, served as a consultant on several of the areas encompassed in the first section of the report on prevention research and epidemiology.

In addition to Drs. Putnam and Saltz, several other consultants to the study provided assistance that was greatly appreciated:

John Buckner, School of Hygiene and Public Health, The Johns Hopkins University

Mary R. Casement, Rockville, Maryland

Diana Cassady, University of California at Berkeley

Zelig Dolinsky, University of Connecticut Health Center

Michael Hofmann, Commission on Hospitals and Health Care, Hartford, Connecticut

Jonathan Howland, Boston University School of Public Health

The committee benefitted from the guidance offered by Barbara Filner and Ruth Bulger of the Institute of Medicine's Division of Health Sciences Policy; they initiated and supervised this project in its early phases. Special thanks also are due Kenneth Warren, Director, Office of Scientific Affairs, National Institute on Alcohol Abuse and Alcoholism (NIAAA). In his capacity as NIAAA project officer for this study, Dr. Warren has been both personally and professionally very supportive of the committee's efforts.

INDEX

Abstinence
  biological markers and, 155
  and cognitive function, 275–276
  from concomitant substance use, 258
  group meeting attendance and, 186
  and hypertension, 319
  and organ damage, 267, 281
  and sleep, 274
  and treatment efficacy, 232
  as treatment goal, 13, 61, 65,
    218–220, 223
Abstinence syndrome, 169
Acetaldehyde, 40, 221
Active treatment, 169, 170
Acupuncture, 189
Addiction Research Foundation of
 Ontario, 173
Addiction Severity Index (ASI), 150, 152
Adenylate cyclase, 156
Adolescents
  automobile accidents, 88
  circumvention of minimum purchase
  age, 91
  community prevention research, 109
  identification of risk in, 47, 53
  peer groups and, 55
  pregnancy, 3, 8, 40, 119–120
  primary prevention and, 121, 123
  public information campaigns and,
    84
  smoking prevention research,
    118–119
  suicide, 78
  television and, 87
  treatment, evaluation of, 187
  treatment matching, 237
  treatment research needs, 299–300
  verbal reporting, 154
Adult children of alcoholics. *See* Children
 of alcoholics
Adult Children of Alcoholics (ACOA),
 179
Advertising
  alcohol industry spending on, 27, 85
  in cancer prevention, 117–118

influences on drinking behavior, 6,
  82, 85–86
  treatment recruitment, 10, 143, 162
Aerobic exercise, 183
Aftercare. *See* Relapse prevention
Age
  alcohol price and consumption by,
    77, 81
  and cognitive function recovery, 276
Agent. *See* Alcohol
Age-graded influences, 48
Aggregate-level descriptive studies,
 161–162
Aggressive behavior, 4, 52, 54
AIDS research, 39, 313, 316
Alanine aminotransferase (SGPT),
 155–156
AlAnon, 179, 181–182, 194
Alaproclate, 173
AlaTeen, 181–182
Alcohol. *See also* Alcohol dependence;
 Alcohol-related problems; Alcohol
 use
  administration in therapies, 176, 274
  alternatives to, 117, 254
  carbimide reactions, 172
  cardiovascular effects, 278–279
  disulfiram reactions, 171
  effects on sleep, 273–275
  emotional effects, 60
  ingestion, testing for, 33
  metabolism of, 33, 34, 40, 155
  neuromuscular effects, 35
  physiological and behavioral effects,
    31–32
  in public health model, 2, 24–25, 27
  withdrawal, 169, 253–254, 268–275
Alcohol, Drug Abuse and Mental Health
 Administration (ADAMHA), 309, 313,
 316, 317, 319
Alcohol Clinical Index, 222
Alcohol dependence. *See also* Alcoholics;
 Alcohol use
  as clinical entity, 24, 131, 222
  comorbidity with drug use, 14, 144,
    158

conceptualization, vi, 10, 149
genetic determinants of, 66
intensity of treatment, 189
labeling, 223
moderation as treatment goal, 61
nicotine dependence comorbidity, 260
prevalence of, 144
progression of, 61
public perceptions of, 141
risk for, 145
severity, classification of, 150–151
severity of, 13, 234, 235, 241, 269
social learning of, 58
subtypes, 152
treatment effectiveness, 198
Alcohol Dependence Scale, 152
Alcohol expectancy questionnaire, 63, 152
Alcoholic amnestic disorder, 275
Alcoholic beverage control (ABC) commissions, 75, 76, 90
Alcoholic beverage industry
advertising, 27, 85
health promotion and, 117
Alcoholic dementia, 275
Alcoholics. *See also* Alcohol dependence;
Children of alcoholics
concomitant depression, 177, 178
denial of problems, 252
health care costs, 292–293
reinforcement and, 60–61
spouses of, 181
subpopulations of, 189
Alcoholics Anonymous (AA), 9–10, 142, 143, 191, 247
adolescent treatment, 300
attribution for change, 249
effectiveness of, 196, 197
meeting attendance, 186, 194, 239, 240
relapse prevention, 184
research on, 178–179
treatment, evaluation of, 187
treatment effects, 158, 159, 186
Alcoholism. *See* Alcohol dependence
Alcoholism, Alcohol Abuse and Related Problems: Opportunities for Research (IOM), vi
Alcohol and Public Policy: Beyond the Shadow of Prohibition (NRC), vii, 20, 24
Alcohol-related cues, 258

Alcohol-related disorders, 235
Alcohol-related problems
in assessment, 151
conceptualization, 10, 149, 223
continuum model of, vi, 1–2, 10, 23
diversity of, 144
epidemiology, 2–3, 31, 44
implications of public health research, 121–123
in primary care, 224
progression of, 222
public health model of, 2, 24–27
secondary prevention of, 215
Alcohol use
attitudes about, 247
biological markers of, 153, 155–157
and blood pressure, 278–279
community prevention research, 109–110
concomitant drug use, 235, 238, 258
consumption rates
advertising and, 85
availability and, 6, 75, 76–77, 128
context and setting effects, 6, 91, 92
minimum purchase age and, 6, 78–80
prices and, 6, 76, 77–78, 81, 129, 130–131
zoning and conditional-use permits and, 80
costs of, 23
cultural drinking behavior, 60, 92, 129
health consequences, 15, 267
historical patterns, 128
identification of at-risk individuals, 47
mortality, vi, 1, 23
periodic problem drinking, 53
severity of, 13, 234
smoking and, 247–248
in smoking prevention studies, 119
social learning of, 58–59
testing for, 11, 155-7
Alcohol Use Inventory, 152
Alpha-2 adrenergic agonists, 268
Alzheimer's disease, 278
American Hospital Association Annual Survey, 161
American Medical Association, 176

American Psychiatric Association, 10, 150, 235, 247
Amethystic agents, 267
Angiotensin converting enzyme antagonists, 279
Antabuse. *See* Disulfiram therapy
Antidepressant medication, 173, 174, 197, 259—260
Antidipsotropic medication, 170—172, 239
Anti-Drug Abuse Act (1986), 315, 320
Anti-Drug Abuse Act (1988), 41
Antipsychotic medication, 174, 259
Antisocial behavior, 4, 52, 54
Antisocial personality disorder
    comorbidity with alcoholism, 144
      and treatment, 13, 234, 235, 241, 257
Anxiety, 170, 183
    effect of alcohol on, 36
Anxiolytics, 259
Apneic aversion therapy, 175
Apoliprotein A-I and A-II, 156
Aspartate aminotransferase (SGOT), 155—156
Assertiveness training, 183
Assessment technology, 150—158
Attention-span deficit, 54
Attribution for change, 249
Australia, 89, 115
Automobile accidents
    alcohol and, 3, 23, 31, 33, 35, 78
    alcohol prices and, 77
    blood alcohol level in, 88
    drunk driving laws and, 6, 89, 90
    epidemiology, 34
    minimum purchase age and, 79
    risk for, 88
    seat belt use and, 116
Autopsy, 33
Autoregression, 129
Aversion therapies, 11—12, 175, 191, 253
Baltimore, 120
Bars, 26, 92
Bartenders, 131
Beer consumption
    advertising and, 85
    decline in, 145
    pitcher sales and, 91
    price and, 77
    purchase age and, 78, 79—80
Behavioral development, 48
Behavioral risk factors, 49, 215

Behavioral self-control training, 180—181, 215
    effectiveness of, 11—12, 196
    and moderation outcome goals, 219
Behavioral therapy, 253
Behavior change
    attribution for, 249
    education and, 120
    legislation and, 116
    motivation for, 12, 63—64, 65, 193—195, 235, 251—252
    readiness to, 5, 63—64, 65, 235, 248
    smoking cessation, 253, 261
    stages of, 248
Behavior change theory, 123
Benzodiazepines, 259, 268, 270, 271, 272
Beta blockers, 268, 279
Biochemical imbalances, 57
Biochemical tests, 221
Biofeedback-assisted relaxation training, 183
Biological markers, 11, 66, 153, 155—157, 221—222
Biological vulnerabilities, 57, 149
Biomedical research, 8, 132
Bipolar affective disorder, 174
Birth defects, maternal drinking and, 40
Bisexuals, 39
Blacks
    cancer in, 117
    hypertension in, 278—279
    smoking rate, 255
Blood alcohol concentrations (BAC), 221
    in automobile accidents, 88
    biological markers of, 11, 155
    in falls, 35—36
    self-monitoring of, 62
    and sleep, 273
Blood-gas exchange, 36
Blood pressure, 111, 115, 278—279
Bone, 282
Border effects, 79
Boston City Hospital, 218
Breath analysis, 11, 89, 159
Broadening the Base of Treatment for Alcohol Problems (IOM), vii
"Cafeteria" matching strategy, 13—14, 232, 233, 242
CAGE questions, 221
Calcium carbimide, 172
Calcium channel blockers, 267, 268, 279
California, 76

alcohol zoning in, 80
  community prevention research, 82,
    110, 112
Cancer, 23
  heavy drinking and, 282
  mortality, blacks, 255
  prevention studies, 8, 117—118, 133
  research, 316
  treatment, 196
Carbohydrate-deficient transferrin, 156
Carbon disulfide breath analysis, 159
Carbon monoxide, 37
  testing, 114, 118
Cardiac arrhythmias, 278, 279—280, 316
Cardiomyopathy, 278, 282
Cardiovascular collapse, 36
Cardiovascular disease
  community prevention studies, 7, 27,
    111—115, 133
  mortality, blacks, 255
  smoking and, 118
Cardiovascular effects, 278—280
Caroverine, 268
Carrier Foundation, 186
Case finding, 221
*Causes and Consequences of Alcohol
  Problems* (IOM), vi, 1, 5, 20, 24, 47,
    66, 267, 275, 282
Centers for Disease Control, 310
Central nervous system, 54, 267, 272,
  275—278
Cesium fluoride, 156
Chemical aversion therapy, 175, 191
Child abuse, alcohol and, 3, 38
Childhood factors, 53
Children of alcoholics, 145
  coping skills training, 64
  family dynamics and, 54—55
  risk for, 5, 66
  therapy groups, 181—182
  treatment matching, 146, 237
Chlordiazepoxide, 170, 270, 274
Cholesterol levels, 111, 115
Chromosomal markers, 5, 66
Citalopram, 173
Clinical decision making, 233
Clinical examinations, 150
Clinical Institute Withdrawal Assessment
  for Alcohol (CIWA-A), 269
Clinical trials
  difficulties of, 291, 314
  early intervention, 221

multicenter, 160, 162
Clinical Trials Cooperative Groups, 316
Clonidine, 252, 268
Cocaine
  craving, 258, 259
  dependence, 259, 260, 272
  dependence treatment, 256, 319, 320
Cocaine-alcohol dependency, 235, 238
Codependence, 145, 146
Cognitive-behavioral mediators, 65
Cognitive-behavioral processes, 57
Cognitive-behavioral therapy, 177, 184
Cognitive impairment, 15, 178, 267,
  275—277
Cognitive restructuring, 5, 62—63, 177,
  183, 277—278
Cognitive variables, 248—249
Cohort effects, 48, 55—56
College prevention programs, 129
Communication-behavior change model,
  112
Communication-persuasion model, 112
Community
  change, 114
  initiatives, 311
  mental health centers, 143
  reinforcement, 183, 197
  as risk factor, 49, 50
Community Mental Health Centers Act,
  141
Community organization model, 112, 113
Community-wide prevention, 7—8, 64, 130
  alcohol, 109—110, 128
  cardiovascular disease, 7, 27,
    111—115
  cost of data collection, 133
  implications from other public
    health fields, 121—123
  NIAAA and, 309
CompCare, 185
Compliance, 12, 193—194
  with disulfiram therapy, 159, 171
Composite International Diagnostic
  Interview, Substance Abuse Module
  (CIDI-SAM), 150
Comprehensive Drinker Profile, 150
Computerized assessments, 154, 157
Computer modeling, 129, 132, 133—134
Conditioned response, 58, 60—61, 257—258
  counterconditioning, 175
Condoms, 39
Confounding variables, 161

Confrontational therapy, 177, 181–182, 194
Conjoint therapy, 11–12, 181–182
Connecticut, University of, 313
Constructive confrontation, 194
Contamination, 130
Contemplation phase, 63
Contraceptive use, 120
Controlled trials
  importance of, 169, 198
  intensity and duration of treatment, 12, 88
  treatment evaluation, 187
  in treatment matching studies, 232
Cooperative agreements, 316, 317, 318–319
Coping skills, 5
  deficits in, 58, 250
  training, 61–62, 63, 65
Coronary artery disease, 278
Cost containment, 296
Cost-effectiveness
  Alcoholics Anonymous, 179
  prevention, 9, 134
  treatment, 16, 188, 289, 294–295
Cost offset effect, 15–16, 292–296, 299
Counterconditioning, 175
Counties, 76
Couples therapy, 12, 181-2
Court conviction rates, drunk-driving laws, 88–89
Covariance analysis, 161
Covert sensitization, 176–177, 191, 258
Craving, 149, 152
  antidipsotropics and, 172
  cognitive, 58
  drug, 257–258, 259
Criminal behavior, 38, 52
Criminal justice programs, 142
Critical conditions, 191
Cross-cultural research, 151
Cue exposure, 184, 185
Cultural change, 64
Data collection
  automation of, 157–158
  cost of, 133
  longitudinal, 56
Death. *See* Mortality
Deglycosylated transferrin, 156
Delirium tremens, treatment of, 271, 272
Demography, 10, 143–144
Denial, 252

Depression, 170
  comorbidity with alcoholism, 144, 174, 177, 178
  in drug dependence, 259–260
  effect of alcohol on, 36
  and smoking cessation, 250
Desialotransferrin, 156
Desipramine, 259, 260
Detection, 221
Detoxification, 169, 236
  cocaine, 256
  and sleep, 274
Developmental epidemiology, 27, 51
Dexamethasone, 272
Diagnosis, 150–151
Diagnostic Interview Schedule (DIS), 150, 152
Diagnostic and Statistical Manual of Mental Disorders (DSM-III), 10–11, 150, 151
Diagnostic and Statistical Manual of Mental Disorders, revised (DSM-III-R), 150, 151, 235, 247
Diary procedures, 155
Diazepam, 268, 270, 272
Diet, 8, 117, 123, 275
Differential assessment, 11, 151–153
Diffusion theory, 112
Diphenylhydantoin, 270–271
Distilled spirits
  consumption, advertising and, 85
  consumption, price and, 77
  decline in consumption of, 145
Disulfiram therapy, 143, 158, 170–172, 239, 316
  compliance with, 159, 171
Diuretics, 279
Doxepin, 259
Dram shop laws. *See* Server liability
Driving-while-intoxicated (DWI)
  behavioral self-control training and, 180–181
  deaths from accidents, 23, 34, 78
  drinking context and, 26, 93
  education programs, 10, 84, 142
  legal environment, 6, 87–90, 129
  public interest groups on, 145
  treatment programs, 194
  and vehicular injuries, 34, 35
Drowning, 3, 31, 36
Drug use
  alcohol use and, 88

community prevention research, 109, 119

comorbidity with alcoholism, 14, 144, 258

conditioned responses, 257—258

during pregnancy, 40

placebo therapy, 217

school-based prevention programs, 27

psychopathology and, 174

psychopharmacological treatments, 259—260

psychotherapy, 256—257

and sexual activity, 39

treatment effectiveness, 300

verbal reporting, 154

withdrawal, 174

Drug-use stress, 57

Early identification, 13, 215, 221

Ecological fallacy, 131

Economic environment, 24, 90, 131

Economic Opportunity Act, 141

Edgehill Newport, 186

Educational intervention, 11—12, 178
pretesting of, 113

Effect-altering medications, 170, 173—174

Electrical aversion therapy, 175

Emetic drugs, 175

Emotions, 54, 58

Empathy, 192

Employee assistance programs, 10, 16, 194—195, 215, 224
and cost research, 297, 298

Encainide, 279

Endocrine organs, 282

Environment, 20
change in, 114
context and setting, 91—93
controls on alcohol availability, 75—80
individual interactions with, 6—7, 23, 26, 57
influences on drinking behavior, 81—93
legal, 24, 87—91, 122, 123, 310
and moderate drinking, 24
normative, 82—87
in public health model, 2, 24—25
risk factors in, 50
treatment and, 149

Epidemiological catchment area studies, 144, 162, 298

Epidemiology
adolescent pregnancy, 40
alcohol-related problems, 2—3, 31, 144
child abuse, 38—39
crime, 38
developmental, 27, 51
fetal alcohol syndrome, 40—41
injuries, 31—37
sexually transmitted diseases, 39—40
suicide, 38

Esophagus, 282

Ethanol. See Alcohol

Ethnic groups, 52, 60—61

Ethnographic methods, 128

Etiology, 151
genetic factors, 49
methodology and, 32
preventive trials and, 25
prospective research opportunities, 55—56

Expectancies, learned, 5, 60, 62—63, 152

Experimental designs, methodology, 159, 160

Extinction procedures, 258

Falls, 3, 23, 31, 35, 36

Family
genetic studies, 66
history of alcoholism, 5, 234, 235, 241
as risk factor, 49, 50, 54—55
and social learning, 58
and treatment, 10, 144, 234, 235

Family therapy, 12, 181—182, 197, 240—241

Federal employees alcohol program, 142

Feedback designs, 233, 242

Females
alcohol-related problems in, 144
fire death risks, 37
inhibition of risk in, 55
pregnant, interventions with, 13, 142, 217—218
in prospective research, 52
in public information campaigns, 84
remission of problem drinking in, 53
and smoking cessation, 255
television and, 87
treatment matching, 237, 238

Fermentation, 34

Fetal alcohol effects, 3, 13, 41, 217—218

Fetal alcohol syndrome (FAS), 3, 13,

Indiana, 109
Indicated interventions 2, 26, 53
    treatment as, 140
Individual
    behavior change, 114, 120, 123, 131
    consumption history, 131
    development of, 47, 55, 132
    environmental interaction, 3—5, 26,
        47, 50, 57, 75
    in public health model, 2, 24—25
    risk factors in, 49
Individual therapy, 159, 177, 239,
    240—241, 257
Injuries
    epidemiology of, 3, 31—37
    falls, 23, 31
    methodological problems in
        studying, 32—34
    vehicular, 34, 35, 88
Inoculation, social, 84, 132
Inpatient treatment, 9—10, 142, 143, 170
    costs, 291
Insight-oriented therapy, 177
Insomnia, 273—275
Institute of Medicine (IOM), vi, vii, 1, 5,
    24, 47, 231, 267
Insurance Institute for Highway Safety, 88
International Classification of Diseases
    (ICD-10), 150, 151
Interrupted time-series analysis, 129
Intoxication
    environmental interaction and, 23,
        26
    estimating, 130
    health consequences, 267
    risk of other problems, 215
    social norms and, 60
Investigator-initiated grant, 16, 142, 309,
    313, 314, 319
Job performance, 221
JWK Corporation, 290
Kaiser-Permanente, 278, 298
Kansas, 109
Kellogg Company, 8, 117
Labeling, 223
Laboratory research, 8, 128, 130—131
Labyrinthitis, caloric, 36
Laryngospasm, 36
Least-squares regression, 129
Legal environment, 24, 87—91, 121, 123,
    310
Liability insurance, 91

Life-course development, 4, 132
    identification of risk factors, 47—50
    and readiness to change, 64, 65
Liquor. *See* Distilled spirits
Liquor by the drink (LBD), 76
Lithium, 174, 267
Liver. *See also* Hepatic cirrhosis;
Hepatitis
    disease, 23
    dysfuntion, 37
    effects of alcohol on, 15, 280—281
    enzymes, 155—156, 216
    transplantation, 281
Lofexidine, 268
Longitudinal research, 133, 146
    data bases, 56
    methodological problems, 295
Lorazepam, 270
Los Angeles, 119
Maine, 89—90, 129
Males
    alcoholic fathers and, 54
    comorbidities in, 235
    remission of problem drinking in, 53
    risk factors, 4, 37, 52
Managed care, 16, 296, 298
Mandated treatment, 12, 145, 194—195
Marijuana, 34
    community prevention research, 109
    in smoking prevention studies, 119
Marital conflict, 4, 52
Marital therapy, 181—182, 197
Massachusetts
    drunk driving laws, 89
    minimum drinking age, 78—79
Media
    alcohol advertising, 6, 85—86
    in community prevention studies, 7,
        111, 117, 128
    fictional depictions of alcohol use, 6,
        86—87
    public information campaigns, 6,
        82—85, 88, 89
    in smoking prevention, 119
    social learning and, 58, 60
    treatment recruitment, 143, 162, 223
Medication, 196
    abuse and dependence, 174
    in smoking cessation, 252
Meditation, 183
Memory, 154, 275—276
    training, 277

Men. *See* Males

Mental health, 63

Mental retardation, maternal drinking
  and, 40

Meprobamate, 268

Meta-analysis, 290, 291, 292

Methadone maintenance, 170, 181, 259

Methodology
  cost research, 295
  patient-treatment matching, 231—233
  policy analysis, 290—292
  prevention research design,
    8—9,128—134
  problems with self-reported data, 11
  problems in studying alcohol-related
    injuries, 3, 32—34
  problems in treatment evaluation,
    186—187
  proxy variables, 120
  treatment research, 159—163

Michigan
  minimum drinking age, 79
  seat belt law, 116

Michigan Alcoholism Screening Test
  (MAST), 152, 221

Midwestern Prevention Project (MPP),
  109

Minimum purchase age, 6, 75, 76, 78—80,
  87

Minnesota Heart Health Study, 115, 130

Minnesota Multiphasic Personality
Inventory, 234

Minnesota treatment model, 185

Minorities
  in prospective research, 52
  television and, 87

Missouri, 109

Model Alcoholic Beverage Retail
Licensee Liability Act (1985), 90

Moderate drinkers, 23
  biological markers in, 156
  differentiation of, 131
  and environmental factors, 24
  in treatment outcome, 219—220

Moderation, as treatment goal, 13, 61,
  218—220, 223

Moral deficiencies, 57

Mortality
  alcohol availability and, 76, 77
  alcohol use, vi, 1, 23
  automobile accidents, 23, 34, 78
  cardiovascular disease, 112, 255

cirrhosis and hepatitis, 15, 77, 267,
  280

drowning, 36

early intervention and, 224

falls, 35

fire and burns, 37

injuries, 3, 31

Mothers Against Drunk Driving, 87, 110

Motivation for change, 12, 63—64, 65,
  193—195, 235, 251—252

Movie theaters, 84

Multistage sampling, 56

Multivariate analysis, 55, 129, 131, 161,
  232

Muscle, 282

Music Television, 84

Mutual help groups, 11—12, 119, 178—180

Naloxone, 267

Naltrexone, 259

Narcotics Anonymous, 186, 300

National Alcoholism and Drug Abuse
Program Inventory (NDAPI), 161

National Alcoholism Program
  Information System (NAPIS), 142

National Association of Alcoholism
Treatment Programs, 161

National Cancer Institute (NCI), 8, 17,
  117, 309, 310, 313, 316

National Drug and Alcoholism Treatment
  Utilization Survey (NDATUS),
  161—162

National Health Interview Survey, 144

National Heart, Lung, and Blood
  Institute (NHLBI), 17, 309, 310, 313,
  316, 319

National Highway Traffic Safety
Administration, 80, 92

National Institute on Alcohol Abuse and
  Alcoholism (NIAAA), vi, vii, 1, 9, 20
  aggregate-level studies, 161
  Alcohol Research Centers, 17—18,
    315, 318
  and community prevention study,
    110, 133
  cooperative research, 316
  and diagnosis, 150
  Division of Clinical and Prevention
    Research, 9, 17, 142, 309, 313
  intramural research, 142
  and longitudinal data bases, 56
  preventive research funding, 16, 309
  prevention research

recommendations, 310, 311, 312
treatment funding, 16, 141—142, 146, 290
treatment research funding, 313, 318, 319, 320
National Institute of Mental Health (NIMH), 141, 316, 319
Treatment of Depression Collaborative Research Program, 318
National Institute on Allergy and Infectious Diseases, 313, 316
National Institute on Drug Abuse (NIDA), 17, 110, 146, 310, 314, 315, 318, 319
National Institutes of Health (NIH), 309—310, 313, 316, 317
National Research Centers Program, 142
National Research Council, vii, 20, 24
Native Americans, 40, 237
Naturalistic studies, 92—93, 131, 291
Natural raters, 49, 50
Nausea, induced, 175, 176
Needs analysis, 113—114, 121
Nerves, peripheral, 282
Neurophysiological variables, 49
Nevada, 76
New Hampshire, 76
Newspapers, 87
New York, 79
Nicotine chewing gum, 253
Nicotine fading, 253—254
Nootropic drugs, 278
Norepinephrine reuptake, 173
Normative environment, 24, 26, 48, 82—87
North Carolina, 76
North Karelia Project, 115
Norzimelidine, 173
Nutrition education, 115
Observational learning, 59—60
Observational studies, 128
Occupational alcohol programs, 142
Office of Economic Opportunity, 141
Office of Substance Abuse Prevention (OSAP), 17, 309, 310, 311, 313
Omnibus Anti-Drug Abuse Act (1986), 309
Ontario, Canada, 76, 77
Ontario Detoxication System, 269
Ontogenetic influences, 48
Operating-under-the-influence. See Driving-while-intoxicated

Opiate
abuse, 258, 272, 319
antagonists, 173
withdrawal, 259
Organ damage, 154, 155, 267
Osteoporosis, 35
Outcome. See Treatment: effectiveness of
Outpatient treatment, 183, 216
costs, 291, 293
patient-treatment matching, 239, 240, 241
social supports and, 13, 234
Oxazepam, 269—270
Pancreas, 282
Paranoia, 272
Partial correlation, 161
Path-analytic procedures, 132
Patient-treatment matching, 13—14, 149—150, 237—241
methodology, 231—233
patient measurement, 233—235, 241
readiness to change and, 248
recommendations, 241—242, 315
treatment measurement, 235—236
Pavlovian learning theory, 191
Pawtucket Heart Health Study, 115, 129
Peer groups
coping skills training and, 61, 119
as risk factor, 49, 50, 55
social learning and, 58, 60
Pennsylvania, 115
Per se laws, 87, 88
Personality tests, 234
Personality variables, 49
Pharmacotherapies, 11—12, 170—175, 261
alcohol withdrawal, 268—269
drug dependence, 259—260
Phenobarbital, 271
Phenothiazine, 312
Physical deformities, maternal drinking and, 40
Physician counseling, 254
Physiological indicators of susceptibility, 66
Placebo therapy, 217
Planned Approach to Community Health, 310
Platelet monoamine oxidase, 156
Point-of-purchase components, 115
Police enforcement, 88—89, 131
Policy development, vii, 9, 15—16, 20, 133—134

Time-line follow-back, 155
Tissue damage, 15, 156, 157
Tourism, 76
Transferrin, 221
Treatment. *See also* Patient-treatment
  matching
  alcohol withdrawal, 268–275
  assessment of, 158–159
  brief interventions, 12, 13, 216–217,
    221, 224, 235, 239
  broad-spectrum strategies, 11–12,
    182–184
  cognitive impairment and, 276
  cost of, 15, 143, 188, 290, 291, 292
  cost-benefit analysis, 289–290
  cost-effectiveness analysis, 16, 289,
    294–295
  cost offset effect, 15–16, 292–296,
    299
  demography and epidemiology,
    143–145
  early intervention, 215–216, 221, 224
  effectiveness, 195–198, 289–290,
    299–300
      evaluation of, 8, 11–12,
        121, 142, 149–150, 237, 310
      outcome expectancies,
        248–249
      outcome objectives,
        multiple, 120
      outcome research,
        169–170, 218–220
      outcome variables, 159
  efficacy, 231, 242, 313–314
      mechanisms of, 190–191
  efficiency, 290
  funding, 9, 17–18, 141–142, 313–320
  historical factors in, 9–10
  implementation, 224
  as indicated intervention, 140
  intensity and duration of, 12, 14,
    188–189, 239
  methodology, 159–163
  phases of, 169
  process, 12, 158, 159, 190–195,
    197–198, 248–252
  recruitment, 9–10, 223
  research methodology, 159–163
  research recommendations, 9–16,
    146
  setting, 315
  smoking cessation, 253–254

  traditional programs, evaluation of,
    185–187
  trends in, 142–143, 145
  variables, 158
Treatment centers, data reporting,
  161–162
Tryptophan, 278
Uncontrolled studies, 169
  treatment evaluation, 12, 186, 187
Unemployment rates, and drunk driving,
  88
Universal interventions, 2, 26, 53, 64
Urine markers, 11, 155, 280–281
United States
  Air Force, 290
  Coast Guard, 36
  Congress, vi, 1, 142, 185, 315
  Department of Defense, 311, 316,
    319
  Department of Education, 311
  Department of Health and Human
    Services, 311
  Department of Transportation, 89,
    311, 319
  Navy, 91
Ventricular fibrillation, 279
Verbal report methods, 11, 153–155
Vermont, 76
Veterans Administration, 141
  clinics, 170
  collaborative study, 18, 174
  funding, 16
  hospitals, 143
  prevention research, 311
  treatment research funding, 313,
    316, 318, 319, 320
Videocassettes, 84
Violence, 3, 33, 38
Viqualine, 173
Vitamins, 275
Vulnerability. *See* Risk factors
Warning labels, 41
Washington, D.C., 76, 117
Washington, University of, 40
Wernicke-Korsakoff syndrome, 275
Wine consumption, advertising and, 85
Women. *See* Females
Women for Sobriety, 179
Work setting, as risk factor, 49, 50, 93
Work site prevention trials, 128, 130